Analgesia, Anaesthesia and Pregnancy

A Practical Guide
Third Edition

Analgesia, Anaesthesia and Pregnancy

A Practical Guide
Third Edition

Steve Yentis
Consultant Anaesthetist, Chelsea and Westminster Hospital, London, UK

Surbhi Malhotra
Consultant Anaesthetist, St Mary's Hospital, London, UK

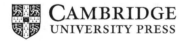
CAMBRIDGE
UNIVERSITY PRESS

CAMBRIDGE UNIVERSITY PRESS
Cambridge, New York, Melbourne, Madrid, Cape Town,
Singapore, São Paulo, Delhi, Mexico City

Cambridge University Press
The Edinburgh Building, Cambridge CB2 8RU, UK

Published in the United States of America
by Cambridge University Press, New York

www.cambridge.org
Information on this title: www.cambridge.org/9781107601598

First edition published 2000
Second edition published 2007
Reprinted 2008
Third edition published 2013

Printed and bound in the United Kingdom by the MPG Books Group

A catalogue record for this publication is available from the British Library

Library of Congress Cataloguing in Publication data

Yentis, S. M. (Steven M.)
   Analgesia, anaesthesia, and pregnancy : a practical guide / Steve Yentis,
Surbhi Malhotra. – 3rd ed.
     p. ; cm.
   Includes bibliographical references and index.
   ISBN 978-1-107-60159-8 (Paperback : alk.paper)
   I. Malhotra, Surbhi, Dr.   II. Title.
   [DNLM: 1. Analgesia, Obstetrical.   2. Anesthesia, Obstetrical.
WO 450]
   617.9'682–dc23

                                                                    2012036026

ISBN 978-1-107-60159-8 Paperback

Contents

III – Operative delivery and third stage

IV – Anaesthetic problems

V – Problems confined to obstetrics

VI – Problems not confined to obstetrics

VII – The neonate

Section 3 – Puerperium and after

Section 4 – Organisational aspects

Preface

The first edition of this book was written in order to provide useful, practical information and advice to obstetric anaesthetists, in the form of a ready and easily accessible guide to obstetric anaesthesia and analgesia. The book was aimed primarily at trainees, both those starting in the maternity suite and their more experienced colleagues preparing for anaesthetic examinations. We also hoped the book would be of use to more senior anaesthetists and those of all levels involved in teaching obstetric anaesthesia, as well as non-anaesthetists working in the maternity suite.

In this third edition, we have reviewed and revised each section but kept to the original aims, structure and format, since we are convinced that the need for a short, practically based text still exists. In doing so, we have attempted to bridge the gaps between routine obstetric anaesthesia and analgesia and the care of women with co-existing medical conditions, and between anaesthetic care and advice before pregnancy and that during pregnancy itself.

As before, we have assumed basic anaesthetic knowledge and thus do not include topics such as anaesthetic equipment and drugs, etc., except where there are areas of specific obstetric relevance. We have tried to base the advice given on what we believe would be considered standard UK practice, supported by evidence wherever possible, although we have deliberately not included supporting references for each point made since this would, in our view, detract from the readability and ease of use of this book; readers wishing to obtain such reference lists are directed to the many larger, more comprehensive texts that are currently available. (N.B. Website addresses are given for non-journal documents that are available online; we apologise if, in time, some of these may become incorrect.)

We hope that the layout of the book is easy to follow and that any repetition and inconsistencies in structure are not too irritating. We have tried to provide a brief list of pertinent further reading where possible; often this has meant that very large topics have been left relatively unreferenced, since there are few journal reviews broad enough in scope. Finally, we gratefully acknowledge the contributions of Dr D. Bogod, Dr D. Brighouse and Dr C. Elton to the first edition, and Dr A. May to the first and second editions.

Chapter

Assisted conception

The treatment of infertility has developed rapidly, and the anaesthetist may be involved in many aspects of the patient's treatment, which may be complex. The harvesting of oocytes needs to take place within a defined period of time, or ovulation may have occurred and oocytes will be lost. Couples presenting for infertility treatment are generally anxious and often the women are emotional at the time of oocyte retrieval. It is therefore particularly important for the anaesthetist to understand the couple's anxieties, and to be able to explain the effects of the anaesthetic technique that is to be used.

Problems/special considerations

All of the techniques involve extraction of oocytes from the follicles, either laparoscopically or, with the development of transvaginal ultrasonography, via the transvaginal route (ultrasound directed oocyte retrieval, UDOR). The techniques differ in the site of fertilisation and/or replacement of the gamete/zygote:

- *In vitro fertilisation (IVF):* This term is often (incorrectly) used to encompass all aspects of infertility treatment. However, the process involves fertilisation in the laboratory and the developing embryo is transferred into the uterus via the cervix, usually 48 hours after oocyte retrieval. Embryo transfer is performed with the patient awake, although there are occasions when the help of the anaesthetist may be required to provide sedation. The success rate is approximately 15–25%.
- *Gamete intrafallopian transfer (GIFT):* This involves retrieval of oocytes which are placed together with sperm into the fallopian tube, laparoscopically, although an ultrasound-guided transvaginal procedure may sometimes be used. The success rate is approximately 35%.
- *Zygote intrafallopian tube transfer (ZIFT) or pronuclear stage transfer:* This process involves oocyte retrieval and IVF, with the zygote then being placed in the fallopian tube as for GIFT. The success rate is approximately 30–40%.
- *Intracytoplasmic sperm injection (ICSI):* Fertilisation occurs in the laboratory via injection of sperm into the oocytes, and the developing embryo is transferred into the uterus as for IVF. This technique is used for male infertility. The success rate is approximately 30%.

The main considerations for laparoscopy are the type of anaesthesia, the pneumoperitoneum and the effects of the anaesthetic agents on fertilisation and cell cleavage. The length of exposure to the drugs is also important. The effects of nitrous oxide and volatile anaesthetic agents on fertilisation and cleavage rates have been extensively examined. It is generally recognised that all volatile agents and nitrous oxide have a deleterious effect, although opinion is divided as to the extent of the problem. It is also recognised that the carbon dioxide used for the pneumoperitoneum causes a similar effect, and it is difficult to separate the effects of the anaesthetic agents from those of the carbon dioxide.

Of the intravenous agents, the effect of propofol on fertilisation and cleavage appears to be minimal. Propofol accumulates in the follicular fluid, and the amount in the follicular fluid may become significant if there are a large number of oocytes to retrieve. Propofol decreases the fertilisation rates but there is no significant effect on the cell division rates.

All assisted conception techniques carry the risk of ovarian hyperstimulation (see Chapter 2, Ovarian hyperstimulation syndrome), and multiple or ectopic pregnancy.

Management options

Most women who present for assisted conception techniques are healthy and in their 30s–40s. However, it is now recognised that some women may also have a number of associated comorbidities with increasing age. Therefore, a multidisciplinary approach is necessary.

It would be logical to use regional anaesthesia whenever possible, although this is not well suited for laparoscopy. The development of the transvaginal route for oocyte retrieval has increased the possibility of using regional anaesthesia.

For patients requiring laparoscopy, it would seem sensible to minimise the use of drugs. This has led to the increased use of propofol as the main agent in total intravenous anaesthesia.

For UDOR, which has become the most common method used for oocyte retrieval, the main anaesthetic techniques are intravenous sedation and regional anaesthesia. It is important to remember that patients requiring UDOR are day cases and the basic principles of day-case anaesthesia apply. There has been a considerable amount of work to date on the use of propofol with alfentanil, and this combination of drugs would appear to be the technique of choice for intravenous sedation. Propofol may be administered by intermittent boluses or by continuous infusion, with the patient breathing oxygen via a Hudson mask. Many anaesthetists find that they are using levels of sedation close to anaesthesia. It is essential that the sedation is administered in a suitable environment with resuscitation facilities and anaesthetic monitoring. Often the assisted conception unit is some distance from the main theatre suite; therefore it may be difficult for the staff working in an isolated environment to maintain their skills in resuscitation.

The aim of minimising the drugs administered to women undergoing ultrasound-guided techniques has led to the use of regional anaesthesia. The main problem has been to develop techniques that allow the woman to go home the same day. Epidural and spinal anaesthesia have both been used with success, particularly where early ambulation is not essential. The low-dose spinal that is used for labour analgesia has been shown to give good operating conditions and to satisfy the criteria needed for day-case anaesthesia; it may be some way to achieving an ideal in this difficult group of patients.

Analgesia following the procedure may be provided with a combination of codeine and paracetamol. Non-steroidal anti-inflammatory drugs such as diclofenac are considered less suitable as these are thought to interfere with embryo implantation, owing to a disruption in prostaglandin levels.

Key points

- Oocyte retrieval may involve laparoscopy requiring general anaesthesia, although intravenous sedation and regional anaesthesia are suitable for transvaginal ultrasound-directed techniques.
- Couples are usually very anxious and require constant reassurance.

Further reading

Tsen L. Anesthesia for assisted reproductive technologies. *Int Anesthesiol Clin* 2007; 7: 99–113.

Vlahos NF, Giannakikou I, Vlachos A, Vitoratos N. Analgesia and anesthesia for assisted reproductive technologies. *Int J Gynaecol Obstet* 2009; **105**: 201–5.

Yasmin E, Dresner M, Balen A. Sedation and anaesthesia for transvaginal oocyte collection: an evaluation of practice in the UK. *Hum Reprod* 2004; **19**: 2942–5.

Chapter

2 Ovarian hyperstimulation syndrome

Ovarian hyperstimulation syndrome is a complication of ovarian induction that may be caused by any agent that stimulates the ovaries. Over the last ten years, the incidence has increased owing to the development of IVF treatments, where the ultimate goal is to produce enough oocytes and embryos. The condition may become severe enough to warrant intensive care admission.

Ovarian hyperstimulation syndrome occurs 3–8 days after treatment with human chorionic gonadotrophin (hCG), and the effects continue throughout the luteal phase. The active ingredient causing the syndrome via increased capillary permeability is thought to be secreted from the ovaries, and both histamine and prostaglandins have been implicated.

Problems/special considerations

Clinical manifestations of the syndrome are:

- Enlargement of the ovaries
- Pleural effusion
- Ascites.

Table 2.1 Grading of ovarian hyperstimulation syndrome

Grade	Features	Incidence
1	Abdominal distension and discomfort	8–23%
2	Grade 1 plus nausea, vomiting and diarrhoea	
3	Grade 2 plus ascites (detected by ultrasonography)	1–8%
4	Grade 3 plus clinical ascites and shortness of breath	
5	Grade 4 plus clinical hypovolaemia, haemoconcentration, coagulation defects, decreased renal perfusion – therefore urea and electrolyte disturbance, thromboembolic phenomena	1–1.8%

Additional complications that may occur are:

- Hypovolaemic shock
- Renal failure
- Acute lung injury
- Thromboembolism
- Cerebrovascular disorders.

Women undergoing ovarian stimulation who develop ovarian hyperstimulation syndrome may be classified by placing them in one of five grades according to presenting symptoms and signs (Table 2.1).

Management options

When a large number of eggs (> 20) have been retrieved ovarian hyperstimulation should be suspected and the patient monitored. This may involve hospital admission.

Once suspected, the diagnosis of ovarian hyperstimulation syndrome can be confirmed by:

- A rapid increase in plasma oestradiol concentration
- The presence of multiple ovarian follicles on ultrasound examination
- An increase in body weight.

Immediate treatment is to stop hCG administration and to aspirate the enlarged follicles. Mild forms of ovarian hyperstimulation syndrome will be self-limiting, but those women graded 3 or worse will require intravenous fluids to correct the hypovolaemia and haemoconcentration. The intravenous administration of 1000 ml of human albumin is recommended at the time of oocyte retrieval if hyperstimulation is suspected.

In women graded 4 and 5, dopamine has been given to improve renal perfusion. In addition, it may be advisable to drain the ascitic fluid and to consider anticoagulation. Ultrafiltration and intravenous reinfusion of ascitic fluid has been used in severe cases.

Monitoring is tailored to the severity of the syndrome, and the following progression is recommended:

- Urea and electrolytes
- Full blood count and packed cell volume
- Plasma/urine osmolality
- Clotting screen

- Chest radiography
- Central venous pressure if large volumes of fluids are needed.

Key points

- Hyperstimulation comprises ovarian enlargement, pleural effusion and ascites, which may be relentless.
- Severe protein loss may result in shock and renal failure.
- The most severe form occurs in 1–2% of cases treated with human chorionic gonadotrophin.

Further reading

Budev M, Arroliga A, Falcone T. Ovarian hyperstimulation syndrome. *Crit Care Med* 2005; **33**: S301–6.

Royal College of Obstetricians and Gynaecologists. The management of ovarian hyperstimulation syndrome. *Green-top 5*. London: RCOG 2011, http://www.rcog.org.uk/womens-health/clinical-guidance/management-ovarian-hyperstimulation-syndrome-green-top-5.

Sansone P, Aurilio C, Pace MC, *et al*. Intensive care treatment of ovarian hyperstimulation syndrome (OHSS). *Ann N Y Acad Sci* 2011; **1221**: 109–18.

Chapter

3

Anaesthesia before conception or confirmation of pregnancy

Many women will require anaesthesia when they are pregnant and many will be unaware that they are pregnant at the time of the anaesthetic, especially in the first 2–3 months of their pregnancy. The thalidomide catastrophe initiated the licensing arrangements for new drugs and their use in pregnancy; the current cautious stance of the pharmaceutical industry is reflected in the *British National Formulary*'s statement that no drug is safe beyond all doubt in early pregnancy. The anaesthetist should have a clear knowledge of the time scale of the developing fetus in order to balance the risks and benefits of any drug given to the mother. A *teratogen* is a substance that causes structural or functional abnormality in a fetus exposed to that substance.

Problems/special considerations

The possible effect of a drug can be considered against the stage of the developing fetus:

- *Pre-embryonic phase (0–14 days post-conception):* The fertilised egg is transported down the Fallopian tube and implantation occurs at around 7 days post-conception. The conceptus is a ball of undifferentiated dividing cells during this time and the effect of drugs on it appears to be an all-or-none phenomenon. Cell division may be slowed with no lasting effects or the conceptus will die, depending on the severity of the cell damage.

- *Embryonic phase (3–8 weeks post-conception):* Differentiation of cells into the organs and tissues occurs during this phase and drugs administered to the mother may cause considerable harm. The type of abnormality that is produced depends on the exact stage of organ and tissue development when the drug is given.
- *Fetal phase (9 weeks to birth):* At this stage, most organs are fully formed, although the cerebral cortex, cerebellum and urogenital tract are still developing. Drugs administered during this time may affect the growth of the fetus or the functional development within specific organs.

Management options

The anaesthetist should always consider the possibility of pregnancy in any woman of child-bearing age who presents for surgery, whether elective or emergency, and should specifically enquire in such cases. If there is doubt, a pregnancy test should be offered. If pregnancy is suspected, the use of nitrous oxide is now generally considered acceptable, despite its effects on methionine synthase and DNA metabolism, as there is little evidence that it is harmful clinically. Similarly, although the volatile agents have been implicated in impairing embryonic development, clinical evidence is lacking. Some drugs cross the placenta and exert their effect on the fetus, e.g. warfarin, which may cause bleeding in the fetus.

Key points

- The possibility of pregnancy should be considered in any woman of childbearing age.
- No drug is safe beyond all doubt in pregnancy.

Further reading

Allaert SE, Carlier SP, Weyne LP, *et al.* First trimester anesthesia exposure and fetal outcome. A review. *Acta Anaesthesiol Belg* 2007; **58**: 119–23.

Chapter

4

Ectopic pregnancy

There are approximately 11 000 ectopic pregnancies per year in the UK (just over 1% of all pregnancies), and the incidence is thought to be increasing as a result of pelvic inflammatory disease. There are many risk factors, with tubal pathology and/or surgery and the use of an intrauterine device the most important; other risk factors are infertility, increased maternal age and smoking. About 3–5 women die as a consequence in the UK per year, representing about 3–6% of all direct maternal deaths (~1 per 2500 ectopics). Most ectopic pregnancies occur in the Fallopian tube, but up to 5% occur elsewhere within the genital tract or abdomen. Typically, the tube initially expands to accommodate the growing zygote, but when it is unable to do so any more, there may be bleeding from the site of implantation or even rupture of the tube.

Problems/special considerations

The main risk of ectopic pregnancy is sudden severe haemorrhage, which may be intra-abdominal and thus concealed until sudden decompensation and collapse occur. A common theme in deaths associated with ectopic pregnancy is the failure to consider the diagnosis before collapse. Ectopic pregnancy may present with non-specific abdominal signs including diarrhoea or constipation, thus mimicking other intra-abdominal conditions (e.g. appendicitis). Mortality rates from misdiagnosis of an ectopic pregnancy have risen since 1997 and the Confidential Enquiries into Maternal Deaths report recommends that an ectopic pregnancy should be considered as a diagnosis in any women of reproductive age who presents with severe gastrointestinal symptoms.

Diagnosis may be difficult. Signs and symptoms of an ectopic pregnancy vary; early symptoms include a brown discharge, bleeding that can be light to heavy – although a significant proportion of women do not have any bleeding (20%) – and abdominal pain. Most ectopic pregnancies present early in pregnancy and thus many of the physiological changes of pregnancy are absent or mild – the patient may even be unaware that she is pregnant. However, even at this early stage there may be features of the physiological changes of pregnancy. Abdominal ultrasound has low specificity and transvaginal ultrasound has been shown to be better. If ultrasound is not convincing, then diagnosis is aided by blood tests and laparoscopy. Serum levels of human chorionic gonadotrophin (hCG) and progesterone are often measured but these measurements often resemble those levels seen in a normal pregnancy. Previously, the gold standard for diagnosis of an ectopic pregnancy was a laparoscopy; however, its accuracy in diagnosing an ectopic pregnancy has been questioned.

The implications for the current and future pregnancies pose a great psychological stress on the patient and her partner. There may be a previous history of ectopic pregnancy since its occurrence is itself a risk factor for subsequent ectopics.

Management options

Initial management is directed at treating and preventing massive haemorrhage; thus the patient requires at least one large-bore intravenous cannula and careful observation at least until the diagnosis has been excluded. Similarly, once the decision to operate has been made, it needs to occur as soon as possible, since the risk of tubal rupture is always present.

Operative management usually involves laparoscopy unless there is severe haemodynamic instability, in which case laparotomy is performed. Traditionally, laparoscopy was performed purely for diagnostic purposes, but laparoscopic removal of the zygote with or without tubal resection has become routine in many units.

Anaesthetic management is as for any emergency surgery, given the above considerations. Haematological assistance and admission to the intensive care unit should be available if required. In severe cases, anaesthesia must proceed as for a ruptured aortic aneurysm: full preoperative resuscitation may be impossible and the patient is prepared and draped before induction of anaesthesia, which may be followed by profound hypotension.

In some countries, medical management is increasingly used as the first-line treatment of early ectopic pregnancies, with intramuscular methotrexate, and guidelines regarding the use of methotrexate have been published by the American College of Obstetricians and Gynecologists. The drug antagonises folic acid and prevents further growth of the trophoblast, which is especially vulnerable at this early stage. Similar outcome to that following surgical management has been claimed. Local injection of hyperosmolar glucose, prostaglandin and potassium chloride have also been used. Finally, expectant management has been used in selected patients, although women whose pregnancies are self- limiting cannot yet be identified reliably.

Key points

- Ectopic pregnancy accounts for 3–6% of all direct maternal deaths in the UK.
- Severe haemorrhage and/or cardiovascular collapse is always a risk.

Further reading

American College of Obstetricians & Gynecologists. Medical management of ectopic pregnancy. Washington (DC): ACOG 2008, www.guidelines.gov/content.aspx?id=12625.

Confidential Enquiry into Maternal and Child Health (CEMACH). Saving mothers' lives: reviewing maternal deaths to make motherhood safer: 2006–2008. The eighth report of the Confidential Enquiries into Maternal Deaths in the United Kingdom. *BJOG* 2011; **118** (Suppl 1): 1–203.

Jurkovic D, Wilkinson H. Diagnosis and management of ectopic pregnancy. *BMJ* 2011; **342**: 3397.

Chapter

5

Evacuation of retained products of conception

Evacuation of retained products of conception (ERPC) may be required at any stage of pregnancy, but it occurs most commonly in early pregnancy following incomplete miscarriage or early fetal demise. It is also required during the puerperium following retention of placental tissue (see Chapter 38, Removal of retained placenta and perineal suturing).

Problems/special considerations

- ERPC following spontaneous abortion at 8 weeks' gestation may be a minor routine gynaecological emergency for the anaesthetist, but the mother may have lost a much-wanted baby.
- The urgency of the procedure varies greatly. The majority of ERPCs are performed as scheduled emergencies in fit young women, and this may lull the inexperienced anaesthetist into a false sense of security. Death may occur from spontaneous abortion; blood loss may be heavy and is frequently underestimated.
- The possibility of co-existing uterine or systemic sepsis must always be considered, especially in postpartum ERPC or in a repeat procedure following incomplete evacuation.

Management options

- Diagnostic ultrasound scanning is frequently used to confirm a non-viable early pregnancy or the presence of retained placental tissue. Transabdominal and transvaginal ultrasonography are now considered to be complementary to each other, with most women requiring a transvaginal ultrasound. Most units now operate a policy of fully assessing mothers on the day of admission in an early pregnancy advisory unit (EPAU), allowing them home and re-admitting them the following day for planned ERPC. This facilitates planning of medical and nursing staffing levels, reduces prolonged periods of waiting and starvation for the mother, and can be economically advantageous. Medical treatment is increasingly used and this enables women to be allowed home after treatment with prostaglandin analogues to await events. Some of these women will need surgical management if the products of conception are not fully expelled.
- Preoperatively, a full assessment is required. Assessment of blood loss may be difficult; fit young women may lose a significant proportion of their blood volume without becoming hypotensive. Tachycardia should alert the anaesthetist to possible hypovolaemia. Signs of sepsis should be sought, and prophylactic antibiotics may be considered.
- General anaesthesia is most commonly used in the UK, although in the absence of uncorrected hypovolaemia or other contraindications, regional anaesthesia is entirely

9

suitable. The puerperal mother in particular may wish to stay awake if offered a choice, and she should be advised to do so if at risk of regurgitation.

- Rapid sequence induction of general anaesthesia is indicated for the non-fasting mother requiring urgent surgery (uncommon) and for the mother who is at risk of regurgitation (see Chapter 54, Aspiration of gastric contents). Anaesthesia using a laryngeal mask airway or facemask using any standard day-case anaesthetic technique is appropriate for the majority of women needing ERPC. Sedative premedication is rarely needed. Intravenous anaesthesia, e.g. with propofol or inhalational anaesthesia, is acceptable, though if the latter is used high concentrations of volatile anaesthetic agents (> 1 minimum alveolar concentration) should be avoided because of the uterine relaxation that may ensue.

- Oxytocic drugs may be requested by the surgeon, although there is little evidence for their efficacy at gestations of less than 15 weeks. A single intravenous bolus of 5 U Syntocinon usually suffices. Ergometrine causes increased intracranial and systemic pressure, and nausea and vomiting, and should not be used routinely.

- Spinal anaesthesia produces more rapid and dense anaesthesia than epidural anaesthesia, and an anaesthetic level of at least T8 is recommended. Clinical experience shows that the traditionally taught anaesthetic level of T10 is insufficient to prevent pain occurring when the uterine fundus is manipulated or curetted.

- Postoperatively, the aim is rapid recovery and discharge home. Requirement for postoperative analgesia rarely exceeds simple non-opioid drugs. Non-steroidal anti-inflammatory agents may be beneficial in relieving uterine cramps. Routine administration of antiemetics should be considered since these women are at risk of postoperative nausea and vomiting.

Key points

- A sensitive and sympathetic approach to the mother is necessary.
- Prolonged preoperative waiting and starvation reflects poor communication and inefficiency.

Further reading

Royal College of Obstetricians and Gynaecologists. Early pregnancy loss, management. *Green-top 25*. London: RCOG 2006, http://www.rcog.org.uk/womens-health/clinical-guidance/management-early-pregnancy-loss-green-top-25.

Termination of pregnancy

Termination of pregnancy in the UK is undertaken under the terms and conditions of the Abortion Act 1967. For the consideration of anaesthetic procedures and potential problems, patients presenting for a termination of pregnancy broadly fall into two groups:

1. The presence of a maternal problem, the most commonly stated reason being danger to the mental or physical health of the mother.
2. Severe fetal congenital abnormality or early fetal death.

Problems/special considerations

When caring for women who are to undergo a termination of pregnancy, it is important to consider the physiological changes of pregnancy, the psychological state of the woman and the need for routine preoperative assessment of the patient.

Those women in the first group above are usually scheduled to have termination of pregnancy on a gynaecological operating list. The second group of patients are often looked after in the maternity unit.

Some members of staff may express conscientious objection to performing or being involved in termination of pregnancy and this must be respected. They cannot be made to participate in such procedures, although they do have a duty to find other staff who will, if that is the patient's wish.

Management options
Termination for maternal indications

Termination of pregnancy is usually a day-case procedure, and routine preoperative assessment is undertaken immediately preoperatively. Assessment should be conducted sympathetically as these women are often very distressed.

Gestation is usually less than 15 weeks and these women can usually be regarded as non-pregnant with respect to gastric emptying and acid aspiration unless they have symptoms of reflux.

An anaesthetic technique suitable for day-case anaesthesia should be employed, e.g. induction with propofol followed by nitrous oxide/oxygen and maintenance with propofol or a volatile anaesthetic agent. There has been concern about concentrations of volatile anaesthetic agents greater than one minimum alveolar concentration causing uterine relaxation unresponsive to oxytocics. For a termination of pregnancy at less than 15 weeks, standard concentrations of volatile anaesthetic agents do not appear to pose a risk and may be used to maintain anaesthesia. Analgesia may be provided by intravenous fentanyl or alfentanil, with rectal diclofenac (100 mg) at the end of the procedure.

The gynaecologist may request that 5–10 U Syntocinon is administered to aid uterine contraction. There is no clear evidence that this is helpful at this stage of pregnancy.

Termination for fetal abnormality or death

Women who present for termination of pregnancy because of fetal abnormality or intrauterine death present a difficult clinical problem. Induction of labour is usually required, and this may be a long and tedious process involving the use of prostaglandin pessaries and Syntocinon infusion (see Chapter 70, Intrauterine death).

Termination of a pregnancy at less than 28 weeks is often associated with the retention of products of conception, for which surgical evacuation and anaesthesia are required. Either regional or general anaesthesia may be offered to the woman, balancing the risks and benefits of each depending on the clinical condition and whether epidural analgesia is already in place. Rapid sequence induction and tracheal intubation may be appropriate.

Key points

- Women may present for termination of pregnancy because of maternal reasons or fetal abnormality/death.
- Such women are distressed and should be dealt with sympathetically.
- Early termination is usually performed as a day-case general anaesthetic procedure.
- Issues surrounding late terminations are as for intrauterine death.

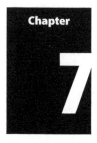

Chapter 7

Cervical suture (cerclage)

Cervical suture (Shirodkar or McDonald cerclage) is performed to reduce the incidence of spontaneous miscarriage when there is cervical incompetence. Although it can be done before conception or as an emergency during pregnancy, the procedure is usually performed electively at 12–16 weeks' gestation; it generally takes 10–20 minutes and is performed transvaginally on a day-case basis. A non-absorbable stitch or tape is sutured in a purse-string around the cervical neck at the level of the internal os; this requires anaesthesia since the procedure is at best uncomfortable, although the suture can usually be removed easily without undue discomfort (usually at 37–38 weeks' gestation unless in preterm labour); spontaneous labour usually soon follows.

In patients with a grossly disrupted cervix, e.g. following surgery, placement of the suture via an abdominal approach may be required. Delivery is usually by elective caesarean section in these cases.

Problems/special considerations

Women undergoing cervical suturing may be especially anxious since previous pregnancies have ended in miscarriage. Otherwise, anaesthesia is along standard lines, bearing in mind the risks of anaesthesia in the pregnant woman and the possible effects of drugs on the fetus (see Chapter 8, Incidental surgery in the pregnant patient).

Cerclage may be difficult if the membranes are bulging; the head-down position and/or tocolysis may be required to counteract this.

Management options

Many authorities advocate spinal anaesthesia as the technique of choice since only a small amount of drug is administered, although epidural anaesthesia is also acceptable. If spinal or epidural anaesthesia is chosen, standard techniques are used. The procedure itself requires a less extensive block than caesarean section (from T8–10 down to and including the sacral roots) and thus smaller doses are required; however, the reduction is offset by the greater requirements at this early stage of pregnancy compared with the term parturient. Thus the doses required for regional anaesthesia are in the order of 75% of those used for caesarean section. Low-dose techniques have also been used, as for caesarean section; the women have more sensation (though painless) but have less motor block.

General anaesthesia may also be used; an advantage is the relaxing effect of volatile agents on the uterus, but it does usually involve administration of several drugs, and the effects on the fetus of many agents in current use are not clear. There may also be an increased risk of regurgitation and aspiration of gastric contents, depending on the gestation and severity of symptoms (see Chapter 54, Aspiration of gastric contents).

Paracervical and pudendal block and/or intravenous analgesia/sedation may also be used, but most authorities would recommend avoiding paracervical block because of the potential adverse effects on uteroplacental perfusion.

Key points

- Cervical suture is usually performed at 12–16 weeks' gestation.
- Patients may be especially anxious because of previous miscarriage.
- Standard techniques are used; spinal anaesthesia may be preferable.

Further reading

Royal College of Obstetricians and Gynaecologists. Cervical cerclage. *Green-top 60*. London: RCOG 2011, http://www.rcog.org.uk/womens-health/clinical-guidance/cervical-cerclage-green-top-60.

Incidental surgery in the pregnant patient

Pregnant women may present with the same surgical conditions as the non-pregnant population, or with problems related to their pregnancy. Most pregnant women are relatively young and fit, although there is an increasing number of women with systemic disease who are becoming pregnant because of advances in medical or surgical management of their condition. Points of particular relevance to anaesthetists are therefore any under-lying condition in addition to the reason for surgery, the effects of pregnancy on its management and the effect upon the fetus.

Problems/special considerations

- Surgical diagnosis of the acute abdomen may be difficult because of the physical presence of the gravid uterus. Non-specific signs such as white cell count may be unreliable (up to $15\,000 \times 10^6/l$ in normal pregnancy). The differential diagnosis may also include obstetric conditions such as placental abruption and HELLP (haemolysis, elevated liver enzymes and low platelet count) syndrome. Surgical technique may be hindered by the pregnancy, and the operation itself may be more difficult than in the non-pregnant patient; e.g. laparoscopic procedures may be impossible.

- The risks of aortocaval compression, difficulties with airway management and aspiration of gastric contents are present as for any pregnant woman, and depend to a certain extent on the stage of pregnancy and the reason for surgery (see Chapter 54, Aspiration of gastric contents).

- Surgery that normally requires the non-supine position, e.g. back surgery, may pose particular problems.

- Since surgery is generally withheld during pregnancy unless absolutely necessary, patients who do present for surgery tend to be more severely affected; thus careful preoperative assessment and management are especially important. Problems of emergency surgery include inadequate preparation and investigation and an increased incidence of vomiting and dehydration.

- The fetus is at risk from the primary effects of the mother's illness (e.g. dehydration, sepsis), the possible teratogenic effects of any drugs that are given to the mother, especially during the first trimester (see Chapter 3, Anaesthesia before conception or confirmation of pregnancy), alterations in uteroplacental blood flow or oxygenation during anaesthesia and surgery, and possible premature onset of labour provoked by the illness, drugs or surgery itself.

Management options

In general, surgery is delayed until the second trimester if possible, because the major fetal organs will have already developed; in addition, the risk of premature labour is lower and the surgery easier than in the third trimester.

Perioperative management requires attendance by senior surgical and obstetric staff, with investigations and scans as required.

Anaesthetic management includes preoperative assessment of the airway and antacid administration. The supine position should be avoided at all times, although the efficacy of lateral tilt when the uterus is still small is uncertain. Particular attention should be paid to general assessment as for emergency surgery in any patient. The disadvantages of regional anaesthesia (e.g. hypotension, increased peristalsis, problems with managing the block during difficult or prolonged surgery) must be weighed against those of general anaesthesia (airway problems, risk of awareness, etc.). Although general anaesthesia involves administration of more drugs with possible effects on the fetus, it also allows administration of volatile agents that relax the uterus. In general, drugs with good safety records during pregnancy should be used; most anaesthetic drugs do not have licences for use in pregnancy (mainly because of the costs involved in extending their licences), but newer drugs should probably be avoided until more is known about their actions. The only standard anaesthetic drug that has excited controversy in recent years is nitrous oxide, because of its effects on methionine synthase and DNA metabolism. Although there is a theoretical risk of its affecting the fetus, there is no evidence to support this clinically and many authorities, if not most, would now consider its use acceptable. General anaesthetic management would thus usually consist of rapid sequence induction with standard agents, tracheal intubation and maintenance of anaesthesia with a volatile agent, as for any emergency general anaesthetic. Other drugs would be used as standard, but those that might increase uterine tone (e.g. ketamine, β-blockers) or vasoconstriction should be avoided if possible. Many obstetricians would request prophylactic administration of tocolytic drugs perioperatively. Certain drugs given near to delivery may cross the placenta and affect the fetus, e.g. non-steroidal anti-inflammatory drugs (which can prevent the ductus arteriosus from closing).

Traditional fears about the detrimental effects of high levels of maternal oxygen by causing uteroplacental vasoconstriction are now known to be unfounded, and fetal arterial partial pressure of oxygen increases (up to a maximum of about 8 kPa (60 mmHg)) as maternal arterial oxygen content increases, so long as maternal hypotension is avoided. Maternal arterial partial pressure of carbon dioxide should be kept in the normal (pregnant) range during controlled ventilation.

The fetus must be monitored preoperatively and postoperatively and, if possible, intra-operatively too. Intraoperative monitoring may be difficult if the surgery is abdominal; it may be possible to use a sterile sleeve over an ultrasonic/Doppler probe. It may be difficult to arrange appropriate midwifery and surgical nursing care both before and after surgery, and the most appropriate area for the mother's postoperative care needs careful consideration.

Key points

- Surgical diagnosis and management may be difficult.
- Maternal risks are those of anaesthesia in the pregnant state.
- Fetal risks are related to the mother's condition, maternal drugs and the premature onset of labour.

Further reading

Cheek TG, Baird E. Anesthesia for nonobstetric surgery: maternal and fetal considerations. *Clin Obstet Gynecol* 2009; **52**: 535–45.

Melnick DM, Wahl WL, Dalton VK. Management of general surgical problems in the pregnant patient. *Am J Surg* 2004; **187**: 170–80.

Reitman E, Flood P. Anaesthetic considerations for non-obstetric surgery during pregnancy. *Br J Anaesth* 2011; **107** (Suppl 1): i72–8.

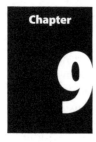

Chapter

9

Intrauterine surgery

Fetal surgery is an attractive option in cases where an isolated abnormality would be otherwise fatal to the fetus or neonate, and is clearly amenable to correction, e.g. neck tumours with airway obstruction, sacrococcygeal teratomas, obstructive uropathy and diaphragmatic hernia. However, results of intrauterine surgery have been conflicting and there is no clear consensus on its place. Simpler measures, e.g. intrauterine blood transfusion in haemolytic disease, are more widely accepted.

Problems/special considerations

Each procedure must be assessed on a risk–benefit basis, since there is a risk of up to 50% fetal loss associated with premature labour, haemorrhage, abruption and infection. For open procedures, vertical uterine incision is required, with caesarean section to deliver the baby if pregnancy proceeds. Maternal thromboembolism has been reported. Thus each lesion must be carefully defined and a chromosomal abnormality or other malformation excluded. For example, intrauterine placement of intraventricular shunts is no longer considered suitable for treatment of hydrocephalus, since the risk–benefit ratio cannot be calculated for individual fetuses because of the difficulty in predicting outcome antenatally. Since most conditions that might be amenable to intrauterine surgery are rare or uncommon and already associated with poor outcome, it is difficult to demonstrate that outcome after fetal surgery is better than that after conventional postpartum therapy, because any expected improvement will be small.

Surgery is technically difficult because of the small size of the fetus and its mobility when small, but leaving the surgery until later may result in increased end-organ damage caused by the malformation. The optimal timing for most procedures is uncertain, although most open ones have been performed at around 18–24 weeks. Percutaneous procedures, e.g. transfusions, may be performed later or at intervals. The EXIT procedure (ex utero intrapartum therapy), for airway obstruction, is also done later and involves delivery of the fetal head through an open hysterotomy and tracheal intubation or tracheostomy while the fetus is oxygenated by the placenta. The fetus may then be delivered and undergo corrective surgery.

Postoperatively, the mother may be confined to bed and receive β_2-agonists, with the risks of deep-vein thrombosis and pulmonary oedema respectively.

Management options

Anaesthetic management is along the lines of that for incidental surgery during pregnancy. Local anaesthetic infiltration of the abdominal wall may be adequate for percutaneous procedures, although there may be a need for emergency caesarean section if fetal bradycardia occurs, and so adequate preparation and facilities are required for this. Regional anaesthesia is a suitable alternative if extensive percutaneous procedures are required.

Fetal and maternal general anaesthesia for corrective surgery is administered by using standard techniques. Fetal injection of a neuromuscular blocking drug may be required to stop fetal movement. Analgesics may also be injected into the fetus – there is increasing evidence that the fetus can 'experience' pain although the significance of this is disputed. Uterine relaxation has been achieved by using one or more of volatile agents, magnesium sulphate or glyceryl trinitrate. Fetal monitoring may be difficult but pulse oximetry, ultrasonography and cardiotocography have been used. Bleeding may be excessive in prolonged open procedures.

Key points

- The place of intrauterine surgery is uncertain.
- To be suitable, malformations must be clearly defined, fatal if untreated and amenable to corrective surgery.
- General principles of anaesthesia are as for incidental surgery during pregnancy.

Further reading

De Buck F, Deprest J, Van de Velde M. Anesthesia for fetal surgery. *Curr Opin Anesthesiol* 2008; **21**: 293–7.

Garcia PJ, Olutoye OO, Ivey RT, Olutoye OA. Case scenario: anesthesia for maternal–fetal surgery: the Ex Utero Intrapartum Therapy (EXIT) procedure. *Anesthesiology* 2011; **114**: 1446–52.

Tran KM. Anesthesia for fetal surgery. *Semin Fetal Neonatal Med* 2010;**15**: 40–5.

Chapter

10

Anatomy of the spine and peripheral nerves

Although not exclusive to obstetric anaesthesia, a sound knowledge of the anatomy pertinent to epidural and spinal anaesthesia is fundamental to obstetric anaesthetists. In addition, knowledge of the relevant peripheral nerves is important in order to differentiate central from peripheral causes of neurological impairment.

The structures involved in obstetric neuraxial anaesthesia comprise the vertebrae and sacral canal, vertebral ligaments, epidural space, meninges and spinal cord. The important peripheral aspects are the lumbar and sacral plexi and the muscular and cutaneous supply of the lower part of the body.

Vertebrae (Fig. 10.1)

The vertebral column has two curves, with the cervical and lumbar regions convex anteriorly and the thoracic and sacral regions concave. Traditionally, T4 is described as the most posterior part (most dependent in the supine position), although T8 has been suggested by recent imaging studies. L3–4 is the most anterior part (uppermost in the supine position), although this curve may be flattened by flexing the hips. In the lateral position, the greater width of women's hips compared with their shoulders imparts a downward slope from the caudal end of the vertebral column to the cranial end.

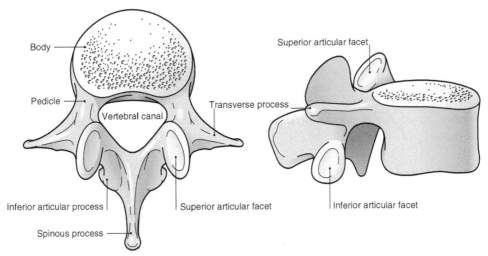

Fig. 10.1 A lumbar vertebra, seen from superior and lateral aspects. Reproduced with permission from Yentis, Hirsch & Smith: *Anaesthesia and Intensive Care A–Z*, 3rd edn; Churchill Livingstone. © Elsevier 2009.

There are seven cervical vertebrae, twelve thoracic, five lumbar, five fused sacral and three to five fused coccygeal. A number of ligaments connect them (see below). Vertebrae have the following components:

- *Body:* This lies anteriorly, with the vertebral arch behind. It is kidney-shaped in the lumbar region. Fibrocartilaginous vertebral discs, accounting for about 25% of the spine's total length, separate the bodies of C2 to L5. Each disc has an outer fibrous annulus fibrosus and a more fluid inner nucleus pulposus (the latter may prolapse through the former: a 'slipped disc'). The bodies of the thoracic vertebrae are heart-shaped and articulate with the ribs via superior and inferior costal facets at their rear. The bodies of the sacral vertebrae are fused to form the sacrum, which encloses the sacral canal; the coccygeal vertebral bodies are fused to form the triangular coccyx, the base of which articulates with the sacrum.

- *Pedicles:* These are round in cross section. They project posteriorly from the body and join the laminae. Each intervertebral foramen is formed by the pedicles of the vertebra above and below.

- *Laminae:* These are flattened in cross section. They complete the vertebral arch by meeting in the midline at the spinous process. The superior and inferior articular processes bear facets for articulation with adjacent vertebrae; those of the thoracic vertebrae are flatter and aligned in the coronal plane, whereas those of the lumbar vertebrae are nearer the sagittal plane.

- *Transverse processes:* In the lumbar region they are thick and pass laterally. The transverse processes of L5 are particularly massive but short. The transverse processes of thoracic vertebrae are large and pass backwards and laterally; they bear facets that articulate with the ribs' tubercles (except T11 and T12).

- *Spinous process:* These project horizontally backwards in the lumbar region; in the thoracic region they are longer and inclined at about 60° to the horizontal. The spinous process of T12 has a notched lower edge.

The cervical vertebrae have a number of features that distinguish them from the others, including the foramen transverarium in the transverse processes, bifid spinous processes and the particular characteristics of C1 and C2.

A line drawn between the iliac crests (Tuffier's line) usually crosses the L3–4 interspace (slightly higher than in the non-pregnant state because of rotation of the pelvis), although this is unreliable, and it has been shown that even experienced anaesthetists can be one or more interspaces lower (or more commonly, higher) than that intended.

Sacral canal (Fig. 10.2)

The sacral canal is 10–15 cm long, triangular in cross section, runs the length of the sacrum and is continuous cranially with the lumbar vertebral canal. The fused bodies of the sacral vertebrae form the anterior wall, and the fused sacral laminae form the posterior wall. The sacral hiatus is a deficiency in the fifth laminar arch, has the cornua laterally and is covered by the sacrococcygeal membrane. Congenital variants are common, possibly contributing to unreliable caudal analgesia.

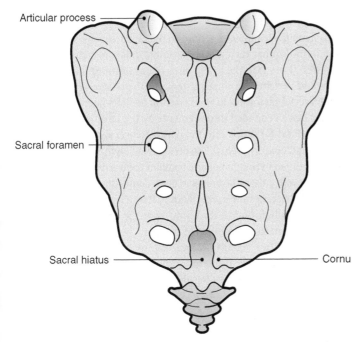

Articular process

Sacral foramen

Sacral hiatus — Cornu

Fig. 10.2 Sacrum. Reproduced with permission from Yentis, Hirsch & Smith: *Anaesthesia and Intensive Care A–Z*, 3rd edn; Churchill Livingstone. © Elsevier 2009.

Vertebral ligaments (Fig. 10.3)

- *Anterior longitudinal ligament:* This is attached to the anterior aspects of the vertebral bodies, and runs from C2 to the sacrum.
- *Posterior longitudinal ligament:* This is attached to the posterior aspects of the vertebral bodies, and runs from C2 to the sacrum.
- *Ligamentum flavum (yellow ligament):* This is attached to the laminae of adjacent vertebrae, forming a 'V'-shaped structure with the point posteriorly. It is more developed in the lumbar than thoracic regions.
- *Interspinous ligament:* This passes between the spinous processes of adjacent vertebrae.
- *Supraspinous ligament:* This is attached to the tips of the spinous processes from C7 to the sacrum.

In addition, there are posterior, anterior and lateral sacrococcygeal ligaments. Other ligaments are involved in the attachments of C1 and C2 to the skull.

The ligaments may become softer during pregnancy because of the hormonal changes that occur.

Epidural space

- *Boundaries:* The space extends from the foramen magnum to the sacrococcygeal membrane. It is triangular in cross section in the lumbar region, its base anterior; it is very thin anteriorly and up to 5 mm wide posteriorly. It lies external to the dura mater of the spinal cord and internal to the ligamenta flava and vertebral laminae posteriorly, the posterior longitudinal ligament anteriorly and the intervertebral foramina and vertebral pedicles laterally. Magnetic resonance imaging suggests the space is divided into segments by the laminae. The space may extend through the intervertebral foramina into the paravertebral spaces.
- *Contents:* These include epidural fat, epidural veins (Batson's plexus), lymphatics and spinal nerve roots. The veins become engorged in pregnancy as a result of the hormonal changes and any aortocaval compression. Connective tissue layers have been demonstrated by radiology and endoscopy within the epidural space, in some cases dividing it into right and left portions.
- *Pressure:* A negative pressure is usually found in the epidural space upon entering it; the reason is unclear but may involve anterior dimpling of the dura by the epidural needle, sudden posterior recoil of the ligamentum flavum when it is punctured, stretching of the dural sac during extreme flexion of the back, transmitted negative intrapleural pressure via thoracic paravertebral spaces and/or relative overgrowth of the vertebral canal compared with the dural sac. Occasionally a positive pressure is found.

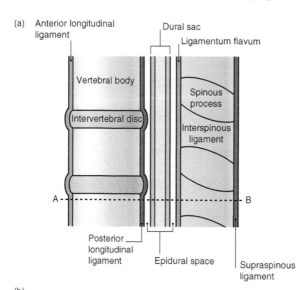

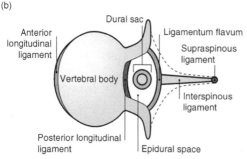

Fig. 10.3 Vertebral ligaments: (a) longitudinal section and (b) transverse section through A–B. Reproduced with permission from Yentis, Hirsch & Smith: *Anaesthesia and Intensive Care A–Z*, 3rd edn; Churchill Livingstone. © Elsevier 2009.

Meninges

- *Pia mater:* This delicate and vascular layer adheres closely to the brain and spinal cord. Between it and the arachnoid mater is the cerebrospinal fluid (CSF) within the subarachnoid space containing blood vessels, the denticulate ligament laterally along its length and the subarachnoid septum posteriorly. The pia terminates as the filum terminale, which passes through the caudal end of the dural sac and attaches to the coccyx.
- *Arachnoid mater:* This membrane is also delicate and contains CSF internally. It lies within the dura externally, the potential subdural space containing vessels, between them. It fuses with the dura at S2.
- *Dura mater:* This fibrous layer has an outer component, which is adherent to the inner periosteum of the vertebrae and an inner one that lies against the outer surface of the arachnoid. The dura projects into the epidural space, especially in the midline. It ends at about S2.

Spinal cord

The spinal cord ends inferiorly level with L3 at birth, rising to the adult level of L1–2 (sometimes T12 or L3) by 20 years. Below this level (the conus medullaris) the lumbar and sacral nerve roots (comprising the cauda equina) and filum terminale occupy the vertebral canal. The main ascending and descending tracts are shown in Fig. 10.4.

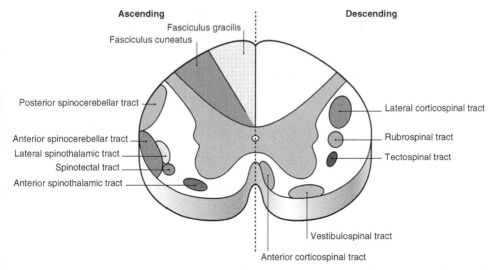

Fig. 10.4 Ascending and descending tracts, spinal cord. Reproduced with permission from Yentis, Hirsch & Smith: *Anaesthesia and Intensive Care A–Z*, 3rd edn; Churchill Livingstone. © Elsevier 2009.

The blood supply of the spinal cord is of relevance to obstetric anaesthetists, since cord ischaemia may result in neurological damage:

- *Anterior spinal artery:* This descends in the anterior median fissure and supplies the anterior two thirds of the cord. The anterior spinal artery syndrome (e.g. arising from profound hypotension) thus results in lower motor neurone paralysis at the level of the lesion, and spastic paraplegia, reduced pain and temperature sensation below the level and normal joint position sense and vibration sensation.

- *Posterior spinal arteries:* These descend along each side of the cord, one anterior and one posterior to the dorsal nerve roots.
- *Radicular branches:* These arise from local arteries (from the aorta) and feed the spinal arteries. Those at T1 and the lower thoracic/upper lumbar level (artery of Adamkiewicz – usually unilateral) are the most important. The cord at T3–5 and T12–L1 is thought to be most at risk from ischaemia. The conus medullaris and cauda equina are supplied by a vascular plexus arising from the artery of Adamkiewicz above and pelvic vessels below. In 15% of the population, the latter are the main source of arterial blood to the conus medullaris and cauda equina; compression during delivery may result in permanent paraplegia.

Venous drainage is via the internal iliac, intercostal, azygos and vertebral veins.

Peripheral nerves of the lower body

The lumbar and sacral plexi are shown schematically in Fig. 10.5. They form at the posterior of the pelvis, and their branches pass round the interior of the pelvis where they may be exposed to pressure during labour and delivery (Figs 10.6; see also Chapter 48, Peripheral nerve lesions following regional anaesthesia).

Peripheral cutaneous innervation may be characterised according to the dermatomal distribution or peripheral nerves (Figs 10.5 & 10.7, Table 48.1). Both representations may vary considerably between individuals. Peripheral motor innervation may also be considered according to myotomal innervation or peripheral nerves (Table 10.1).

Dermatomal innervation of the upper body is also important when determining the upper extent of regional blockade.

Table 10.1 Motor innervation of lower limbs by myotomes and peripheral nerves

Joint	Movement	Myotomes	Nerve supply
Hip	Flexion	L1–3	Lumbar plexus
		L2–4	Femoral nerve
	Extension	L5–S2	Sacral plexus
		L5–S2	Sciatic nerve
	Abduction	L5–S2	Sacral plexus
	Adduction	L2–4	Obturator nerve
Knee	Extension	L2–4	Femoral nerve
	Flexion	L5–S2	Sciatic nerve.
		S1–2	Tibial nerve*
Ankle/foot	Dorsiflexion	L4–5	Deep peroneal nerve[†]
	Eversion	L5–S1	Superficial peroneal nerve[†]
	Plantar flexion	S1–2	Tibial nerve*
	Inversion	L4–5	Tibial nerve*

* Branch of sciatic nerve
[†] Branch of common peroneal nerve, itself a branch of the sciatic nerve

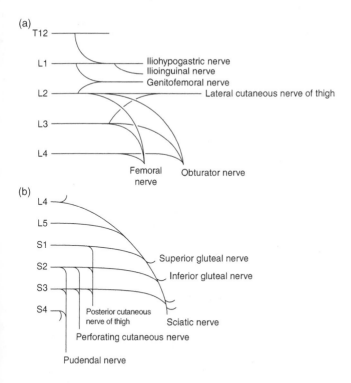

(a)

T12
L1 — Iliohypogastric nerve
Ilioinguinal nerve
Genitofemoral nerve
L2 — Lateral cutaneous nerve of thigh
L3
L4
Femoral nerve   Obturator nerve

(b)

L4
L5
S1
S2 — Superior gluteal nerve
Inferior gluteal nerve
S3
S4
Posterior cutaneous nerve of thigh   Sciatic nerve
Perforating cutaneous nerve
Pudendal nerve

Fig. 10.5 Plan of (a) lumbar and (b) sacral plexi. Reproduced with permission from Yentis, Hirsch & Smith: *Anaesthesia and Intensive Care A–Z*, 3rd edn; Churchill Livingstone. © Elsevier 2009.

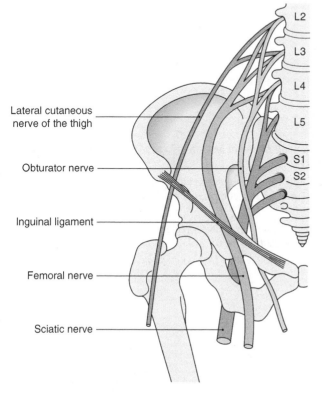

L2
L3
L4
L5
S1
S2

Lateral cutaneous nerve of the thigh

Obturator nerve

Inguinal ligament

Femoral nerve

Sciatic nerve

Fig. 10.6 Relationship of peripheral nerves with the pelvis. Adapted with permission from Holdcroft & Thomas: *Principles and Practice of Obstetric Anaesthesia*; Blackwell Science Ltd. © John Wiley & Sons Ltd 1999.

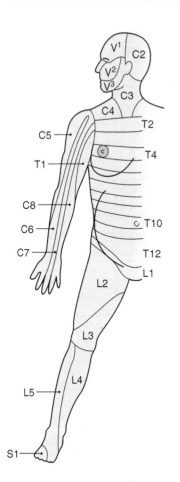

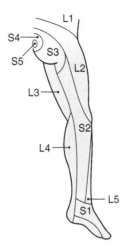

Fig. 10.7 Dermatomes of lower body. Reproduced with permission from Yentis, Hirsch & Smith: *Anaesthesia and Intensive Care A–Z*, 3rd edn; Churchill Livingstone. © Elsevier 2009.

Futher reading

Broadbent CR, Maxwell WB, Ferrie R, *et al.* Ability of anaesthetists to identify a marked lumbar interspace. *Anaesthesia* 2000; **55**: 1122–6.

Capogna G, Celleno D, Simonetti C, Lupoi D. Anatomy of the lumbar epidural region using magnetic resonance imaging: a study of dimensions and a comparison of two postures. *Int J Obstet Anesth* 1997; **6**: 97–100.

Harrison GR. Topographical anatomy of the lumbar epidural region: an in vivo study using computerized axial tomography. *Br J Anaesth* 1999; **83**: 229–34.

Richardson J, Groen G. Applied epidural anatomy. *CEACCP* 2005; **5**: 98–100.

Physiology of pregnancy

Pregnancy is associated with major physiological changes throughout the body. These are caused by both hormonal factors (influential from conception onwards) and the mechanical changes caused by the enlarging uterus (of increasing significance as pregnancy progresses). It is important to understand the normal physiological changes occurring during pregnancy in order to predict the risks and effects of analgesic and anaesthetic intervention, and also to anticipate the impact of pregnancy on any co-existing medical condition.

Hormonal changes

Following fertilisation, the corpus luteum in the ovary secretes progesterone, oestrogens and relaxin, and these hormones are secreted by the placenta when it takes over the function of the corpus luteum from 6–8 weeks' gestation onwards. The placenta also secretes human chorionic somatomammotrophin (hCS; previously known as human placental lactogen and chorionic growth hormone-prolactin).

Human chorionic gonadotrophin (hCG) can be measured by radioimmunoassay and detected in the blood 6 days after conception and in the urine 2–3 weeks after conception. It is therefore a useful early diagnostic test of pregnancy. It is produced by the syncytiotrophoblast, and levels rise rapidly during the first 8 weeks of pregnancy, falling to a plateau thereafter.

Progesterone is responsible for most of the hormonally mediated changes occurring during pregnancy. It causes:

- Smooth muscle relaxation
- Generalised vasodilatation
- Bronchodilatation
- Dilatation within the renal tract
- Sluggish gastrointestinal tract motility and constipation.

It is thermogenic, causing an increase in basal temperature during pregnancy. It may be responsible for the nausea and vomiting that are common in early pregnancy. Progesterone is a neurotransmitter and, together with increased endogenous endorphins, is implicated in the elevated pain threshold experienced by pregnant women. It also decreases the minimum alveolar concentration of inhalational anaesthetic agents. Progesterone has also been demonstrated to enhance conduction blockade in isolated nerve preparations, and it is therefore thought likely to play a role in the decreased requirement for local anaesthetic agents for spinal and epidural anaesthesia.

Progesterone levels return to pre-pregnancy values over a period of 3–4 weeks after delivery, and thus hormonally mediated changes do not reverse immediately in the puerperium.

Mechanical changes

The uterus enlarges as pregnancy progresses. The fundus is palpable:

- Abdominally by the beginning of the second trimester
- At the umbilicus by 20 weeks' gestation
- At the xiphisternum by 36 weeks.

If the fetal head engages in the maternal pelvis at the end of pregnancy the fundal height decreases and this may alleviate some symptoms attributable to mechanical factors. In multiple pregnancies, the uterus expands to a greater extent and more rapidly, and therefore the mechanical effects are usually greater.

Following delivery the uterus involutes rapidly, and should not be palpable above the maternal umbilicus. It has usually returned to within the pelvis by 72 hours after delivery.

Cardiovascular and haemodynamic changes

Pregnancy

- Blood volume increases throughout pregnancy, to approximately 45–50% more than pre-pregnant values by term (see below).
- Cardiac output, heart rate and stroke volume all increase as pregnancy progresses. Cardiac output increases by approximately 40–50% by term, with most of the increase occurring by 20 weeks' gestation. The increased blood flow is distributed primarily to the uterus, where blood flow increases from approximately 50 ml/minute at 10 weeks' gestation to 850 ml/minute at term. Approximately 1 litre of blood is contained within the uterus and maternal side of the placenta.
- Renal blood flow increases by 80% over non-pregnant levels, and this level is achieved by the middle of the second trimester. Glomerular filtration rate and creatinine clearance increase by 50% during pregnancy.
- Systemic vascular resistance falls (peripheral vasodilatation mediated by progesterone, prostacyclin and oestrogens), and there is a decrease in both systolic and diastolic blood pressures, which reach a nadir during the second trimester and then increase gradually towards term, although remaining lower than pre-pregnancy values.
- Aortocaval compression can occur from the middle of pregnancy onward if the supine position is adopted. This is due to mechanical compression of the aorta and inferior vena cava. Venous return is dependent on the competence of collateral circulation via the azygos and ovarian veins. Studies have demonstrated that uterine blood flow decreases primarily as a result of aortic rather than venous compression.
- Central venous and pulmonary arterial pressures are unchanged during normal pregnancy.

Labour and delivery

- Cardiac output increases by 25–50% in labour, with an additional 15–30% increase during contractions. This increase in cardiac output is mediated through increased sympathetic nervous system activity, and is therefore significantly attenuated by epidural analgesia.
- Central venous pressure increases during contractions, partly due to sympathetic activity and partly from the transfer of up to 500 ml of blood from the intervillous space.

The latter is unaffected by epidural analgesia, as is the increase in central venous pressure which occurs when the Valsalva manoeuvre is performed during pushing.
- Autotransfusion of blood (from the placenta) occurs during the third stage. The effect of this may be significant in women with cardiac disease.
- After delivery there is a sustained increase in cardiac output and central venous pressure for several hours, which is associated with hypervolaemia. The implications of these changes for women with cardiac disease are significant (see relevant sections).

Respiratory changes
Pregnancy
- Progesterone increases the sensitivity of the respiratory centre to carbon dioxide and also acts as a primary respiratory stimulant. These effects are enhanced by oestrogens, and the combined hormonal effect causes an increase in minute ventilation of 45–50%.
- The partial pressure of carbon dioxide in arterial blood (P_aCO_2) is re-set to approximately 4 kPa during the first trimester and remains at that level throughout pregnancy. A partially corrected respiratory alkalosis is found in normal pregnant women.
- Functional residual capacity decreases to 80% of pre-pregnancy values as pregnancy progresses, caused by increased intra-abdominal pressure and upward displacement of the diaphragm by the enlarging uterus. Total lung capacity remains unchanged. Functional residual capacity remains greater than closing capacity throughout pregnancy whilst the woman remains in an upright position, but falls when a recumbent position is adopted. It has been estimated that airway closure within normal tidal ventilation may occur in as many as 50% of all supine pregnant women during the second half of pregnancy.
- Oxygen consumption increases progressively during pregnancy to 35% above pre-pregnancy levels.

Labour and delivery
- Massive hyperventilation occurs during labour (unless there is effective analgesia), with minute ventilation increasing by 3–4 times pre-labour values.
- P_aCO_2 falls to below 2 kPa in some women. This respiratory alkalosis is associated with a metabolic acidosis, since maternal aerobic requirement for oxygen (increased by hyperventilation, hyperdynamic circulation and uterine activity) cannot be met, resulting in a progressive lactic acidosis.
- Effective epidural analgesia abolishes these effects during the first stage of labour but not during the second, when the additional uterine activity and work of pushing produce a further oxygen demand that cannot be met.

Gastrointestinal changes
Pregnancy
- Lower oesophageal sphincter pressure is reduced because of the smooth muscle relaxant effect of progesterone.
- Intragastric pressure rises as a mechanical consequence of the enlarging uterus.

- The overall effect of these changes is a decrease in gastro-oesophageal barrier pressure, with a concomitant increase in risk of regurgitation and aspiration of gastric contents.
- 75–85% of pregnant women complain of heartburn during the third trimester, and a significant number will have a demonstrable hiatus hernia.
- Gastric emptying is not delayed during pregnancy.
- There is some evidence that gastric volume is increased, and the pH of the intragastric volume may be lower than in the non-pregnant individual.

Labour and delivery

- Gastric emptying is now thought to be normal in labour in most cases, unless opioids have been given.
- Opioid analgesia (regardless of route of administration) delays gastric emptying.
- Studies suggest that gastric volume (but not acidity) may remain elevated for 48 hours after delivery.

Haematological changes

Total blood volume increases by approximately 1.5 l during pregnancy, with plasma volume increasing by 30–50% and red cell mass increasing by 20–30% (thus causing the so-called 'physiological anaemia' of pregnancy). The magnitude of the increase is greater in women with multiple pregnancy and greatly reduced in women with pre-eclampsia. Plasma volume changes are maximum by mid-pregnancy, returning to normal by approximately 6 weeks postpartum. The haemoglobin concentration falls by 1–2 g/dl by mid-pregnancy; the red cell indices remain approximately constant apart from a small increase in the mean cell volume, unless women become iron/folate deficient. The haemoglobin concentration usually takes up to 4–6 weeks to reach pre-pregnancy levels.

The white blood cell count increases, peaking at $10–15 \times 10^9$/l around mid-pregnancy and increasing further in labour (to up to 30×10^9/l), returning to normal non-pregnant levels by 6–7 days postpartum. Most of the increase is in neutrophils. (N.B. The use of steroids in preterm labour can also increase white cell count.)

The platelet count usually remains within the normal range in pregnancy although population mean counts are slightly lower, with the lower normal limit usually given as approximately $100–120 \times 10^9$/l.

Pregnancy represents a state of increased coagulability; there is increased hepatic production of coagulation factors, especially fibrinogen (increases by approximately 50%) and factor VIII (approximately doubles), but others also increase (II, X and von Willebrand factor). Resistance to activated protein C also increases. Fibrinolytic inhibitors decrease, as do factor XI and protein S activity.

Management options

Positioning

- It is the anaesthetist's responsibility to exercise vigilance, with special attention being paid to the hips and back. The pregnant woman has increased ligamentous laxity, and may be particularly at risk of musculoskeletal trauma if she has received epidural analgesia. This risk is considerably increased if she has received either regional or general anaesthesia, when she is unable to safeguard her position.

- No pregnant woman should lie in the unmodified supine position at term (it is rare to find a mother who will voluntarily adopt this position). The wedged supine position and the use of lateral tilt are compromises and do not reliably relieve aortocaval compression. Women should be encouraged to remain sitting upright or in the full lateral position whenever possible. Walking and standing in labour should also be encouraged.
- Obstetricians and midwives should be asked to perform fetal scalp blood sampling and vaginal examinations with the woman in the left lateral, or at least tilted, position.
- Closing volume may occur within tidal volume when the semi-recumbent position is adopted, and consideration should be given to continuous administration of oxygen to women particularly at risk (e.g. those who are obese, and those with respiratory disease).

General anaesthesia

- Pregnant women have increased oxygen consumption and decreased oxygen reserves. They are therefore at greatly increased risk of hypoxia during periods of apnoea.
- The risk of pulmonary aspiration of gastric contents means that rapid sequence induction of general anaesthesia, preceded by measures to reduce the acidity of the gastric contents, may be required, depending on the gestation and severity of symptoms (see Chapter 54, Aspiration of gastric contents).

These topics are discussed further elsewhere.

Chapter

12

Antenatal care

Antenatal care includes a wide range of functions, including:

- Provision of information to mothers about the importance of diet and lifestyle, and about choices available to them during their pregnancy.
- Screening for pre-existing maternal conditions and risk factors.
- Assessment of maternal wellbeing during pregnancy and screening for development of pregnancy-specific and non-specific conditions.
- Screening for fetal anomalies and assessment of fetal growth and wellbeing.

Table 12.1 Checklist for antenatal anaesthetic referral

Obstetric	Placenta accreta/percreta Three or more fetuses
Cardiovascular/respiratory/ neurological	All except mild, without functional limitation, and without history of previous surgery
Haematological	Coagulopathy including anticoagulant therapy Sickle disease and variants
Musculoskeletal	Severe back or neck problems Spina bifida
Anaesthetic	Previous difficulties e.g. intubation
Other	Severe obesity Severe allergy to drugs or latex Severe anxiety/needle phobia Severe connective tissue disease Refusal of blood products Inability to give consent

Maternal assessment

Assessment and management of specific maternal conditions are addressed in subsequent chapters. For routine antenatal care in the UK, ten antenatal appointments are currently recommended for nullipara with uncomplicated pregnancies, and seven for multipara, with regular urine and blood pressure checks and further checks (e.g. for anaemia) at specified intervals. Anaesthetic involvement may be ad hoc or via formal clinics, in which anaesthetists can assess women referred to them and arrange further referral/investigations and discuss management options. A checklist for midwives and obstetricians, listing those conditions that warrant anaesthetic referral, is useful (Table 12.1).

Fetal assessment

It is possible to make detailed assessments of fetal wellbeing in the antenatal period. A decision to deliver the baby early may be made on the outcome of these assessments, and the obstetric anaesthetist may be involved in this decision making. The most commonly used tests are serial ultrasonography, serial Doppler flow studies and cardiotocography.

- *Serial ultrasonography:* Routine scanning is offered at 10–13 weeks and 18–20 weeks. The head circumference is measured in association with the abdominal circumference. If the fetus is starving, glycogen stores in the liver will be depleted and there will be an increase in the ratio of head circumference to abdominal wall circumference (asymmetrical growth retardation). There may also be a generalised growth retardation (symmetrical growth retardation). The liquor volume is also used as an indicator of fetal wellbeing and placental function, poor placental function being reflected in a reduced liquor volume. As a measure of this volume, the anterior–posterior distance across the liquor (the liquor column) is measured using a transducer. A column of less than 3 cm is indicative of oligohydramnios and one less than 2 cm represents very severe oligohydramnios. Amniotic fluid index may also be used to measure the liquor volume; this is the sum of the liquor column in each of the four liquor quadrants and is normally 8–20 cm.

- *Serial Doppler flow studies:* Both maternal uterine blood flow and fetal umbilical artery blood flow may be measured using Doppler techniques. The pattern of flow reflects placental function as follows:

  (i) Normal flow continues through systole and diastole, as there is little resistance to flow through the placenta. The systolic:diastolic flow velocity ratio (SD ratio) is widely used to indicate resistance to arterial flow; several other derived indices (e.g. pulsatility index) have also been used to indicate fetal perfusion and oxygenation. The use of these techniques for screening for high risk fetuses is controversial and they may be reserved for monitoring known high risk cases.

  (ii) Just absent end-diastolic flow may indicate the need for delivery of the baby. Wide absence of end-diastolic flow suggests the need to deliver the baby urgently.

  (iii) Reversal of end-diastolic flow suggests the need for immediate delivery of the baby. Plans for timing and mode of delivery of the baby may be based on the evidence of the Doppler studies. The anaesthetist should understand that the anaesthetic management should optimise the placental flow and that meticulous care should be taken to avoid sudden cardiovascular changes and in particular supine hypotension.

  In specialised fetal medicine units, blood flow may also be measured by using Doppler techniques in the fetal abdominal aorta, renal or middle cerebral arteries.

- *Cardiotocography:* This will only record the fetal heart during the time of the trace and cannot provide historical or predictive information. The pattern of the trace may be indicative of fetal compromise and may be used to plan the mode of delivery, e.g. either induction of labour or caesarean section (see Chapter 20, Intrapartum fetal monitoring). It is important that the anaesthetist communicates with the obstetrician and understands how compromised the fetus is when asked to give analgesia or anaesthesia to these mothers. The degree of urgency for the delivery will depend on the condition of the fetus. It should be remembered that women in these circumstances may be very anxious and upset and will need extra support during delivery.

Key points

- Antenatal assessments may identify mothers and fetuses at special risk.
- High-risk mothers should be referred for antenatal anaesthetic assessment.
- Meticulous care should be taken to maintain optimal placental perfusion if investigations indicate fetal hypoxaemia.
- Communication between medical and midwifery staff is crucial.

Further reading

Grivell RM, Alfirevic Z, Gyte GM, *et al.* Antenatal cardiotocography for fetal assessment. *Cochrane Database Syst Rev* 2010; (1): CD007863.

National Institute for Health and Clinical Excellence. Antenatal care: routine care for the healthy pregnant woman. *Clinical Guideline 62.* London: NICE 2008, http://www.nice.org.uk/CG62.

Chapter 3

Aortocaval compression

Aortocaval compression (supine hypotensive syndrome) was first reported in 1931. The inferior vena cava and aorta become compressed by the pregnant uterus (the vena cava may be totally occluded), causing reduction in venous return and cardiac output, thus compromising the mother, fetus or both. Vasovagal syncope may follow aortocaval compression. Maternal symptoms and signs vary from asymptomatic mild hypotension to total cardiovascular collapse, partly dependent on the efficacy of the collateral circulation bypassing the inferior vena cava. Onset of symptoms and signs is associated with lying in the supine or semi-supine position, and is relieved by turning to the full lateral position in most cases.

Problems/special considerations

- Aortocaval compression is not confined to the woman at term. The condition has been reported in the fifth month of pregnancy. Women with multiple pregnancy or hydramnios are at increased risk because of the increased size of the gravid uterus.
- It is important to appreciate that a normal blood pressure and lack of maternal symptoms do not exclude a significant fall in cardiac output and placental perfusion.
- Onset of symptoms may occur within 30 seconds, but may be delayed by 30 minutes. Severity of symptoms is not a reliable guide to the severity of hypotension.
- Slight changes in maternal position may cause significant change in symptoms. A 15° lateral tilt does not always relieve aortocaval compression, and even a 45° tilt does not guarantee abolition of hypotension.
- Catastrophic hypotension, and even cardiac arrest, may occur if general anaesthesia is induced in a woman who is experiencing severe aortocaval compression (e.g. in the supine position). Even mild degrees of aortocaval compression may lead to severe hypotension after spinal or epidural anaesthesia.
- It is impossible to perform effective cardiopulmonary resuscitation on a pregnant woman in the supine position, and the uterus must be displaced off the vena cava and aorta by tilting the pelvis or using manual displacement.

Management options

Women will not voluntarily adopt positions in which aortocaval compression occurs, and therefore the condition is largely iatrogenic, occurring after a woman has been placed in the supine position by her midwifery or medical attendants. A history suggestive of aortocaval compression in late pregnancy may indicate an increased risk of developing the condition during labour and delivery. All healthcare staff must be aware of aortocaval compression and of the need to avoid the supine position. This is particularly important if the woman is unable to change her own position because of administration of analgesia or anaesthesia.

Uterine displacement (usually to the left, although occasionally improved symptomatic relief will be obtained by displacement to the right) must be used during all vaginal examinations and during both vaginal and operative delivery, and is especially important if regional analgesia or anaesthesia is used. This can be achieved manually or by use of table tilt or a wedge under the hip. Use of uterine displacement rather than the full lateral position is a compromise between maternal safety and obstetricians' convenience. Use of the full lateral position for caesarean section has been reported.

Extreme vigilance is necessary when maternal symptoms are abolished by induction of general anaesthesia. During regional anaesthesia for operative delivery, complaints of faintness, dizziness, restlessness and nausea should alert the anaesthetist to the onset of hypotension. Pallor, particularly of the lips, yawning and non-specific feelings of anxiety are also warning signs of aortocaval compression. Continuous fetal monitoring may indicate signs of fetal distress when the mother adopts the supine or semi-supine position, and occasionally this may be the only indicator of the condition. Turning the mother into the full left lateral position should be the first step in the treatment of hypotension or cardiotocographic abnormalities.

Key points

- No pregnant woman should lie supine beyond 16–18 weeks.
- The uterus must be displaced off the aorta and vena cava during vaginal examinations and during caesarean section. This can be done manually, with a wedge under the hip, or by using lateral tilt of the operating table.
- Cardiopulmonary resuscitation will be ineffective if the mother is supine.

Further reading

Cluver C, Novikova N, Hofmeyr GJ, Hall DR. Maternal position during Caesarean section for preventing maternal and neonatal complications. *Cochrane Database Syst Rev* 2010; (6): CD007623.

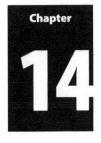

Chapter

14 Gastric function and feeding in labour

Physiological changes in pregnancy affect the volume, acidity and emptying of gastric secretions as well as sphincter mechanisms in the lower oesophagus. Interventions in labour such as analgesia may also affect these changes adversely. General anaesthesia is occasionally necessary in emergency situations, and the presence of a full stomach (and thus the risk of aspiration of gastric contents) should always be assumed in such patients (see Chapter 54, Aspiration of gastric contents). The increasing incidence of obesity in the pregnant population has raised concerns that these patients may be at more risk of aspiration should they need a general anaesthetic for operative delivery.

Problems/special considerations

Increased circulating progesterone associated with pregnancy relaxes smooth muscle and causes relaxation of the lower oesophageal sphincter, whereas placental gastrin increases the volume and decreases the pH of gastric contents. The enlarging uterus increases intragastric pressure and there is an increase in small and large bowel transit time. However, evidence suggests that gastric emptying per se is not affected by pregnancy, although it may be decreased in labour if opioids are given.

Epidural analgesia with local anaesthetic solutions in labour is associated with normal gastric emptying, whereas subarachnoid or epidural opioids (fentanyl or diamorphine) in large doses cause a modest decrease in gastric emptying. Systemic opioid analgesia causes a much greater and prolonged decrease in gastric emptying. There are some randomised trials that have demonstrated large gastric volumes and a high incidence of vomiting in women allowed to eat solid food, even when pain was adequately controlled with a low-dose fentanyl/bupivacaine epidural. Previous studies suggested that oral intake of food during labour may be associated with a longer duration of labour and also possibly an increase in caesarean section rate, but recent evidence suggests this to not be the case.

Plasma progesterone concentrations return to non-pregnant values within 24 hours of delivery, and gastroesophageal reflux is considerably reduced within 48 hours of delivery. The period of risk of aspiration thus extends to a poorly defined time after delivery, and appropriate general anaesthetic management in the early postpartum period is somewhat controversial.

Routine withholding of food and fluids in labour has been challenged by a number of authors, particularly those who are not anaesthetists. They point out that absolute starvation is not popular with mothers, that aspiration associated with emergency general anaesthesia nowadays is uncommon owing to the increase in use of regional anaesthesia, and that there may be risks associated with prolonged starvation. On the other hand, there is little evidence that a period of starvation during labour is harmful, although it may be unpleasant. Starvation is associated with ketosis, but this has not been found to affect the duration or outcome of labour.

Management options

There are three approaches to the treatment of feeding in labour. The traditional approach is to assume that all women in labour are at risk of an event in labour that will require emergency general anaesthesia, and that they are therefore at risk of aspiration of large volumes of acid gastric contents. As a consequence of this assumption, all women in labour are starved, allowed only sips of water to drink and given regular H_2-antagonists and antacids (see Chapter 54, Aspiration of gastric contents). This regimen has become less common in recent years for the reasons discussed above. In addition, women who know that a unit's policy is not to allow any oral intake are more likely to 'binge' before admission in labour, potentially negating any benefit from the policy.

Another approach is to assume that women in labour require food and fluid and to give these liberally. Often no H_2-blockers are given.

A more rational approach is to stratify management on the basis of risk. Women at high risk of requiring general anaesthesia are advised to have only clear fluids and receive regular H_2-blockers. In addition, for those who do eat and drink during labour, substances that are associated with slower gastric emptying (those with high fat or sugar content) should be discouraged in favour of protein-based snacks and isotonic drinks.

If intravenous water is required in labour, the most sensible fluid to provide might be 5% or 10% dextrose. Unfortunately this has been associated with fluid overload in the mother and hyponatraemia in the neonate. However, modest volumes (< 1 litre) do not significantly affect neonatal plasma sodium concentrations. Many units give relatively low volumes of intravenous saline, dextrosesaline or Hartmann's solution when intravenous fluid is considered necessary.

Key points

- Solid food ingested during labour is not predictably absorbed.
- Women treated with epidural analgesia may have normal gastric emptying unless large boluses of opioid are given.
- Opioids given parenterally markedly decrease gastric emptying.
- Acid aspiration prophylaxis should be given to all women at risk of intervention in labour.

Further reading

O'Sullivan G, Liu B, Hart D, Seed P, Shennan A. Effect of food intake during labour on obstetric outcome: randomised controlled trial. *BMJ* 2009; **338**: b784.

Singata M, Tranmer J, Gyte GM. Restricting oral fluid and food intake during labour. *Cochrane Database Syst Rev* 2010; (1):CD003930.

Toohill J, Soong B, Flenady V. Interventions for ketosis during labour. *Cochrane Database Syst Rev* 2008; (3): CD004230.

Chapter

15

Drugs and pregnancy

Pregnancy may interact with drugs in a number of different ways. Firstly, the pregnant state confers alterations in both pharmacokinetics and pharmacodynamics; secondly, the fetus may be affected by drugs administered to the mother, and in many cases this may restrict the use of certain drugs; and thirdly there may be further passage of certain drugs to the neonate in breast milk (see Chapter 151, Drugs and breastfeeding). Because of these considerations, special licensing requirements exist for drugs to be used in pregnancy, which have not been met by many drugs in current use.

Pharmacokinetics

Each of the traditional components of pharmacokinetics may be altered in the pregnant, as opposed to the non-pregnant, state.

- *Absorption of drug:* This depends on the route of administration and, in general, is little affected by pregnancy. However, absorption of enterally administered drugs may be affected by pregnancy-associated gastrointestinal upsets including vomiting. Owing to the increased minute ventilation and cardiac output, absorption of inhalational agents is more rapid.
- *Distribution of drug:* This is affected by the increased blood volume and body fluid and altered plasma protein profile. The former two result in a greater volume of distribution. In addition, the fetus represents an additional compartment to which drugs will distribute, depending on their lipid solubility, pKa and protein binding. The increased cardiac output will tend to redistribute drugs more quickly unless they are extensively bound to the tissues. During labour, acute changes in plasma pH (e.g. acidosis associated with maternal exhaustion or alkalosis associated with pain-induced hyperventilation) may affect both protein binding and degree of dissociation of drug.
- *Metabolism of drugs:* Drugs broken down by the major organs (usually the liver) should be handled normally in pregnancy, unless there is hepatic impairment, e.g. in HELLP (haemolysis, elevated liver enzymes and low platelet count) syndrome. Some drugs are metabolised by plasma cholinesterases and may thus have longer duration of action if the protein concentration is reduced, e.g. suxamethonium.
- *Elimination:* Since glomerular filtration rate is increased in pregnancy, clearance of many drugs is increased unless renal function is impaired, e.g. in pre-eclampsia. Another route of elimination is in breast milk, although this represents a relatively small amount of total drug elimination. Inhalational agents are excreted via the lungs more rapidly in the pregnant than non-pregnant state.

Pharmacodynamics

The effects of most drugs are unchanged in pregnancy. However, notable and important exceptions are anaesthetic agents. Thus the minimum alveolar concentration of inhalational agents is reduced as is the minimal blocking concentration of local anaesthetics. The cause of this decrease in anaesthetic requirement is thought to be progesterone and/or a metabolite thereof. In addition, a given amount of epidural local anaesthetic solution produces a more extensive block than in non-pregnant subjects, possibly related to the reduction in epidural space caused by epidural venous engorgement, although progesterone has also been suggested as a cause.

Fetal effects of drugs

Drugs may affect the fetus at any stage of pregnancy. During the first trimester the developing organ systems and overall body structure are especially at risk, particularly between the third and tenth weeks; administration of certain drugs during this period may result in congenital malformations. During the second and third trimesters, the growth and development of fetal tissues may be affected. Finally, drugs given before delivery may affect fetal oxygenation indirectly (e.g. by causing maternal hypotension or respiratory depression), may affect labour (e.g. β-agonists), or may have neonatal effects after birth (e.g. opioids). Many drugs are known to be harmful when given during pregnancy, but for many others, precise information is not always available. Thus, in general, drugs are not prescribed unless the benefits are felt to outweigh any possible risk, especially during the first trimester. Where possible, older drugs of which clinicians have greater experience are preferred over newer ones, and this is also true of anaesthetic agents.

Licensing of drugs in pregnancy

Many drugs, including anaesthetic agents, are not licensed for use in pregnancy, mainly because of the prohibitive costs to the manufacturer of performing the appropriate studies required and the relatively limited addition such licensing would make to the market. For example, the data sheets of etomidate, alfentanil and fentanyl contain the sentence 'safety in human pregnancy has not been established' or words to that effect, whilst those of propofol and fentanyl specifically warn against their use in obstetrics. Even in the case of thiopental, the data sheet merely states that there is 'epidemiological and clinical evidence' of its safety in pregnancy, whereas that of atracurium, vecuronium and suxamethonium state that they should only be used in pregnancy 'if the potential benefits outweigh any potential risks'.

Key points

- Pharmacokinetics and pharmacodynamics in pregnancy may be altered from those in the non-pregnant state.
- Most drugs administered to the mother will pass to the fetus to a degree.
- Many drugs pass into breast milk.
- Most anaesthetic drugs are not licensed for use in pregnancy.

Further reading

Henderson E, Mackillop L. Prescribing in pregnancy and during breast feeding: using principles in clinical practice. *Postgrad Med J* 2011; **87**: 349–54.

Howell PR, Madej T. Administration of drugs outside of product licence: awareness and current practice. *Int J Obstet Anesth* 1999; **8**: 30–6.

World Health Organization. Breastfeeding and maternal medication: Recommendations for Drugs in the Eleventh WHO Model List of Essential Drugs: WHO 2002, http://whqlibdoc.who.int/hq/2002/55732.pdf.

Chapter 16

Placental transfer of drugs

The placenta is a complex structure composed of both maternal and fetal tissues. Nevertheless, it is basically a semi-permeable biological membrane and as such obeys the laws that govern transport across such membranes. Virtually all transfer of drugs across the placenta occurs by simple diffusion, and all drugs administered to the mother will reach the fetus, albeit to a variable extent depending upon the factors discussed below.

Factors determining placental transfer

Molecular weight and lipid solubility

The molecular weight of the drug, its degree of ionisation, its lipid solubility and the degree to which it is protein bound will all affect the readiness with which it will cross the placenta. The majority of anaesthetic drugs are small (molecular weights of less than 500) and lipid soluble; thus they cross the placenta readily. The main exceptions are the neuromuscular blocking drugs, which are less lipid soluble, more highly ionised quaternary ammonium compounds, and in the doses used in normal clinical anaesthesia do not cross the placenta to any significant extent. However, if used in large doses or over a prolonged period of time (e.g. to facilitate artificial ventilation in the intensive care unit) they do reach the fetal circulation in doses that may have a clinical effect necessitating ventilatory support.

Changes in maternal or fetal pH may alter the degree of ionisation and protein binding of a drug, and thus alter its availability for transfer. This is most likely to occur if the pKa of a drug is close to physiological pH, and becomes clinically relevant in the acidotic fetus. Once drug transfer to the fetus has occurred, acidosis results in increased ionisation of the drug, which is then unable to equilibrate with the maternal circulation by diffusion back across the placenta. This results in drug accumulation in the fetus ('ion trapping'), and is particularly relevant for local anaesthetics, which all have a pKa > 7.4.

Maternal drug concentration

Drug transfer occurs down a concentration gradient (which is usually from mother to fetus but can also occur from fetus to mother). The drug concentration on the maternal side depends on the route of administration, total maternal dose, volume of distribution and drug clearance and metabolism. The highest maternal blood concentration of a drug will be achieved following intravenous administration; epidural and intramuscular administration result in similar maternal blood concentrations. Systemic drug absorption will be greater from more vascular tissues, such as the paracervical region.

The increase in blood volume and cardiac output that accompanies normal pregnancy has an effect on maternal drug concentration; the volume of distribution and plasma clearance of drugs such as thiopental is increased.

Placental factors

The area of placenta available for transfer is important. Physiological shunting occurs in the placenta, and in maternal disease such as pre-eclampsia the placenta itself may present an increased barrier to transfer. Although there is evidence that some drug metabolism occurs within the placenta itself, this is not clinically significant.

Fetal drug concentration

Once a drug has reached the fetus it is subject to redistribution, metabolism and excretion. The fetus has less plasma protein binding capacity and less mature enzyme systems than the mother, and will therefore eliminate drugs less effectively. Some transfer of drugs occurs back across the placenta to the mother if the maternal concentration falls below that in the fetus (unless ion trapping occurs – see above).

Uteroplacental blood flow

This is the other major factor influencing placental transfer. Any reduction in blood flow to the placenta will inevitably reduce transfer of drugs (and nutrients) to the fetus. Reduction in uteroplacental flow may occur as a result of generally reduced maternal blood flow (hypotension, reduced cardiac output states, aortocaval compression, generalised vasoconstriction) or direct obstruction of flow (aortocaval compression, uterine contraction, umbilical cord compression).

Problems/special considerations

All general anaesthetic agents cross the placenta readily; and in normal clinical practice their effects on the fetus are only of significance immediately after delivery. The compromised fetus, or one in whom the uterine incision to delivery interval has been prolonged, may be depressed at birth, but rarely requires more than simple resuscitative measures.

Pethidine (and all other opioids) crosses the placenta readily. It has maximal effect in the fetus 3–4 hours after maternal administration and minimal effect if given to the mother within an hour of delivery. (This is contrary to traditional midwifery teaching, which recommends that pethidine is not given if delivery is expected within 2–3 hours.) Both pethidine and its active metabolite norpethidine have prolonged half-lives in the fetus and cause respiratory depression and reduced sucking ability. Opioid side effects are reversed by naloxone.

Local anaesthetics cross the placenta by simple diffusion, but the extent of placental transfer is also dependent on maternal plasma protein binding (bupivacaine and ropivacaine are highly protein bound, and therefore cross less readily than lidocaine, which is less protein bound).

Key points

- The major determinants of transfer by simple diffusion are the maternal–fetal drug concentration gradient, molecular weight of the drug, lipid solubility, degree of drug ionisation and extent of protein binding.
- Uteroplacental blood flow is also important.
- Opioids given to the mother for labour analgesia cross the placenta freely and may cause fetal respiratory and neurobehavioural depression, which are reversible with naloxone.

Further reading

Littleford J. Effects on the fetus and newborn of maternal analgesia and anesthesia: a review. *Can J Anesth* 2004; **51**: 586–609.

Chapter

17 Prescription and administration of drugs by midwives

In the UK, regulations for prescription and administration of drugs by midwives fall under the responsibility of the Nursing and Midwifery Council (NMC; previously the UK Central Council for Nursing, Midwifery and Health Visiting (UKCC)), which issues codes and standards relating to the practical application of acts such as the Medicines Act 1968, Misuse of Drugs Act 1971, and Medicinal Products: Prescription by Nurses Act 1992, and their subsequent amendments. Many of the NMC's publications on the matter are not legally binding but would be taken into account if there were to be medicolegal or regulatory action concerning administration of drugs. Against this background of central control, the setting up of, and adherence to, local policies is strongly encouraged, in recognition of the differing requirements from unit to unit.

Problems/special considerations

A compromise must exist between: (i) supporting the midwife's role as an independent practitioner; (ii) reducing the workload on, and requirement for, medical staff to treat common and relatively minor conditions; (iii) permitting the rapid administration of drugs that may have real benefits to mothers and reduce morbidity or mortality; and (iv) restricting the use of potentially harmful drugs or reducing the incidence of adverse effects. Whether a particular drug should be allowed to be given thus depends on the incidence, importance and potential severity of the condition for which it is indicated and the efficacy, method of administration and safety profile of the drug concerned. In

Table 17.1 Sample standing orders for drugs that may be prescribed and administered by midwives without medical prescription

Analgesics	Opioids (usually pethidine, up to two intramuscular doses)
	Paracetamol/codydramol/cocodamol
	Entonox
	Diclofenac
Local anaesthetics	Lidocaine for infiltration/local application
Gastrointestinal	Liquid antacids
	Ranitidine/cimetidine
	Laxatives
	Antiemetics
Oxytocics	Oxytocin/ergometrine
Sedatives	Temazepam
Haematological	Iron/folate preparations
	Subcutaneous heparin
	Anti-D
	Vitamin K (neonatal)
Other	Naloxone (neonatal)
	Topical clotrimazole

N.B. Midwives can also administer TENS.

recent years, many NHS trusts have developed strategies for improving safety in administering drugs, along with improved methods of assessing competency for nursing and midwifery staff.

Drugs that midwives can administer without medical prescription

There is regional variation according to local policies, and individual trusts bear ultimate responsibility for approving drug policies within their maternity services. However, the drugs that midwives are allowed to prescribe and administer generally fall into a number of categories (Table 17.1). Local regulations are usually decided by a panel including representatives of midwives, pharmacists and obstetricians; anaesthetic staff may also be involved, e.g. in helping with analgesic or local anaesthetic drug policies.

Midwives in different units may interpret the NMC's guidelines differently, especially with regard to epidural top-ups; for example, midwives in certain units may be prepared to administer epidural drugs prescribed by a doctor (i.e. anaesthetist) whereas those in others may not. This is rarely a problem with local anaesthetic drugs alone but has been problematic with mixtures of local anaesthetics and opioids, e.g. fentanyl, which are both controlled drugs and unlicensed for epidural use. Recently, in the UK, there has been stricter attention to the proper handling of all preparations containing controlled drugs, even the dilute mixtures used for epidural analgesia. Interpretation of current UK law has led to suggestions that each single top-up with such mixtures constitutes a separate administration and thus requires the syringe to be kept in a locked cupboard between top-ups, with double-checking and double-signing before each top-up. This has led some units to change from midwife-administered boluses to infusions or patient-controlled epidural analgesia. In all cases, midwives' willingness to give epidural drugs is only on the understanding that ultimate responsibility for administering the drug is with the anaesthetist.

The regulations are regularly reviewed, with recent attention being paid to administration of intravenous fluids to reflect (i) the widespread competence of midwives in venous cannulation and (ii) the number of women choosing to deliver at home and therefore the potential for severe haemorrhage away from hospitals.

Key points

- The Nursing and Midwifery Council (NMC) issues professional guidelines and codes for administration of drugs by midwives.
- Midwives are able to administer several drugs without a doctor's prescription, according to the NMC's recommendations and local policies.
- Midwives may administer certain drugs unlicensed for use in labour, e.g. epidural fentanyl, if covered by local policies and on the written prescription of a doctor.

Further reading

Nursing and Midwifery Council. *Standards for Medicines Management*. London: NMC 2008, http://www.nmc-k.org/Documents/Standards/nmcStandardsForMedicinesManagementBooklet.pdf.

Chapter

18 Local anaesthetics

Bupivacaine, lidocaine, ropivacaine and levobupivacaine (the S-enantiomer of bupivacaine) are all licensed for obstetric epidural use in the UK, although heavy (hyperbaric) 0.5% bupivacaine is the only local anaesthetic licensed for obstetric spinal use (levobupivacaine is licensed for non-obstetric spinal anaesthesia). These local anaesthetics are all amides. There are no local anaesthetics in the ester group in use in British obstetric anaesthesia.

Pharmacology

Local anaesthetics act by reducing permeability of the nerve cell membrane to sodium, and thus preventing development of a propagated action potential. The local anaesthetic binds to receptor sites within the sodium channels of the nerve membrane.

Increasing lipid solubility allows the local anaesthetic drug to penetrate the nerve membrane more readily, and is associated with increased potency (bupivacaine and levo-bupivacaine have greater lipid solubility than lidocaine and ropivacaine).

Increased capacity for protein binding increases duration of action of the local anaesthetic. Bupivacaine and levobupivacaine are 95% protein bound and ropivacaine is 94% protein bound, and these drugs therefore have a longer duration of action than lidocaine, which is only 64% protein bound.

The speed of onset of local anaesthetic activity is related to the degree of ionisation of the drug. The non-ionised form of the drug diffuses across the nerve sheath to reach the nerve membrane. The degree of ionisation is dependent on the pKa of the drug. Bupivacaine, ropivacaine and levobupivacaine all have a pKa of 8.2 and are therefore more ionised (and thus have a slower onset of anaesthetic action) at body pH than lidocaine, which has a pKa of 7.7. Addition of bicarbonate to local anaesthetic solutions speeds onset time and may improve the quality of the block.

The development of the minimum local analgesic concentration/dose (MLAC/D) technique, using an up–down sequential allocation model, has enabled relative analgesic potency ratios to be determined for epidural analgesia (and to a lesser extent, spinal analgesia/ anaesthesia). In this technique, the first patient in a study group is given a set volume of a certain concentration (MLAC) or a set volume containing a certain dose (MLAD). If the target response is achieved (e.g. pain scores < 1 cm on a scale of 0–10 cm), the next patient receives a 20% decrease in concentration/dose; if the target response is not achieved the next patient receives a 20% increase. The process is repeated and the ED_{50} may be derived from the resultant graph of responses. This technique has allowed the potencies of different local anaesthetics, and the effect of additives (e.g. opioids) to be compared.

The amide local anaesthetics are metabolised by the liver and excreted via the kidney.

Toxicity

Systemic toxicity of local anaesthetics is manifest as central nervous system excitability (caused by inhibition of inhibitory fibres) resulting in convulsions. This progresses to central nervous system depression if the local anaesthetic dose is increased further. Local anaesthetics also affect the cardiovascular system. Toxic doses cause depolarisation of cardiac cell membranes and systemic vasodilatation; this may lead to cardiovascular collapse. Resuscitation of the pregnant patient is notoriously difficult. In recent years, lipid rescue has become established as the treatment of choice in local anaesthetic toxicity; experience in pregnancy is limited but its use is generally advocated in parturients as for non-pregnant patients.

The safety margin (i.e. the difference between systemic concentration of local anaesthetic causing central nervous system symptoms and signs and that causing cardiovascular signs) is smaller for bupivacaine than for the other local anaesthetic agents in clinical use, and it is this problem that has stimulated the development of newer local anaesthetics. Bupivacaine appears to be particularly cardiotoxic in pregnancy, causing ventricular arrhythmias and asystolic cardiac arrest. Both ropivacaine and levobupivacaine appear to have a wider safety margin than bupivacaine.

The addition of adrenaline to lidocaine reduces its systemic absorption and therefore permits administration of larger doses (up to 7 mg/kg body weight compared with 4 mg/kg if adrenaline is not used). This is not the case with bupivacaine, the maximum dose of which is 2 mg/kg.

Amide local anaesthetics have a minimal chance of causing allergic reactions, unlike the ester group.

Differential block

The ideal local anaesthetic for obstetric analgesia would provide complete sensory analgesia of rapid onset and long duration without any motor blockade. Although bupivacaine provides long lasting sensory block, this is accompanied (especially at increasing dosage) by motor blockade. Ropivacaine has similar action at higher concentrations, but at lower concentrations is claimed to produce differential sensory block by preferential action on C fibres. The extent to which this is clinically significant is still unproven, and the increasing use of very low concentrations of local anaesthetic combined with opioids for labour analgesia may make any difference clinically irrelevant.

Key points

- All the local anaesthetics used in British obstetric anaesthetic practice are amides.
- Anaesthetic potency is proportional to lipid solubility.
- Duration of action is proportional to extent of protein binding.
- Speed of onset of action is proportional to the amount of non-ionised drug present.
- Systemic toxicity is manifest by central nervous system excitability followed by cardiovascular depression. The margin of safety between central nervous system and cardiovascular toxicity is lowest for bupivacaine. Lipid rescue is recommended for local anaesthetic toxicity.

Further reading

Association of Anaesthetists of Great Britain & Ireland. *Management of Severe Local Anaesthetic Toxicity*. London: AAGBI 2010, http://www.aagbi.org/sites/default/files/la_toxicity_2010_0.pdf.

Bern S, Weinberg G. Local anesthetic toxicity and lipid resuscitation in pregnancy. *Curr Opin Anesthesiol* 2011; **24**: 262–7.

Chapter

19

Normal labour

A large number of pregnant women are assessed as being 'low risk' and are predicted to have a normal labour, but the diagnosis of normal labour is retrospective.

The parameters for normal labour are:

- Contractions once in every 3 minutes, lasting 45 seconds
- Progressive dilatation of the cervix

- Progressive descent of the presenting part
- Vertex presenting with the head flexed and the occiput anterior
- Labour not lasting less than 4 hours (precipitate) or longer than 18 hours (prolonged)
- Delivery of a live healthy baby
- Delivery of a complete placenta and membranes
- No complications.

A labour record is kept to measure and record the vital signs of the mother and fetus, together with the progress of labour. It also serves as a record of events should an adverse outcome occur, especially if there is subsequent medicolegal involvement (see Chapter 159, Medicolegal aspects; Chapter 160, Record keeping). A list of items recorded would normally include:

- Fetal heart rate every 15 minutes
- Cervical dilatation at least every 4 hours
- Descent of the presenting part
- Colour of the liquor
- Fetal pH if relevant
- Amount of oxytocics given
- Strength and frequency of uterine contractions
- All drugs administered, including those for the epidural
- Maternal blood pressure, pulse rate and temperature
- Urine volume and analysis for ketones, protein or glucose
- Fluid input.

The most commonly used means of charting the progress of labour is the partogram, which presents the data in a graphical form. 'Normal' curves are printed on the partogram, obtained from large numbers of healthy primigravidae and multigravidae, against which it is easier to assess the progress of labour. An example of a partogram is shown in Fig. 19.1.

First stage of labour

During the latent phase, the cervix effaces then cervical dilatation begins. The rate of cervical dilatation should be around 1 cm per hour for a primiparous woman and 2 cm per hour for a multigravid woman.

It is standard practice to perform a vaginal examination every 4 hours to assess the dilatation of the cervix, or more frequently if there is cause for concern.

The fetal heart may be monitored intermittently by auscultation using Pinard's stethoscope or by cardiotocographic monitoring (see Chapter 20, Intrapartum fetal monitoring). The cardiotocogram (CTG) is recorded either intermittently or continuously depending on the condition of the fetus. Continuous recording of fetal heart rate may be done using either an abdominal transducer or a clip applied to the fetal head. Radiotelemetry is available in some units and this allows the woman to be mobile while her baby is monitored. Uterine contractions may be monitored externally by an abdominal transducer or internally by an intrauterine catheter. The fetal heart rate and the uterine contractions are recorded together.

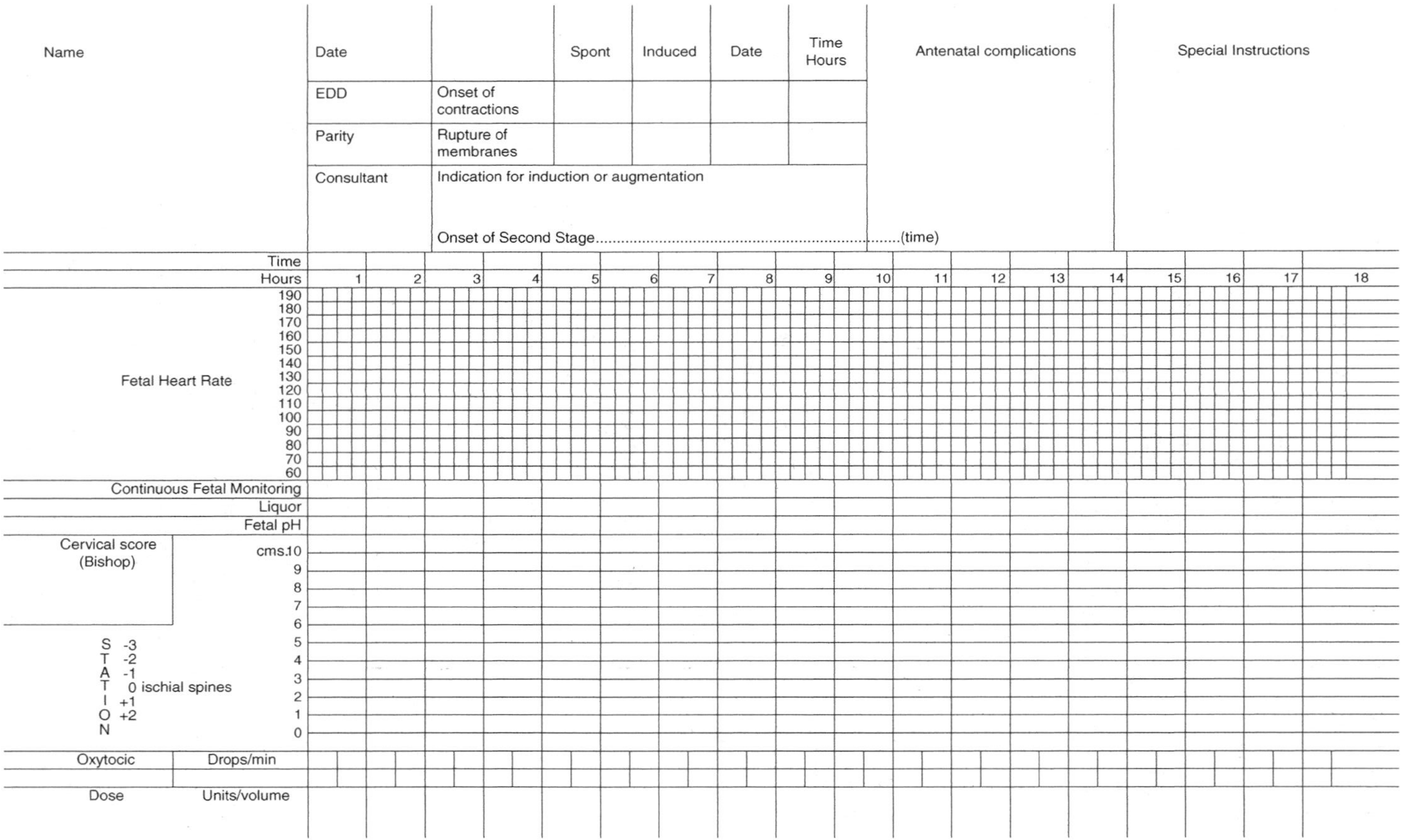

Fig. 19.1 Example of a partogram for assessing and recording progress of labour.

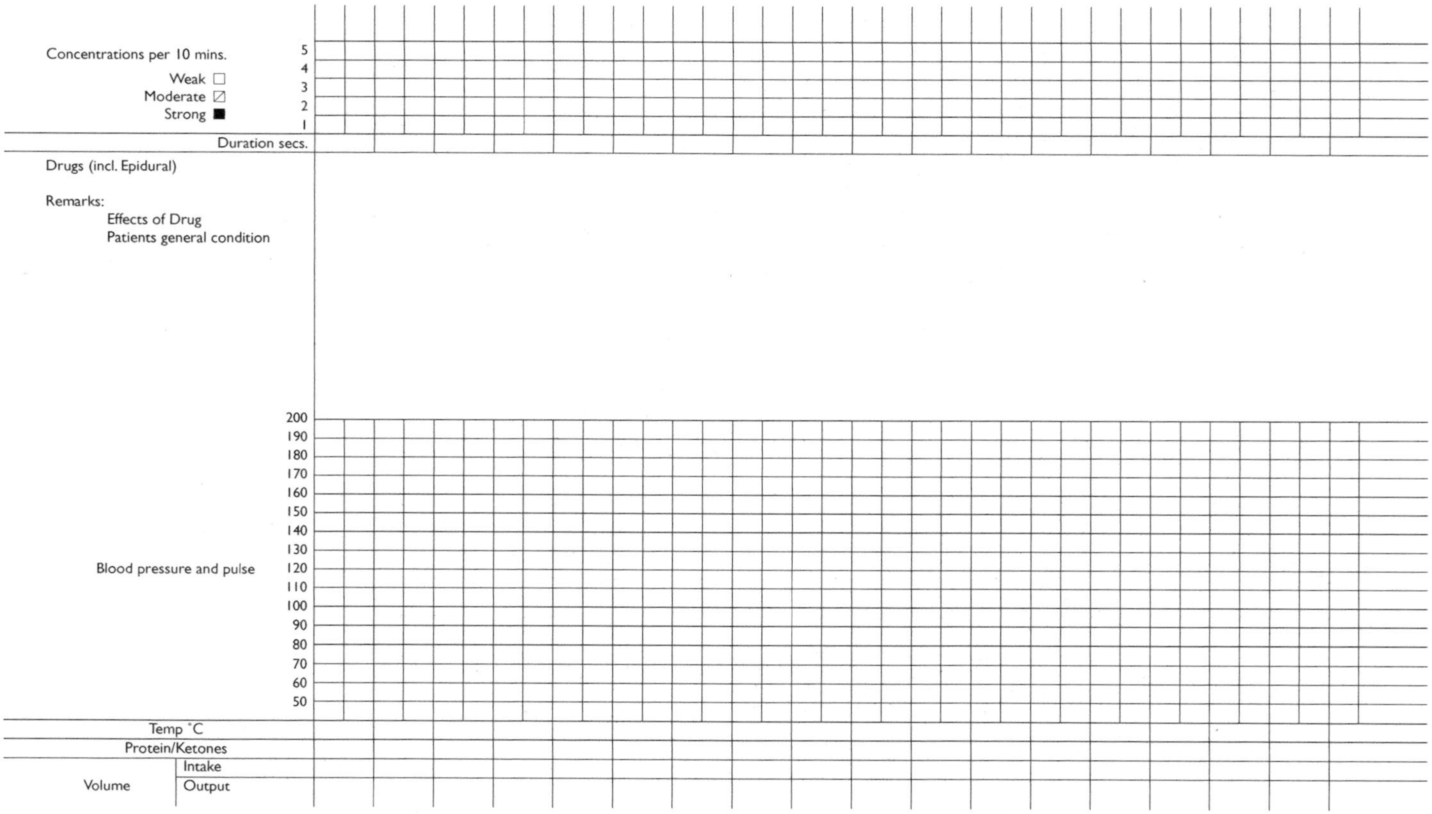

Concentrations per 10 mins.

Weak ☐
Moderate ◪
Strong ■

5
4
3
2
1

Duration secs.

Drugs (incl. Epidural)

Remarks:

Effects of Drug
Patients general condition

Blood pressure and pulse

200
190
180
170
160
150
140
130
120
110
100
90
80
70
60
50

Temp °C

Protein/Ketones

Intake

Volume

Output

Fig. 19.1 *(cont.)*

Second stage of labour

The second stage of labour commences at full dilatation of the cervix and terminates at the delivery of the baby.

At full dilatation of the cervix, the character of the contractions changes and they are usually, but not invariably, accompanied by a strong urge to push. In normal labour, there is an increase in circulating oxytocin secondary to Ferguson's reflex, with consequent increased strength of uterine contractions at full dilatation. Higher-dose epidural analgesia is thought to diminish the effect of this reflex.

The second stage of labour can be divided into passive and active stages and this is particularly relevant when epidural analgesia is used. With epidural analgesia, especially using older, higher-dose techniques, the labouring woman may not have the normal sensation at the start of the second stage of labour. Therefore, the active stage of pushing should only commence when the vertex is visible or the woman has a strong urge to push. In normal labour, the active stage usually commences at full dilatation. Traditionally, the second stage is limited to 2 hours because of the risk of fetal acidosis; up to 3 hours is often allowed in the presence of epidural analgesia in recognition of the slower descent of the fetal head. It is difficult for a woman to push efficiently for more than one hour, and after this time fetal acidosis is felt to be more likely. If there is not good progress, the advice of the obstetrician should be sought. At the delivery of the anterior shoulder, intramuscular oxytocics (e.g. Syntometrine) are given to hasten the delivery of the placenta and to stimulate uterine contraction.

Third stage of labour

The third stage of labour is the complete delivery of the placenta and membranes and the contraction of the uterus. It is usually managed actively by administering an oxytocic as above, but it may also be managed physiologically without oxytocics. This may prolong the third stage and increase the risk of postpartum haemorrhage.

During the third stage of labour there is a major redistribution of (and increase in) maternal circulating blood volume. This is potentially dangerous to those women who have cardiac disease and who may be precipitated into heart failure immediately postpartum.

Key points

- Normal labour can be anticipated but can only be diagnosed after delivery.
- Routine recording of labour is a standard of care in maternity units.
- The partogram is used to chart labour and for reference should a bad outcome or legal proceedings occur.
- The first stage comprises cervical effacement and dilatation.
- During the second stage, the baby passes through the birth canal.
- The placenta and membranes are delivered during the third stage.

Further reading

Ferguson E, Owen P. The second stage of labour. *Hosp Med* 2003; **64**: 210–13.

Ferguson E, Owen P. National Institute for Health and Clinical Excellence. Intrapartum care: care of healthy women and their babies during childbirth. *Clinical Guideline 55*. London: NICE 2007, http://www.nice.org.uk/CG055.

Steer P, Flint C. Physiology and management of normal labour. *BMJ* 1999; **318**: 793–6.

Chapter 20

Intrapartum fetal monitoring

Fetal monitoring is an important part of intrapartum care since labour is a stressful event for the fetus, and the ability of the fetus to maintain oxygenation is tested with each uterine contraction. Fetal wellbeing can be monitored routinely using the following methods:

- Assessment of liquor colour
- Fetal heart auscultation
- Fetal heart cardiotocography (CTG)
- Fetal electrocardiography (ECG) waveform analysis
- Fetal blood sampling and oximetry.

Special considerations

The pregnancy and labour can be assessed as either low- or high-risk. A low-risk pregnancy uncomplicated by any obstetric or medical problems will need a low level of fetal monitoring during labour, whereas a high-risk pregnancy (e.g. one complicated by hypertensive disease of pregnancy or poor intrauterine growth) will need careful intrapartum monitoring. The labour itself can be assessed as either low- or high-risk; it is generally recognised that a spontaneous labour is usually low-risk whereas an augmented labour or an induced labour is usually high-risk.

Liquor colour

When the membranes are ruptured, the liquor may be observed for the presence of meconium; this may indicate fetal hypoxia, which can cause the anal sphincter to relax allowing the fetus to pass meconium. Meconium may range from 'light' or 'grade-1' staining (in which a small amount of meconium diluted in a large volume of amniotic fluid gives the latter a greenish or yellowish discolouration), through 'moderate' or 'grade-2' staining (definite green/brown-coloured waters) to 'heavy' or 'grade-3' staining (thick, dark green/black-coloured fluid). Although such grading is commonly used, it has poor consistency between observers and poor predictive value for identifying degrees of fetal compromise. However, the appearance of thick new meconium is an indication for urgent delivery. If meconium is aspirated into the lungs of the neonate, severe lung damage may ensue; therefore, it should be aspirated from the neonate's mouth before intermittent positive pressure ventilation is started. A paediatrician should be present at the delivery if meconium is present. Meconium is more commonly seen in post-term labour.

Fetal heart rate and CTG

Fetal heart monitoring is recommended as follows:

1. *Low-risk (low-risk pregnancy and normal labour):* Intermittent monitoring with a Pinard's stethoscope is said to be as effective as CTG monitoring. Structured intermittent monitoring involves listening immediately after a contraction for a minimum of 60 seconds and repeating this every 15 minutes in the first stage of labour (every 5 minutes in the second stage). It has been suggested that CTG monitoring in the low-risk group may lead to unnecessary intervention and increased anxiety.

2. *High-risk (high-risk pregnancy and induced or augmented labour):* Continuous monitoring of the fetal heart rate is recommended by using a CTG, which records the fetal heart rate and the uterine contractions (and thus the effect of the latter on heart rate). The monitor uses either an external transducer or a 'clip' applied to the fetal head. It is generally recommended that women with epidural analgesia have continuous fetal monitoring, although there is some evidence to suggest that women who have a mobile (low-dose) epidural may not need this. The need for continuous fetal monitoring during epidural analgesia is related to the cardiovascular instability that may follow administration of large doses of local anaesthetic solutions into the epidural space. There is also evidence that epidural or spinal opioids may cause transient fetal bradycardia.

There are four features of the fetal heart rate that are especially important:

- *Baseline rate:* Normally 110–160 beats/min.
- *Variability:* Normally 5–25 beats/min.
- *Accelerations from baseline (> 15 beats/min for 15 s):* Two in 20 minutes are normally present. The significance of absent accelerations on an otherwise normal CTG is uncertain.
- *Decelerations from baseline:* Normally absent. Decelerations are classified as early, variable and late. Early decelerations are synchronous with the contraction; they are benign and may be associated with compression of the fetal head in the pelvis. They mirror the uterine contractions and should be associated with good beat-to-beat variability. Variable decelerations vary in their shape, size and occurrence. They may or may not indicate fetal hypoxia. Late decelerations continue after the contraction has finished and are more ominous, especially if associated with other abnormalities, e.g. reduced variability.

Opioids or other sedative drugs may cause a flat trace with a loss of beat-to-beat variability, which makes interpretation difficult.

National Institute for Health and Clinical Excellence (NICE) guidelines define three categories of CTG patterns (Table 20.1):

- *Normal:* all four of the above features are normal ('reassuring').
- *Suspicious:* one of the features is 'non-reassuring'.
- *Pathological:* two or more of the features are 'non-reassuring' or one or more is classified as abnormal.

Fetal heart rate monitoring has low specificity and sensitivity. Any trace that causes concern, especially in a high-risk pregnancy, is an indication for a fetal blood sample to be taken, unless there is evidence of acute fetal compromise, in which urgent delivery is indicated. The CTG trace should be kept for at least 25 years in case of a later medicolegal claim.

Use of the CTG may be combined with fetal ECG waveform analysis (see below).

Table 20.1 NICE classification of CTG traces

	Reassuring	Non-reassuring	Abnormal
Baseline	110–160 beats/min	100–109 beats/min 161–180 beats/min	< 100 beats/min 180 beats/min Sinusoidal pattern for ≥ 10 min
Variability	≥ 5 beats/min	< 5 beats/min for 40–90 min	< 5 beats/min for 90 min
Decelerations	None	Typical variable decelerations with over 50% of contractions, occurring for > 90 min Single prolonged deceleration for ≤ 3 min	Either atypical variable decelerations with > 50% of contractions or late decelerations, both for > 30 min Single prolonged deceleration for > 3 min
Accelerations	Present*		

* Absence of accelerations is of uncertain significance if the trace is otherwise normal.

Fetal ECG waveform analysis

This requires application of an electrode to the scalp of the fetus following rupture of the membranes. It is thought that ST changes in the fetal ECG are associated with hypoxaemia.

Although this technique has not reduced the caesarean section rate, it is associated with a decrease in interventions during labour. Problems associated with its use include poor signal quality, difficulties in interpretation, poor compliance with guidelines and deterioration in the clinical status of the fetus without any ECG alert. Recently, European guidelines have been agreed with regards to ST waveform analysis.

Fetal blood sampling

When the fetus becomes hypoxic, there is a build up of lactic acid and a reduction in the fetal pH. Fetal blood sampling (FBS) allows a more accurate assessment of fetal wellbeing than the CTG and is likely to be performed whenever there is anxiety about the CTG or when there is meconium in the liquor. It is thought that the use of FBS may help reduce intraoperative interventions. The sample may be taken with the mother in the lithotomy position or the left lateral position. Whichever position is used, care must be taken to avoid aortocaval compression during the procedure. Recommended actions for values of fetal pH are as follows:

- > 7.25 – normal; should be repeated if the fetal heart rate abnormality continues.
- 7.21–7.24 – borderline; should be repeated within 30 minutes, or delivery considered if there has been a rapid fall since the last sample.
- < 7.20 – indicative of significant acidosis and a need for urgent delivery of the baby.

Fetal gas tension measurement and oximetry

Non-invasive continuous transcutaneous measurement of oxygen and carbon dioxide tensions has been developed. This method requires the application of a suction ring to the baby's head; therefore the cervix needs to be dilated. Fetal oxygen saturation may also be measured by using special pulse oximeters; however, the technique is not yet reliable enough for routine use. Preliminary results suggest that fetuses normally have saturations of 30–60%.

These techniques may be influenced by skin contact, uterine contractions, caput on the baby's head and fetal hair.

Key points
- Good communication between anaesthetist, midwife and obstetrician is important.
- Fetal monitoring includes assessment of liquor colour, auscultation, cardiotocography and fetal scalp blood pH measurement.
- Fetal heart rate monitoring has poor specificity and sensitivity but this may be improved by ST analysis.

Further reading

ACOG practice bulletin no. 106. Intrapartum fetal heart rate monitoring: nomenclature, interpretation and general management principles. *Obstet Gynecol* 2009; **114**: 192–202.

Hinshaw K, Ullal A. Peripartum and intrapartum assessment of the fetus. *Anaesth Intensive Care Med* 2010; **11**: 324–32.

National Institute for Health and Clinical Excellence. Intrapartum care: care of healthy women and their babies during childbirth. *Clinical Guideline 55*. London: NICE 2007, http://www.nice.org.uk/CG055.

Chapter

21

Pain of labour

The pain of primiparous labour is said to be one of the most severe pains experienced, reported to be exceeded only by the pains of traumatic amputation and causalgia. Approximately 50% of women report severe or very severe pain during labour. Painless childbirth is a reality for only a small minority of women, although labour pain can be modified by a number of non-pharmacological manoeuvres.

The pain pathways involved in labour and delivery are extensive, involving afferent fibres from T10 down to S4.

Pain pathways

The uterus, lower uterine segment and cervix are all supplied by afferent Aδ and C fibres, which accompany the thoracolumbar and sacral sympathetic outflows. The pain of the first stage of labour is therefore referred to the dermatomes supplied by the same spinal cord segments that receive input from the uterus and cervix: T10–L1 during the first half of the first stage and then the lower lumbar and sacral dermatomes as labour progresses.

The second stage of labour may also involve somatic pain caused by distension and tearing of pelvic structures and by abnormal pressure on perineal skeletal musculature.

Modification of labour pain

Psychological factors

There is considerable evidence that preparation for childbirth can significantly modify the degree of pain experienced. This was the basis of the 'childbirth without fear' movement, which was popular in the 1960s. Although there can be little doubt that fear, fatigue and anxiety enhance pain perception, it is misleading for the majority of mothers to suggest that good antenatal education will lead to painless childbirth. Such expectations may in fact have the reverse effect, since the mother may develop complete loss of self-confidence when she begins to experience significant labour pain.

Women whose pregnancy is unplanned or unwanted are likely to experience more pain, as are those who have no birth partner to support them during labour. Conversely, the continuous presence of a midwife or female birth partner (doula) has been shown to reduce the amount of pain reported.

Cultural factors and ethnic group also have an influence on pain behaviour during labour, although it is likely that women from different cultures and of different racial groups actually experience similar levels of pain.

Promise of a finite duration of labour (as with active management of labour) may improve the ability to tolerate labour pain, although not necessarily reduce the level of pain experienced.

Physical factors

First labours are acknowledged to be more painful than subsequent labours, and older primiparae experience more painful labours than do younger women. Malpresentations, especially occipito-posterior positions, increase the pain of labour. Augmentation of labour by oxytocic drugs is reported to increase labour pain, and obstructed labour is more painful than normal labour. Tiredness is well known to reduce pain tolerance and is likely to occur if either the latent or the active phase of labour is prolonged.

There is a positive correlation between menstrual pain and labour pain, which has been postulated to be caused by excessive prostaglandin production.

Physiological factors

Progesterone may increase pain thresholds, and there is some evidence that in rats there is activation of endogenous opioid systems during late pregnancy. Experimental work in humans appears to confirm this.

Untreated pain causes an increase in circulating maternal catecholamines and other stress hormones. This may be detrimental to the mother with co-existing medical disease, and is also detrimental to the fetus. Maternal pain and acidosis are associated with reduced uteroplacental blood flow and fetal acidosis.

Key points

- Pain of childbirth is one of the most severe pains experienced.
- Pain from afferent Aδ and C fibres is referred to the dermatomes of T10 to S4 and is augmented during the second stage of labour by somatic pain from stretching and tearing of pelvic structures.
- Labour pain may be modified by antenatal education, and by the presence of a supportive partner.

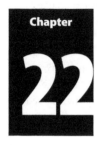

Epidural analgesia for labour

The caudal route was the first approach used for epidural analgesia and anaesthesia in childbirth and was described in 1901. It has now been superseded by the lumbar route, with continuous lumbar epidural analgesia for labour described in the 1940s. The caudal route is rarely used now, but may still have a place e.g. when anatomical abnormalities prevent access via the lumbar approach.

The use of epidural analgesia varies widely between different units in the UK, some small units having no provision and others having an epidural rate of over 50%.

It is generally accepted that epidural analgesia provides the most consistently effective form of pain-relief during labour, and there are other benefits such as the ability to top up for instrumental delivery/caesarean section, and an improved fetal acid–base status, especially if the mother is exhausted. Conversely, side effects and complications do exist, and the provision of a 24-hour epidural service is expensive. There are therefore differing (and often strong) views on the place of epidural analgesia in labour, held by mothers, midwives, obstetricians and obstetric anaesthetists.

Contraindications

The contraindications of epidural analgesia are the same as those in the non-pregnant population, but in the context of the above benefits, especially avoidance of general anaesthesia if an epidural catheter is *in situ*. The most common reasons for being unable to recommend epidural analgesia are coagulation disorders (whether iatrogenic or pathological), sepsis (local or systemic), and spinal neurological abnormality or the presence of metal or other implants around the lumbar region.

Consent

The modern emphasis on informed consent and the placement of mothers at the centre of their care have highlighted the difficulties that can exist when providing epidural analgesia for labour. There are many factors that may impair the usual consenting process, both antenally and during labour itself; these are discussed further in Chapter 158, Consent.

Equipment

Provision of epidural analgesia for labour in the UK virtually always involves the insertion of an epidural catheter, usually with one of a variety of disposable epidural packs available. These usually include a 16 G or 17 G Tuohy epidural needle, a multi-orifice catheter and a filter. Single, end-hole epidural catheters are popular in North America but are rarely used in the UK. Most epidural packs include a loss-of-resistance (LOR) syringe for identifying the epidural space.

If analgesia is to be provided by continuous infusion or patient-controlled epidural analgesia (PCEA), a suitable infusion syringe or pump will be required. Dilute solutions of local anaesthetic and opioid for either intermittent top-up or infusion may be prepared 'in-house' by the hospital pharmacy or may be purchased from an external manufacturer.

In the UK, the National Patient Safety Agency has required all NHS organisations to employ only non-Luer connections for all epidural equipment from April 2013.

Technique

Either a midline or a paramedian technique may be used to approach the epidural space – both techniques are equally possible and acceptable in the lumbar spine, and the final choice of approach is usually determined by personal preference. Ultrasound has been used to assist the location of the epidural space, e.g. by identifying the midline and/or depth of space before needle insertion, but its use is not routine.

The epidural space is usually identified by LOR to the injection of saline (Table 22.1), using a continuous injection technique. The use of LOR to air is no longer advocated as this has been associated with a number of disadvantages including pneumocephalus.

The continuous technique involves the operator's hand exerting a continuous pressure on the syringe plunger as the needle is advanced. When the needle tip lies in the ligament or the ligamentum flavum, there will be resistance to injection, which is lost as the epidural space is entered. With the intermittent technique, usually with air, the plunger is tested after each incremental advance of the needle. However, this technique is used less now as air is not routinely used for LOR; it is also thought that the intermittent technique may be associated with a higher incidence of dural puncture.

Once the epidural space has been identified the epidural catheter is inserted through the needle, leaving 3–5 cm within the epidural space, and is secured to the mother's back. With shorter lengths inserted, the spread of the block is usually better, but there is a greater chance of the catheter's falling out; longer lengths are associated with lower replacement rates but more one-sided blocks.

Table 22.1 Comparison of saline and air for loss-of-resistance (LOR) technique

	Saline	Air
Advantages	Allows the continuous technique of LOR Non-compressible. Thus no 'bounce' of the plunger when pressure is applied against resistance Retrospective surveys suggest a decreased incidence of accidental dural puncture	Compressible, giving the plunger a characteristic 'bounce' Clear fluid dripping from the hub of the needle can only be cerebrospinal fluid
Disadvantages	Saline dripping from the hub of the needle may be confused with cerebrospinal fluid if dural tap is suspected (although testing for glucose etc. will distinguish it)	The intermittent technique must be used Has been associated with a wide range of complications, including subcutaneous emphysema, neck discomfort, air embolism, pneumocephalus, patchy block (thought to be caused by bubbles around the nerve roots) and neurological impairment The injected air is not sterile If pneumocephalus occurs, subsequent general anaesthesia with nitrous oxide may result in expansion of air bubbles

Epidural drugs

In the 1970s–1980s, the only drug used widely in the UK to provide epidural analgesia was bupivacaine, used in concentrations of 0.25–0.5%. During the past 30 years a variety of drug mixtures has been assessed. The most commonly used combination in the UK is now bupivacaine and fentanyl (0.1–0.125% bupivacaine with 2–2.5 μg/ml fentanyl). The reason for adding opioids to local anaesthetic is to enhance the quality of analgesia and to reduce the total dose of local anaesthetic given. Initially it was hoped that this would lead to a reduction in motor block and improved rates of spontaneous vaginal delivery. Although there is a reduction in motor block, this has unfortunately not been accompanied by a dramatic reduction in instrumental delivery rate. In North America, combinations of up to four drugs (bupivacaine, sufentanil, adrenaline and clonidine) have been recommended, but the clinical benefit and wisdom of using such mixtures, given the potential for drug errors, has been questioned. More recently, levobupivacaine (0.1–0.125%) or ropivacaine (0.2%) has been used alone or in combination with opioids.

These 'low-dose' mixtures are given as intermittent top-ups of 10–15 ml, infusions of 10–12 ml/h, or PCEA. For the latter, a wide variety of methods have been described but typical regimens consist of boluses of 8–15 ml with no background infusion, or boluses of 4–6 ml with a background infusion of 4–8 ml/h. Suitable lockout periods are 5–20 minutes.

Infusions and PCEA have been shown to have similar efficacy to intermittent boluses given by the midwife or the anaesthetist. However, the two former techniques have been associated with better maternal satisfaction and less workload for staff compared with intermittent boluses. The main advantage that PCEA has over infusions and intermittent boluses is that the amount of local anaesthetic required, and therefore motor blockade, is reduced with PCEAs. The fact that mothers are also in control of their pain relief may also be a reason that women prefer this technique.

Recently, more sophisticated methods of drug delivery have been explored; these include programmed intermittent bolus administration (in which mandatory boluses are given, e.g. 10 ml low-dose solution every 30 min, instead of boluses on demand) and computer-integrated PCEA (in which basal infusion rates are adjusted according to the woman's demands/usage during the previous hour). A 'programmed intermittent mandatory bolus' technique has also been described, in which mandatory boluses are given unless the woman has received a self-administered bolus within a set time frame. Such techniques have been developed with the aim of reducing drug requirements and/or improving the quality of analgesia. They currently require sophisticated equipment and are not widely used.

Side effects of epidural analgesia

These are listed in Table 22.2.

Table 22.2 Risk of side effects and complications of epidural analgesia (N.B. from several sources)

Side effect/complication	Risk
Backache	Thought to be unchanged
Caesarean section	Thought to be unchanged
Length of first stage of labour	Thought to be unchanged
Second stage of labour	Average increase ~15 min
Need for instrumental delivery	Increased risk ~1.4
Itching	~1:10
Need for adjustment to epidural and/or other analgesia	~1:10
Heavy leg(s)	~1:20
Difficulty passing urine	~1:20
Significant fall in blood pressure	~1:50
Failure of epidural	~1:50
Headache	~1:200
Temporary nerve palsy	~1:2000
Permanent nerve palsy	~1:13 000
Total spinal	~1:15 000
Paraplegia	~1:100 000

Table 22.3 Bromage score for assessing motor power following epidural analgesia

The scoring system has been modified several times from the original one, described in 1965, to account for the less intense motor block that occurs with modern, low-dose techniques.

Score	Original Bromage scoring system	Examples of modified Bromage scoring systems	
1	Unable to move feet or knees	Unable to flex ankles	Unable to move legs at all
2	Able to move feet only	Able to flex ankles but not knees	Able to move legs but unable to raise against gravity
3	Just able to move knees	Able to flex ankles and knees but unable to straight leg raise	Able to raise legs against gravity but not against resistance
4	Able to flex knees and feet fully	Able to sustain straight leg raise	Able to raise legs against gravity and resistance

Epidural local anaesthetics cause sympathetic blockade and hypotension. Administration of intravenous fluids, vasopressor agents, or a combination of both, can prevent and/or treat this. Currently used low-dose combinations of local anaesthetic and opioid cause minimal haemodynamic disturbance, but it is mandatory to establish venous access before initiating epidural analgesia, although routine preloading with intravenous fluids has been abandoned in many units unless there are other indications, e.g. dehydration.

Local anaesthetics also cause motor blockade, commonly graded by using various versions of the Bromage score (Table 22.3). Motor blockade can be minimised by using the lowest concentration of local anaesthetic compatible with adequate analgesia. Addition of opioid facilitates reduction of local anaesthetic dose but motor blockade may still occur.

Epidural opioids may cause nausea, vomiting, urinary retention, itching and respiratory depression. Each of these side effects occurs less commonly with fentanyl than with other opioids.

The effect of epidural opioids on gastric emptying is uncertain. Boluses of fentanyl (50–100 µg) have been shown to delay gastric emptying by up to 45 minutes, but the use of low-dose continuous infusions do not appear to have this effect.

There has been considerable debate about the effect of epidural analgesia on the outcome of labour. Meta-analysis suggests that epidural analgesia may prolong the second stage of labour, with a resultant increase in the need for instrumental delivery, but not caesarean section.

Complications

Epidural analgesia is highly effective but is an invasive technique with the potential for life-threatening complications (Table 22.2). It must not, therefore, be used unless there is adequate care from a suitably trained birth attendant and the ability to access advanced resuscitation facilities rapidly if required.

Complications of epidural administration include:

- Failure to identify the epidural space
- Bloody tap/accidental intravascular injection

- Dural puncture
- Extensive conduction blockade
- Poor quality block
- Neurological complications
- Infectious complications.

These are discussed under the relevant headings elsewhere.

Key points
- Most units in the UK offer a 24-hour epidural service for labour.
- Modern techniques consist of low-dose local anaesthetic (usually bupivacaine) with opioid (usually fentanyl in the UK and fentanyl or sufentanil elsewhere).
- PCEA techniques are associated with reduced usage of local anaesthetic.
- Use of epidural analgesia may prolong the second stage of labour and increase the likelihood of instrumental delivery.

Further reading

Anim-Somuah M, Smyth RM, Jones L. Epidural versus non-epidural or no analgesia in labour. *Cochrane Database Syst Rev* 2011; (12): CD000331.

Halpern SH, Carvalho B. Patient-controlled epidural analgesia for labor. *Anesth Analg* 2009; **108**: 921–8.

Jenkins JG. Some immediate serious complications of obstetric epidural analgesia and anaesthesia: a prospective study of 145,550 epidurals. *Int J Obstet Anesth* 2005; **14**: 37–42.

Loubert C, Hinova A, Fernando R. Update on modern neuraxial analgesia in labour: a review of the literature of the last 5 years. *Anaesthesia* 2011; **66**: 191–212.

Chapter

23

Epidural test doses

The purpose of the epidural test dose is to detect intravenous or subarachnoid placement of the catheter. As such, it must be formulated to produce an easily detected result when in one of these two situations, without compromising the safety of the mother or the fetus.

Problems/special considerations

- As with all screening procedures, the sensitivity and specificity of the test dose are all-important when assessing its ability to protect the mother from the unwanted effects of intravenous or subarachnoid administration. Sensitivity is the ability of the test dose to detect accurately a misplaced catheter; failure to do so represents a false-negative result. Specificity is the ability of the test dose not to produce a false-positive result, i.e. incorrectly alerting the anaesthetist when the catheter is actually in the right place.
- Accidental catheterisation of the epidural veins is common in obstetric practice, since these vessels act as collateral conduits of venous blood from the lower limbs to the heart and are therefore dilated when the inferior vena cava is compressed by the gravid uterus. Venous cannulation occurs about 1 in 20 times and is usually detected before the test dose is given, by the ability to aspirate blood.
- Subarachnoid puncture occurs about 1 in 100 times, with the incidence decreasing as the practitioner becomes more experienced. Again, the vast majority of dural punctures are detected by the free flow of cerebrospinal fluid through the needle or catheter.
- It follows that it is very rare for a test dose to be used in a situation where the catheter is actually intravenous or subarachnoid. This means that, in addition to the sensitivity and specificity of the test, it is also important to know what proportion of positive test results will actually indicate misplacement of the catheter; this is known as the positive predictive value of the test and is often lower than might be expected from the sensitivity and specificity.
- A test dose, designed to improve safety, should not in itself compromise the safety of the mother or fetus. This is a particular problem when trying to detect intravenous placement, as many tests rely on the use of adrenaline to produce tachycardia in these circumstances. Intravenous adrenaline may stress the maternal cardiovascular system and temporarily reduce placental perfusion, so doses must be carefully chosen.
- Although initial confirmation of the correct placement of the epidural catheter is particularly important, the possibility of later catheter migration should not be forgotten. Every top-up given down an epidural catheter that might be dangerous if accidentally injected intravenously or intrathecally should really be regarded as a test dose and should be fractionated if time permits, so as not to produce systemic toxicity or a dangerously high block.
- It is difficult – if not impossible – to design a test dose that will detect subdural, extra-arachnoid placement with any reliability. The possibility of subdural catheterisation must always be borne in mind and suspected when an unusual block pattern emerges.

Management options
Subarachnoid placement

This is usually relatively easy to detect, and it is only necessary to choose a dose of local anaesthetic that will produce a recognisable but safe block. Lidocaine 45–60 mg or bupivacaine 7.5–12.5 mg is suitable; lidocaine has the advantage of a slightly faster onset of block, but many practitioners prefer bupivacaine on the grounds that this will be the drug used for the main dose. Signs of sensory block in the lower lumbar segments and motor block of the legs should be sought after 3 minutes with lidocaine or 5 minutes with bupivacaine. This test is regarded as close to 100% specific and sensitive.

Intravenous placement

Most tests rely on the use of sympathomimetic drugs to produce changes in maternal heart rate and/or blood pressure when administered intravenously. Adrenaline 15 μg or isoprenaline 5 μg has been recommended for this purpose. Intravenous injection of adrenaline has been shown to have a low positive predictive value (55–73%) and it has been associated with significant side effects. Even when an adrenaline-free bupivacaine test dose is used, 12% of patients will demonstrate a rise in heart rate that would count as a positive response. The sensitivity is also low but can be improved by ensuring that the heart rate is measured between contractions and by using the change in peak heart rate (as measured over a 2 minute period before and after the test injection), rather than a simple change from a random baseline rate, as the basis of the test.

Subjective symptoms have also been used to detect intravenous placement, and some test dose regimens rely on this. Fentanyl 100 μg produces obvious sensations of drowsiness within 1 minute when given intravenously, and lidocaine 45–60 mg may cause tingling in the perioral region. These methods are far from reliable and the increased sensitivity of pregnant women to local anaesthetic toxicity should always be borne in mind when using the systemic effects of lidocaine as a test.

Finally, though no longer advocated, 1–2 ml of air has been used as a test for intravenous placement, with a Doppler probe (readily available on the labour suite in the form of a fetal heart monitor) placed over the mother's right ventricle to detect the characteristic sounds of air entering the heart. A safer version of this test is to inject 10 ml agitated saline.

Best practice

It is important to consider the possibility of a misplaced epidural catheter before every top-up. Careful aspiration via the catheter before administering a dose of local anaesthetic and a continuous high index of suspicion are vital adjuncts to an effective test dose policy.

Since no single regimen has been proven to be superior, many obstetric anaesthetists therefore recommend abandoning a formal test dose, instead fractionating all epidural doses. The current practice of using low concentrations of local anaesthetic (usually 0.1–0.125% bupivacaine) means that accidental intravenous or subarachnoid administration is unlikely to produce any serious adverse maternal or fetal effects.

Midwives should be trained to recognise the early signs of local anaesthetic toxicity and fractionate all doses to ensure safety if the catheter migrates through a dural tear.

Key points

- A test dose should be safe with a high sensitivity and specificity; high specificity is difficult to achieve when the condition being sought is uncommon.
- Accidental subarachnoid placement is relatively easy to detect with a test dose, whilst intravenous placement is more difficult to detect.
- Subdural placement cannot be reliably detected with a test dose.
- Catheter migration can occur, and every epidural top-up should be regarded as a test dose.

Further reading

Camorcia M. Testing the epidural catheter. *Curr Opin Anesthesiol* 2009; **22**: 336–40.

Guay J. The epidural test dose: a review. *Anesth Analg* 2006; **102**: 921–9.

Chapter

24

Combined spinal–epidural analgesia and anaesthesia

The combined spinal–epidural (CSE) technique was first described over 60 years ago. Although it is commonly assumed that CSE means a needle-through-needle technique, there are theoretically several ways of instituting CSE:

1. Insertion of an epidural needle into the epidural space, insertion of a long spinal needle through the epidural needle into the subarachnoid space and finally insertion of an epidural catheter through the epidural needle after the spinal needle has been removed. This is the most commonly used technique in the UK.
2. Insertion of an epidural needle (and usually an epidural catheter) into the epidural space followed by separate insertion of a spinal needle into the subarachnoid space, either at the same or at a different lumbar interspace. This is favoured by a minority of UK anaesthetists.
3. Insertion of a spinal needle into the subarachnoid space followed by insertion of an epidural needle and catheter. This is rarely practised other than when the pain of labour is so severe that the mother is felt to be unable to lie/sit still long enough for epidural insertion.
4. Specialised needles that consist of an epidural needle with a side channel, through which the spinal needle is passed. This has theoretical advantages, but is not in widespread use.
5. The use of a single needle to identify and inject drugs into the epidural space, then advancing it through the dura to make a subarachnoid injection. This is not practised today.

CSE offers the certainty and speed of onset of spinal analgesia or anaesthesia and the flexibility and continuity of an epidural catheter. For the needle-through-needle technique, successful aspiration of cerebrospinal fluid (CSF) upon insertion of the spinal needle confirms correct placement of the epidural needle, which may be reassuring in difficult cases.

Problems/special considerations

- Anaesthetists should be entirely familiar with the management of both spinal and epidural analgesic and anaesthetic techniques before considering CSE. Either a needle-through-needle or separate space technique can be used according to the equipment available and the anaesthetist's preference. The separate space technique has the advantage of not requiring special needles but the disadvantage of inflicting two sets of injections upon the woman. The needle-through-needle technique involves only a single injection but requires long (approximately 120 mm) and more expensive spinal needles either singly or as part of specialised CSE kits.

- Any standard Tuohy needle can be used, although most of the leading needle manufacturers produce kits containing specially matched spinal and epidural needles for needle-through-needle CSE. Some of these include locking devices for fixing the two needles together so that once CSF is obtained, the spinal needle cannot move in or out during subarachnoid injection, which might increase the chance of inadequate block; however, these devices may reduce the 'feel' as the spinal needle is advanced through the dura. Typically, an 18 G or 16 G Tuohy needle and a 25 G or 27 G spinal needle are used, as for separate epidural and spinal techniques. It is essential to check that the spinal needle will project beyond the end of the epidural needle by an adequate amount to achieve dural puncture (usually 12–15 mm). Attempts to move towards a completely non-Luer system for neuraxial block in the UK have raised concerns that CSE techniques will become less flexible and more complicated since different manufacturers may not use the same connector dimensions.

Management options

Analgesia

The use of CSE for labour analgesia varies. Some maternity units employ the technique routinely, others never. The benefits include rapid onset of pain relief (usually within 5 minutes) and absence of significant motor block in most cases. There is also evidence to suggest that the presence of a hole in the dura (even without injecting drugs intrathecally) may improve epidural analgesia. The major disadvantage is the additional potential for complications introduced by deliberate dural puncture. The use of a spinal needle in addition to an epidural needle also adds to the cost of labour analgesia.

The original regimen for the spinal component recommended in the UK was 25 μg of fentanyl and 2.5 mg of bupivacaine (1 ml of 0.25% solution), made up to a volume of 2 ml with saline. Further experience has suggested that smaller doses of fentanyl (5–15 μg) may be adequate; 3–5 ml of the standard 'low-dose' epidural mixture (bupivacaine 0.1% with fentanyl 2 μg/ml) may also be suitable and not require a separate ampoule of fentanyl to be obtained from the locked controlled drug cupboard. These combinations will provide approximately 60–90 minutes' analgesia, in most cases with little motor blockade. (Spinal opioids alone are very rarely used in the UK, although they may be considered in some high-risk women with co-existing medical disease. In the USA and continental Europe sufentanil is widely used.) When further analgesia is needed, a low concentration of bupivacaine with fentanyl is given via the epidural catheter, either by intermittent bolus top-ups, an infusion or PCEA.

Those who do not routinely use CSE analgesia point to the above disadvantages and to the fact that epidural analgesia is usually effective within a few contractions. However, many anaesthetists would consider CSE for women who request regional analgesia late in the first stage of labour, or for those needing regional analgesia for instrumental delivery.

Anaesthesia

The use of CSE for caesarean section combines the speed of onset and reliability of spinal anaesthesia with the ability to extend the block and provide postoperative analgesia through an epidural catheter. There are three different techniques of CSE for caesarean section:

1. The spinal injection is performed using a 'full' spinal dose of local anaesthetic, and the epidural catheter is used as a back-up in the event of inadequate anaesthesia, to extend the block if surgery is prolonged and to provide postoperative analgesia.
2. A smaller volume of local anaesthetic (e.g. 1 ml heavy bupivacaine 0.5%) is used intrathecally, with the intention of producing a limited spinal block (usually to about T8–10). Anaesthesia is then extended gradually with local anaesthetic via the epidural catheter. It was thought that this might result in greater haemodynamic stability, but this may not be the case. However, this technique does allow a more controlled and controllable extension of block that may be advantageous in women with systemic disease (e.g. cardiac, respiratory or neurological).
3. A small dose of local anaesthetic (e.g. 1 ml heavy bupivacaine 0.5%) is given intrathecally using a needle-through-needle technique; when the spinal needle is withdrawn approximately 8–10 ml saline is injected through the epidural needle to extend the height of block suitable for surgery, by compressing the dural sac. The epidural catheter is then placed as usual. Proponents of this 'EVE' (epidural volume extension) technique claim greater cardiovascular stability, less motor block, and smaller doses of local anaesthetic. However, although EVE may increase the dermatomal height of the block (between four to eight dermatomes), the quality of block may be less than with larger doses, and it does not necessarily allow a reduction in the amount of local anaesthetic required.

Complications

If specific 'locking' CSE kits are not used, it may be awkward for the inexperienced practitioner to grip the spinal and epidural needles in such a way as to stop the former moving during subarachnoid injection. Possibly as a result of this, or because of the greater time taken to complete the procedure after spinal injection if insertion of the epidural catheter is difficult, it has been claimed that there is a higher failure rate of the subarachnoid component of CSE than with single-shot spinal anaesthesia, but this does not appear to be a problem as experience with the technique is gained.

CSE carries similar risks to both spinal and epidural injection alone. A number of early reports of meningitis following CSE suggested that there might be an increased risk of this complication with CSE compared with a single-shot spinal; however, since CSE is widely used this could equally be an artifact of reporting. There have also been reports of neuropraxia and neurological damage with CSE, presumed to be related to needle length and design. A particular concern relates to the difficulty in identifying the correct lumbar interspace that even experienced anaesthetists may have, and the risk that the chosen level may be above the termination of the spinal cord. In such a case, there should be no extra risk from epidural analgesia in labour, for example, so long as an accidental dural tap does not occur, but if CSE is used, there is a risk of neurological damage from the spinal needle. The 3rd National Audit Project of the Royal College of Anaesthetists (NAP3) found that the incidence of permanent harm associated with obstetric CSEs was approximately six times greater than that with epidurals, and approximately three times greater than that with spinals (see Section 2, Part IV, Anaesthetic problems).

It must be remembered that the epidural catheter is untested at the time of insertion, and there is always the risk of an 'epidural' dose passing into the subarachnoid space, as for any epidural catheter – increased perhaps by the presence of a dural hole (though this complication remains a rarity despite widespread usage of CSE). In addition, the physical compressing effect of epidural solutions on the spread of spinal anaesthesia (as in the EVE technique above) means that should the subarachnoid block be inadequate, small boluses (< 5 ml) of local anaesthetic should be used to top up the epidural catheter.

Key points
- Needle-through-needle combined spinal–epidural (CSE) requires only a single injection but is more expensive than separate space techniques.
- CSE analgesia provides pain relief usually within one or two contractions but is a more invasive and complex technique than epidural alone.
- CSE anaesthesia combines the advantages of spinal anaesthesia (speed of onset and quality of anaesthesia) with the ability to extend the level and duration of anaesthesia via the epidural route.

Further reading

Cook TM. Combined spinal–epidural techniques. *Anaesthesia* 2000; **55**: 42–64.

Loubert C, Hinova A, Fernando R. Update on modern neuraxial analgesia in labour: a review of the literature of the last 5 years. *Anaesthesia* 2011; **66**: 191–212.

McNaught AF, Stocks GM. Epidural volume extension and low-dose sequential combined spinal–epidural blockade: two ways to reduce spinal dose requirement for Caesarean section. *Int J Obstet Anesth* 2007; **16**: 346–53.

Simmons SW, Cyna AM, Dennis AT, Hughes D. Combined spinal–epidural versus epidural analgesia in labour. *Cochrane Database Syst Rev* 2007; (3): CD003401.

Chapter

25

Spinal analgesia

Single-shot spinal analgesia is rarely used alone for labour since its duration is usually much shorter than that of labour itself. However, it may be useful in the later stages of labour when delivery is felt to be imminent, or to provide rapid onset of analgesia in a mother who is desperate and losing control, thus enabling her to cooperate whilst an epidural catheter is inserted.

Use of an intrathecal catheter to allow repeated boluses (or infusion) of local anaesthetic or other mixtures is an attractive concept, since the advantages of spinal block (rapid onset, profound block) are potentially combined with those of epidural block (flexibility, titrated effect). In practice, however, continuous spinal block is uncommon in the UK.

Problems/special considerations

The main considerations for a single-shot spinal are the risk of postdural puncture headache and the choice of solution, given the requirement for maximal analgesia whilst minimising motor block and other side effects (see Chapter 24, Combined spinal–epidural analgesia and anaesthesia).

Modern intrathecal catheters are very fine (e.g. 28–32 G) and thus may be difficult to handle and insert. They are usually supplied in a kit with a spinal needle; originally these needles had cutting tips, but they are now available with pencil-point tips in an attempt to reduce the incidence of postdural puncture headache. However, even with fine catheters, 22–26 G spinal needles are required. Some catheters include a removable wire to make them stiffer for insertion. A catheter-over-needle kit also exists, in which a 27–29 G needle protrudes from the distal end of a 22–24 G catheter; the catheter is slid over the needle into the subarachnoid space whilst advancement of the needle is prevented by a wire attached to its distal end.

A continuous catheter technique may also be used with a standard epidural kit (e.g. 16 G or 18 G catheter), either because specialist kits are unavailable or when an accidental dural puncture has occurred during attempted epidural block. A reduced incidence of headache after placement of an intrathecal catheter has been claimed when this is done, possibly related to inflammation around the dural puncture site, which leads to faster healing; however, this is uncertain since evidence is mostly observational.

The main factor that has led to the withdrawal of microspinal catheters in the USA and that has contributed to the technique's unpopularity in the UK is the association between their use and the development of subsequent cauda equina syndrome. This is thought to be caused by a combination of factors, including the use of lidocaine (more common in the USA), the known neurotoxic effect of high concentrations of lidocaine on neural tissue experimentally (more so than bupivacaine), the pooling of drug around the sensitive nerves of the cauda equina associated with very fine catheters placed caudally and the use of excessive doses of drug in an attempt to extend an inadequately extensive block (resulting in more pooling around the nerves).

Management options

Management after a single-shot spinal is discussed elsewhere (see Chapter 32, Spinal anaesthesia for caesarean section).

For continuous techniques, once the catheter has been inserted, it should be clearly labelled, since accidental injection of an epidural-style dose may be disastrous. For labour analgesia, a standard spinal dose can be given as for a combined spinal–epidural. Subsequent analgesia may be provided with repeated boluses of 0.5–1.5 ml bupivacaine 0.1–0.25% ± fentanyl 10–20 μg as required. Infusions (e.g. 0.1–0.25% bupivacaine ± fentanyl at 1–5 ml/h) have also been used. Unless the technique is commonly used in a particular unit, it is prudent for all top-ups to be given by an anaesthetist, since midwifery and other staff are likely to be unfamiliar with it.

For caesarean section, incremental doses of bupivacaine ± opioid may be given to achieve the required level of block, as slowly as is felt appropriate for the clinical circumstances.

Whatever the indication, directing the catheter caudally should be avoided as should repeated injections of concentrated solutions of local anaesthetic if the block is inadequate. Greater than normal doses of local anaesthetic should not be given.

Key points

- Single-shot spinal analgesia is rarely used alone for labour but may be useful when delivery is imminent, or to provide rapid onset of analgesia before siting an epidural.
- Continuous spinal techniques are acceptable for both labour and operative delivery:
  - Advantages include good quality of block and ability to titrate the dose.
  - Disadvantages include difficulty handling the catheters, risk of postdural puncture headache, cauda equina syndrome, cost and mistaking the catheter for an epidural one.

Further reading

Loubert C, Hinova A, Fernando R. Update on modern neuraxial analgesia in labour: a review of the literature of the last 5 years. *Anaesthesia* 2011; **66**: 191–212.

Palmer CM. Continuous spinal anesthesia and analgesia in obstetrics. *Anesth Analg* 2010; **111**: 1476–9.

Chapter

26

Spinal and epidural opioids

Epidural opioids are widely used in combination with local anaesthetics to provide analgesia both during labour and following caesarean section. Spinal opioids have also been used to enhance surgical anaesthesia and to provide postoperative analgesia, and more recently to provide analgesia for labour (in combined spinal–epidural techniques). Spinal and epidural opioids alone do not provide adequate pain relief for the late first stage and second stage of labour.

All opioids have significant maternal side effects, ranging from mild nausea to life-threatening respiratory depression. These side effects may occur following administration of opioids by any route, although the published literature has tended to focus on adverse effects associated with neuraxial administration. In the UK, fentanyl is the opioid most commonly used to provide labour analgesia, with diamorphine or fentanyl being used for intra- and postoperative analgesia. Epidural morphine is less commonly used because of the greater risk of late respiratory depression, although spinal morphine appears to be very safe.

Sufentanil is used widely in the rest of Europe and in North America, but is not available in the UK.

Site of action

Opioids act at the opioid receptors in the substantia gelatinosa of the spinal cord. Drugs injected into the epidural space have to penetrate the dura to reach the site of action. Ease of dural penetration will depend on lipid solubility and molecular weight, with highly lipid-soluble molecules (such as fentanyl) entering the subarachnoid space most readily. Once the opioid has reached the cerebrospinal fluid (CSF), the more lipid-soluble drugs will fix readily in the spinal cord, whereas less lipid-soluble drugs (such as morphine) remain in the CSF and are carried in a cranial direction with CSF flow, reaching the lateral ventricles in about 6 hours. This accounts for the slow onset of action, higher incidence of nausea, vomiting and pruritus, and late respiratory depression seen with morphine.

The epidural space is highly vascular in the pregnant woman, and there is significant systemic uptake of epidurally administered opioids (with similar blood concentration curves to those seen after parenteral administration). In addition, some opioid is bound to fat in the epidural space and does not reach the spinal cord. The ratio of epidural to spinal dose of opioid is thus in the order of 5–10:1.

Commonly used epidural and spinal bolus doses are:

- Fentanyl: epidural 50–100 μg, spinal 15–25 μg
- Diamorphine: epidural 2–3 mg, spinal 0.2–0.5 mg
- Morphine: epidural 3–4 mg, spinal 75–100 μg

Benefits

Several studies have confirmed that epidural administration of opioids alone provides analgesia for early labour but is inadequate for the later stages of labour. However, the combination of local anaesthetic and opioid is synergistic. This is clearly advantageous, allowing improved quality of analgesia, reduced consumption of local anaesthetic, reduced motor block and reduction in opioid side effects. Typical combinations used consist of 0.1–0.125% bupivacaine with 2–2.5 μg/ml fentanyl.

Improved maternal mobility increases maternal satisfaction with labour analgesia, and improvement in rates of spontaneous vaginal delivery compared with the traditional, higher-dose and opioid-free techniques (e.g. 0.25–5% bupivacaine alone). The mechanism of local anaesthetic/opioid synergy is unclear.

Epidural and intrathecal opioids are claimed to provide superior postoperative analgesia, although there are so many variables involved and different measures of analgesic outcome, that it is difficult to assess this reliably.

Side effects

Side effects of both epidural and intrathecal opioids are dose dependent and are more severe for less lipophilic drugs such as morphine. With the exception of urinary retention (which is not dose related), all the side effects seen after neuraxial administration of opioids may occur following parenteral administration (although itching is only common when opioids are given epidurally or intrathecally). A unique side effect is the potential for reactivation of herpes simplex labialis 2–5 days after the epidural administration of morphine. Several theories have been proposed, but the exact mechanism is uncertain.

Use of an opioid receptor antagonist such as naloxone reliably reverses the side effects of epidural and intrathecal opioids, but reversal of analgesia may occur. This has encouraged symptomatic treatment of individual side effects, e.g. using antihistamines such as chlorphenamine 4 mg orally or 10 mg parenterally for itching. Low doses of propofol (10 mg) and ondansetron have been reported to reduce opioid-induced itching but the evidence for benefit is inconclusive.

Respiratory depression

Fentanyl has the shortest duration of action following epidural or subarachnoid administration (approximately 4 hours) and the lowest potential to cause respiratory depression, although cases have been reported. Epidural morphine is well recognised as being associated with a small risk of respiratory depression for up to 12–24 hours after administration, but will also provide analgesia for a similar period of time. Diamorphine has an intermediate duration of action and there have been no reported cases of delayed respiratory depression, although early cases have occurred – usually in combination with other sedatives.

The potential for this life-threatening side effect of centrally administered opioids has led to a general prohibition on the concomitant use of opioid and sedative drugs by any other route. It has also caused considerable controversy about the intensity and duration of monitoring and nursing care required for patients who have received epidural or spinal opioids. Respiratory depression manifests itself as increasing sedation (due to carbon dioxide retention) rather than reduced respiratory rate; therefore in the absence of facilities for prolonged high-dependency nursing (which few obstetric units possess), it is sensible to nurse the mother in a postnatal bed that can be readily observed from the central nursing station, and in the company of other mothers, rather than in a side room. Many obstetric anaesthetists consider that the small but real risks of late respiratory depression associated with epidural morphine outweigh the benefits of using it in preference to diamorphine or fentanyl, although there are many studies confirming the safety of spinal morphine.

If naloxone is required to reverse respiratory depression it is important to use either repeated doses or an infusion, because of the prolonged action of the opioid compared with its antagonist.

Gastric emptying

This is delayed after epidural or intrathecal boluses of opioids, although there is some evidence that low-dose infusions of fentanyl do not impair gastric emptying.

Placental transfer

Although centrally administered opioids cross the placenta, this occurs in a dose-dependent manner. Administration of an epidural bolus of fentanyl 100 µg 20 minutes before delivery results in umbilical artery concentrations well below those needed to cause neonatal respiratory depression. Similarly, although opioids can be found in breast milk after maternal epidural administration, the amounts are negligible.

Key points

- There is synergy between neuraxial opioids and local anaesthetics.
- Side effects occur following all routes of administration.
- Side effects are dose dependent, with the exception of urinary retention.
- Morphine has a slower onset, longer duration of action and increased incidence of side effects compared with fentanyl; the action of diamorphine is intermediate.

Further reading

Bonnet MP, Mignon A, Mazoit JX, Ozier Y, Marret E. Analgesic efficacy and adverse effects of epidural morphine compared to parenteral opioids after elective Caesarean section: a systematic review. *Eur J Pain* 2010; **14**: 894.e1–9.

Carvalho B. Respiratory depression after neuraxial opioids in the obstetric setting. *Anesth Analg* 2008; **107**: 956–61.

Chapter

27

Inhalational analgesic drugs

The most commonly used agent for inhaled analgesia in the UK is Entonox, which is a mixture of 50% nitrous oxide and 50% oxygen. Its advantages are that it is inexpensive, is almost universally available (including for use in the community), has a long record of safety, and is acceptable to many mothers and midwives. Its low blood solubility means that blood levels rapidly reach a maximum after inhalation and fall once a contraction has passed and inhalation has ceased. It does not appear to have any detrimental effect on the fetus. The main disadvantage of Entonox is that it provides only limited pain relief. In addition, some mothers are phobic about the use of 'gas'.

Volatile anaesthetic agents such as methoxyflurane and trichloroethylene have been used for analgesia in labour, but these drugs have been withdrawn for non-obstetric reasons. They were administered using a draw-over vaporiser and breathing system and provided analgesia of slow onset because of their high blood solubility, with residual effects between contractions. Other volatile agents, more recently sevoflurane, have also been studied, but none are widely used. A premixed preparation of isoflurane and Entonox (Isoxane) has been described but this too is not widely available.

Problems/special considerations

- Nitrous oxide is a relatively weak analgesic, helping 30–50% of mothers who use it but with little effect on actual pain scores. Use of more than 50% nitrous oxide improves analgesic efficacy, but at the cost of increased maternal sedation and decreased inspired concentration of maternal oxygen. The use of the 50:50 mixture of nitrous oxide and oxygen represents a compromise between analgesic efficacy and maternal and fetal safety.
- Entonox is presented as a premixed agent, available in cylinders for community use and piped from central tanks in hospital maternity units. The mixture is stable under most conditions, but at very low temperatures the constituent gases separate out. This is

relevant for community midwives practising in parts of the UK in winter, who must be aware that they need to invert Entonox cylinders several times before use to ensure adequate mixing. The mother administers the gas to herself from a demand valve via either facemask or mouthpiece. Maternal sedation may occur even with 50% nitrous oxide and it is therefore important that, in order to avoid the risk of aspiration, Entonox is self-administered, not administered by the midwife or by the woman's partner.

- Some mothers find inhalation of dry gases unpleasant, and in asthmatics this may provoke bronchospasm. Entonox also causes unacceptable nausea in a small number of women, and dizziness is common.

- The efficacy of Entonox can be improved by instructing the mother to start inhaling as soon as she becomes aware of a contraction, and to continue inhalation until the contraction subsides. It is also important to ensure that if a facemask is used it is applied firmly to the face to avoid entraining air.

- Although Entonox crosses the placenta readily, it is excreted by the neonatal lungs after delivery. Entonox does not have adverse effects on the fetus, but the maternal hyperventilation associated with its use may cause placental vasoconstriction and impair fetal oxygenation in an already compromised fetus. Similarly, the combination of pethidine and Entonox has been associated with a high incidence of maternal arterial oxygen desaturation and should be avoided if there is evidence of fetal compromise.

- There has been recent concern about the pollutant effects of Entonox. Many labour wards do not have any means of scavenging exhaled Entonox, and this is increasingly considered unacceptable. Scavenging equipment is available but obviously has resource implications.

- Volatile anaesthetic agents cause dose-dependent uterine relaxation, although this can be overcome at low concentrations by oxytoxic drugs. They also have cardiorespiratory side effects, although these are usually minimal at low concentrations.

Key points

- Entonox provides acceptable (but incomplete) analgesia to up to half of the mothers who use it. It is appropriate for low-risk mothers in uncomplicated labour and for mothers awaiting regional analgesia.

- Entonox should not be recommended for high-risk mothers or as a supplement to inadequate systemic analgesia.

Further reading

Yentis SM, Clyburn P. The use of Entonox™ for labour pain should be abandoned. *Int J Obstet Anesth* 2001; **10**: 25–9.

Systemic analgesic drugs

A variety of opioid analgesics have been used in the UK to reduce the pain of labour, and none have been found adequate for the majority of mothers. Pethidine is the most commonly used systemic analgesic in England and Wales, whereas in Scotland diamorphine is also common. Shorter-acting opioids such as fentanyl, alfentanil and remifentanil have also been used. All opioid analgesics, given in equianalgesic doses, have similar advantages and disadvantages, and the widespread use of pethidine is largely historical.

The major advantages of systemic opioid analgesia for labour are ease of administration, low cost, midwife autonomy of use and acceptability by many mothers. The major disadvantages are failure to provide adequate analgesia for many women, general opioid side effects for the mother and rapid placental transfer to the fetus.

Problems/special considerations

Dosage and administration

- Midwives in the UK are authorised to give a total of 200 mg pethidine to a labouring mother, provided that the dose is divided, without a doctor's prescription. It is common practice to give 100 mg intramuscularly as the first dose. Blood levels of pethidine following intramuscular injection are unpredictable, and it is not possible to achieve therapeutic levels reliably with this standardised approach to administration. There is also little correlation between the weight of the mother, the amount of pethidine given and subsequent plasma concentration of pethidine.

- Intravenous administration of pethidine, either by medical staff or as patient-controlled analgesia (PCA; e.g. 10–20 mg with a lockout of 10 min), is more likely to achieve therapeutic plasma concentrations of the drug, but the intramuscular route remains the most commonly used.

- Diamorphine is also used in some units, in doses of 5.0–7.5 mg intramuscularly. Despite suggestions that diamorphine might have benefits over pethidine, randomised trials are few and the evidence supporting diamorphine is weak.

- Fentanyl has been used intravenously to provide labour analgesia. Use of bolus doses of 20–50 µg at least 5–6 min apart has been reported to cause less neonatal depression than intravenous boluses of pethidine (25–50 mg). The advantages are a rapid onset and short duration of action. The general risks and benefits of opioid analgesics in labour apply although severe neonatal depression is uncommon.

- Use of intravenous alfentanil via PCA has been described but is rare.

- Remifentanil is a very short-acting opioid that is rapidly hydrolysed by red blood cell and tissue esterases and thus is thought to have the characteristics that are ideal for PCA in labour. Furthermore, studies suggest that fetal/neonatal effects are few since the drug is rapidly metabolised after crossing the placenta. Although analgesia is incomplete (the ideal drug dose and lockout time are unclear but a commonly used regimen, $0.5 \ \mu g.kg^{-1}$ with a 2-min lockout, has been shown to reduce pain scores in labour by $> 85\%$), there exist two groups of women who might particularly benefit from remifentanil PCA: first, those unable to have an epidural sited for medical reasons; and second, those who do not necessarily want to have an epidural, but who just want analgesia that is more effective than the other methods. Apart from incomplete analgesia, disadvantages include the need for one-to-one midwifery care owing to the risk of respiratory depression in the mother, and associated nausea and vomiting.

Side effects

These are common to all opioid drugs. Maternal side effects include:

- Altered respiratory pattern – hypoventilation occurs between contractions, but inadequate analgesia is accompanied by hyperventilation during contractions
- Reduced gastric motility
- Nausea and vomiting
- Sedation, dysphoria and euphoria.

Drugs such as promethazine and promazine are still frequently administered with pethidine in an attempt to reduce the incidence of nausea and vomiting, and these drugs considerably enhance the sedative effects of pethidine, sometimes to the extent that the mother has no clear recall of the events surrounding delivery.

All opioids cross the placenta freely; fetal effects include:

- Loss of heart rate variability – the typical 'flat' cardiotocographic trace that results may make interpretation of any other changes difficult
- Neonatal respiratory depression, especially if given within 2–4 hours of delivery for pethidine or diamorphine (reversible with naloxone, although it is important to remember that naloxone is a short-acting drug and may need to be given either as an infusion or in repeated boluses)
- Depression of neonatal neurobehavioural scores for up to 3 days – the significance of this is not clear
- Smaller likelihood of successful breastfeeding in babies whose mothers have received pethidine in labour, although there may be other psychosocial factors relevant to these findings.

Pethidine has a long-acting metabolite, norpethidine, which accumulates in both the mother and fetus and has significant opioid activity. Its half-life is 21 hours in the mother and 63 hours in the fetus, compared with 3–7 hours and 13–23 hours respectively for pethidine. Norpethidine also has proconvulsant activity, and therefore on theoretical grounds pethidine is not an ideal analgesic for women with epilepsy or pre-eclampsia.

Management options

The advantages of intramuscular opioid analgesia (simplicity of administration, low cost and acceptability to many midwives and mothers) have to be balanced against the disadvantages for both mother and baby, and the fact that the quality of analgesia is generally poor, although it may be useful in very early labour or pre-labour. For mothers with significant medical disease and those at increased risk of operative delivery, regional analgesia is usually preferable. However, women unable to have regional analgesia (e.g. those with coagulation disorders) may benefit from PCA as an alternative.

Women receiving systemic opioid analgesia should be considered at risk of gastric stasis and advised accordingly regarding oral intake. Concurrent administration of H_2-antagonists should also be considered. In some units, metoclopramide is given concurrently to women receiving opioids as a non-sedating antiemetic.

Key points
- Pethidine is the most commonly used opioid analgesic for labour in the UK.
- Other opioids have similar risks and benefits.
- Patient-controlled analgesia may improve efficacy and reduce side effects.
- Systemic opioid analgesia is not advisable for women at increased risk of operative delivery.
- Neonatal respiratory depression and impaired neurobehavioural scores may follow maternal administration of opioids.

Further reading
Hinova A, Fernando R. Systemic remifentanil for labor analgesia. *Anesth Analg* 2009; **109**: 1925–9.

Littleford J. Effects on the fetus and newborn of maternal analgesia and anesthesia: a review. *Can J Anesth* 2004; **51**: 586–609.

Ullman R, Smith LA, Burns E, Mori R, Dowswell T. Parenteral opioids for maternal pain relief in labour. *Cochrane Database Syst Rev* 2010; (9): CD007396.

Chapter

29

Non-pharmacological analgesia

Many women wish to avoid intervention in labour, including use of pharmacological methods of analgesia. The use of psychoprophylaxis ('childbirth without fear') dates from the 1950s, and since that time a variety of relaxation techniques have been introduced. Relaxation techniques, self-hypnosis, acupuncture, aromatherapy, reflexology, water labour/birth and transcutaneous electrical nerve stimulation (TENS) are now widespread.

Problems/special considerations

Fear of the unknown is a major factor in the experience of pain. Provision of antenatal education about the process of labour and the common complications that occur is an essential first step in provision of analgesia for labour. Translations of information leaflets and availability of interpreters must be considered, especially in units delivering a significant number of women for whom English is not their first language. It is desirable to have an independent translator rather than a family member whenever possible. Videos about pain relief in labour are readily available and provide information in a format that is familiar and accessible to the majority of the population. Attendance at parentcraft classes should be encouraged.

Relaxation techniques

These range from simple breathing exercises to formal yoga techniques. There is a vast range of literature in the lay press about such techniques. The association between tension, anxiety and pain is well recognised, and the use of relaxation techniques should be encouraged for all pregnant women.

Self-hypnosis

Practitioners of hypnosis differentiate between a hypnotic state and deep relaxation. Hypnosis has been successfully used not only for pain relief in labour but also to provide anaesthesia for caesarean section. Hypnosis is time-consuming, requires considerable antenatal preparation and is not freely available to the majority of women. However, evidence suggests that women taught self-hypnosis have reduced requirements for pharmacological analgesia including epidurals.

Acupuncture, aromatherapy and reflexology

Acupuncture has much evidence to support its use in certain areas of medicine, but properly conducted studies in obstetric practice are few. What evidence there is mostly concerns manual acupuncture and suggests a beneficial effect on pain and analgesic requirements in labour, including the need for epidural analgesia.

Practitioners of aromatherapy and reflexology are becoming more numerous, and include an increasing number of midwives. The usefulness of such analgesic techniques is dependent on the availability of a practitioner. The available evidence does not suggest a reduction in pain or analgesic requirements with aromatherapy.

Water

The use of the birthing pool has become increasingly popular since the 1980s. Enthusiasts for the pool claim reduced rates of virtually all forms of medical intervention in labour, whereas some obstetricians view the pool as an unnecessary additional hazard for the labouring mother. The evidence regarding the first stage of labour suggests a reduction in labour pain and analgesic requirements with no effect on outcome of labour or neonatal status.

For decades mothers have been advised to have warm baths to help them relax in early labour, and use of the pool for labour analgesia is an extension of this advice. Women who have had a lot of back pain during pregnancy often find the birthing pool particularly helpful. Continuous fetal monitoring is not possible in a birthing pool, and therefore the mother with an at-risk fetus should be advised against using the pool. Similarly, the use of the pool is inadvisable in mothers needing intravenous infusions or any form of continuous maternal monitoring. Mothers requesting pharmacological analgesia should be asked to leave the birthing pool.

TENS

Particular benefit for TENS is claimed for women in early labour, those with backache associated with a posterior position, and for women with a prolonged latent phase of labour.

The advantage of TENS is the absence of any effect on the fetus and the lack of any significant side effects for the mother. Meta-analysis of randomised controlled trials of TENS in labour suggests only limited evidence of its efficacy, but it remains popular with mothers and midwives.

Water blocks

This technique involves injection of small volumes of sterile water (0.1 ml) subcutaneously or more commonly, intracutaneously, over four spots lateral to the lumbosacral spine. Although intensely painful for up to 30 seconds after injection, meta-analysis suggests a reduction in pain scores lasting up to 2 hours. Water blocks are common in certain countries but rarely used in the UK.

Doulas

It is recognised that the constant presence of a supportive and encouraging second person reduces the pain scores of women in labour. Some cultures ban the father from the labour room and provide a female partner for the labouring woman. There has been a resurgence of interest in use of birth partners, or doulas, in both the USA and the UK. The constant presence of the midwife during labour is also thought to reduce demand for analgesia and other interventions.

Management options

Anaesthetists should be aware of the benefits and limitations of non-pharmacological analgesia and be able to advise mothers when use of these methods of pain relief is or is not appropriate. It is important that anaesthetists realise that maternal satisfaction with pain relief in labour is not necessarily related to the degree of analgesia obtained.

Non-pharmacological methods of pain relief have the major advantage of minimal or absent fetal and maternal adverse effects, and as such their use by mothers in normal, uncomplicated labour should be encouraged. Prolonged use of these methods of pain relief by mothers with pregnancy or labour complications may increase the risk of ultimate recourse to general anaesthesia for delivery. For this group of women a change from non-pharmacological to regional analgesia is advisable.

It should be noted that the National Institute for Health and Clinical Excellence (NICE) has recommended that water injections and TENS should not be offered to women in established labour, and that whilst hypnosis and acupuncture should not be provided, women wishing to use them should not be prevented from doing so. NICE does recommend offering women water in which to labour.

Key points

- There is evidence for efficacy of several non-pharmacological methods of analgesia, and many women request them.
- Those techniques for which evidence of efficacy is limited or lacking still have minimal, if any, adverse effects, and women should not be denied them if that is their wish.
- Antenatal education should include all methods of analgesia available in a particular unit.

Further reading

Cluett ER, Nikodem VC, McCandlish RE, Burns EE. Immersion in water in pregnancy, labour and birth. *Cochrane Database Syst Rev* 2004; (2): CD000111.

Dowswell T, Bedwell C, Lavender T, Neilson JP. Transcutaneous electrical nerve stimulation (TENS) for pain relief in labour. *Cochrane Database Syst Rev* 2009; (2): CD007214.

Hodnett ED, Gates S, Hofmeyr GJ, Sakala C, Weston J. Continuous support for women during childbirth. *Cochrane Database Syst Rev* 2011; (2): CD003766.

Mårtensson L, Wallin G. Sterile water injections as treatment for low-back pain during labour: a review. *Aust N Z J Obstet Gynaecol* 2008; **48**: 369–74.

National Institute for Health and Clinical Excellence. Intrapartum care: care of healthy women and their babies during childbirth. *Clinical Guideline 55*. London: NICE 2007, http://www.nice.org.uk/CG055.

Smith CA, Collins CT, Cyna AM, Crowther CA. Complementary and alternative therapies for pain management in labour. *Cochrane Database Syst Rev* 2006; (4): CD003521.

Instrumental delivery

Vaginal delivery may be facilitated by the use of forceps or a suction cup (ventouse). Forceps deliveries can be divided into outlet, low, mid-cavity or high (rotational), although high forceps deliveries are now rarely used, in favour of caesarean section.

In the UK, 10–13% of deliveries are performed with forceps or ventouse, but the figure is very variable in different units and is greatly affected by individual policies with respect to the maximum allowable duration of the second stage, the use of Syntocinon to augment contractions and criteria for caesarean section.

In general, instrumental delivery can be indicated by maternal factors (exhaustion, failure to descend, illness precluding Valsalva manoeuvre) or fetal factors (fetal distress, prematurity). The commonest indication is prolongation of the second stage, often defined as longer than 2 hours for a primigravida (3 hours with an effective epidural), or 1 hour for a multigravida (2 hours with an epidural).

Problems/special considerations
Analgesia
Analgesia produced by low-dose epidural solutions may be adequate for low-outlet ('lift-out') forceps or ventouse delivery, but mid- or high-cavity forceps delivery requires dense surgical anaesthesia. A good pelvic block is essential, and the perineum should be tested before inserting the instrument. For anything other than an outlet forceps or ventouse, the sensory block should extend up to T10. It is advisable for the anaesthetist to be present when anything other than the most straightforward instrumental delivery is being performed, in order to assess the existing block, consider the options, and give (and monitor the effects of) an appropriate top-up.

Trial of forceps
When it is anticipated that instrumental delivery may be difficult, provision should be made for immediate conversion to caesarean section. The procedure should be carried out in the operating theatre and regional anaesthesia should be adequate for rapid operative delivery. Attempted instrumental delivery is more likely to fail if the mother's BMI exceeds 30 kg/m^2, if the baby is large, and if the head is in the occipito-posterior position or mid-cavity or above.

Aftercare
It should be remembered that the extensive episiotomy that usually accompanies instrumental delivery, coupled with the inevitable tissue trauma, often results in significant pain

in the immediate postpartum period. Non-steroidal anti-inflammatory drugs should be used prophylactically if there are no contraindications, and epidural opioids are often required. Significant postpartum haemorrhage can result from cervical or vaginal tears, even more so than a caesarean section, and so vigilance regarding blood loss is essential in these cases.

Instrumental delivery and regional analgesia

There is no doubt that, in most centres, there is a higher rate of instrumental delivery in mothers who opt for regional analgesia. Although it is very difficult to exclude potential confounders (e.g. it is likely that women who need epidural analgesia are those with other factors that predispose to instrumental delivery, such as slow progress, malpresentation, multiple gestation, relative cephalopelvic disproportion), and most randomised trials of epidural analgesia have been complicated by considerable crossover between groups (mostly from non-epidural to epidural), meta-analysis suggests an increased likelihood of instrumental delivery with epidural techniques (relative risk ~1.4). This must be weighed against the improved quality of analgesia compared with alternatives, the beneficial effect of epidural analgesia on fetal acid–base balance, and the ability to avoid general anaesthesia in many cases should caesarean section be required.

Management options

For deliveries other than outlet forceps and ventouse, with a functioning epidural *in situ*, it is usually an easy matter to intensify the block by administering 10–20 ml of 0.5% levobupivacaine, 0.75% ropivacaine or 2% lidocaine with adrenaline and bicarbonate, depending on the anticipated difficulty with delivery and the urgency. Pelvic spread may be encouraged by sitting the mother up, and it is therefore important to establish the block before putting the legs into stirrups.

When no epidural is in place, spinal anaesthesia is most appropriate, using ~1.5 ml of hyperbaric 0.5% bupivacaine in the sitting position, ±10–15 μg fentanyl. However, if caesarean section is anticipated, a spinal or a CSE technique, using the same dose as required for surgical anaesthesia, may be more appropriate.

Pudendal block may be performed by the obstetrician if there is no anaesthetist available, although it has a high failure rate and needs at least 10–20 minutes to become effective. Pudendal block may also be used to supplement an existing epidural with sacral sparing, and infiltration of the perineum with local anaesthetic is a useful adjunctive technique before performing an episiotomy.

In all cases, care must be taken to ensure that aortocaval compression is avoided, e.g. by tilting the mother's pelvis with a wedge.

Key points

- A good pelvic block is essential and should be confirmed by testing.
- Conversion to caesarean section may be required.
- Anaesthesia should be established before elevating the legs.

Further reading

Anim-Somuah M, Smyth RM, Jones L. Epidural versus non-epidural or no analgesia in labour. *Cochrane Database Syst Rev* 2011; (12): CD000331.

Liu EH, Sia AT. Rates of caesarean section and instrumental vaginal delivery in nulliparous women after low concentration epidural infusions or opioid analgesia: systematic review. *BMJ* 2004; **328**: 1410–12.

Royal College of Obstetricians and Gynaecologists. Operative vaginal delivery. *Green-top* 26. London: RCOG 2011, http://www.rcog.org.uk/womens-health/clinical-guidance/operative-vaginal-delivery-green-top-26.

Chapter

31

Caesarean section

The caesarean section (CS) rate in much of the developed world has increased markedly in recent decades; in England the rate has stabilised since about 2007 (Fig. 31.1). (The rates are similar in the devolved countries; in Wales and Scotland the CS rate is currently about 1–2% higher, and in Northern Ireland about 5% higher, than in England.) There is wide variation between units. There has been general concern over increasing CS rates and the associated complications, notwithstanding the benefits that CS might have in individual cases. Since CS is such an important procedure in obstetrics, and anaesthetic-related maternal deaths commonly involve emergency CS, it is important that obstetric anaesthetists have an understanding of the practical aspects relating to obstetric indications and techniques.

Classification and delivery time

Traditionally, CS was classified as elective (i.e. a date is given beforehand) or emergency (the rest). The latter group is thought by many obstetricians and obstetric anaesthetists to be too broad, since it includes cases in which immediate delivery is required (e.g. severe fetal compromise or cord prolapse) as well as cases in which there is little urgency (e.g. early spontaneous labour in a mother with a breech scheduled for elective CS the next day). This led to the reclassification of CS into four grades (Table 31.1); this classification has been adopted by all the major UK bodies involved in this field. Although intended as an audit tool (e.g. to monitor outcomes and allocation of staff), the classification has been used to guide management (e.g. second operating theatre opened for grade-1 cases). However, attempts to link the grades to acceptable maximum times to delivery (e.g. 30 min for grade 1) are hampered by the unwillingness of obstetricians to commit themselves to 'acceptable' delays for grades 2

Table 31.1 Classification of caesarean section

1	Immediate threat to life of woman or fetus
2	Maternal or fetal compromise which is not immediately life-threatening
3	Needing early delivery but no maternal or fetal compromise
4	At a time to suit the woman and maternity team

N.B. Applies to the time of decision to operate; e.g. an episode of fetal compromise caused by aortocaval compression responding to therapy, followed some hours later by caesarean section for failure to progress, would be graded as 3, not 2. Similarly, a case booked as an elective procedure for malpresentation could eventually be classified as grade 3 if the mother goes into labour before the chosen date of surgery. Also applies whether or not the woman is in labour.

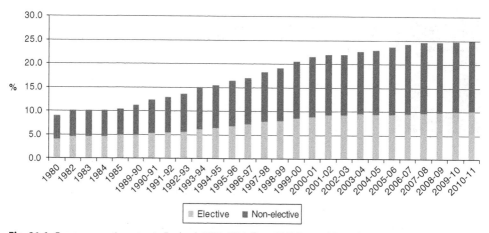

Fig. 31.1 Caesarean section rates in England, 1980–2011 (from NHS Hospital Episodes Statistics).

and 3 in case of a bad outcome. In addition, maximum times to delivery are controversial and not based on good science: the often quoted maximum of 15–30 minutes for fetal compromise is derived largely from work in the 1960s in which animal fetuses were exposed to varying durations of intrauterine hypoxia and the degree of subsequent fetal damage assessed. Most cases of cerebral palsy are now known to be related to factors arising before labour. A number of audits within maternity units have found that meeting the particular standard set is extremely difficult to achieve in practice because of delays at each stage of the process (e.g. calling the anaesthetist/anaesthetic assistant, moving the mother to the operating theatre, preparing the surgical equipment, etc.). Finally, the defined time period itself varies: the time from decision to skin incision; from decision to delivery; and from informing the anaesthetist to skin incision or delivery have all been quoted in various recommendations or guidelines.

Analysis of data from the Royal College of Obstetricians and Gynaecologists' Sentinel audit of CS in the UK in 2000 suggests that poorer maternal and neonatal outcomes were associated with decision-to-delivery intervals exceeding 75 minutes, but not intervals of 31–75 minutes. Recent guidance from the Joint Standing Committee of the Royal College of Obstetricians and Gynaecologists and Royal College of Anaesthetists reiterated that all maternity units in the UK should be using the same classification for CS, that every individual woman in labour should be

Table 31.2 Indications for caesarean section

Previous caesarean section
   Elective
   Following trial of labour
   Other

Maternal disease
   Worsening pre-existing disease, e.g. cardiac
   Associated with pregnancy, e.g. pre-eclampsia

Placenta praevia or abruption

Maternal exhaustion/choice

Obstructed labour/failure to progress

Malpositions

Multiple pregnancy

Fetal compromise

Cord prolapse

considered to have a continuum of risk, and that the 30-minute interval should be considered as an 'audit standard' and not the 'gold standard' in which to deliver a baby in an emergency. Updated guidance from the National Institute for Health and Clinical Excellence (NICE) states that category 1 and 2 CS should be performed 'as quickly as possible' and that for category 2, within 75 minutes 'in most situations'. Further, delivery times of 30 minutes for category 1, and both 30 and 75 minutes for category 2 CS, should be used as audit standards for the unit and not to judge performance for any individual CS.

Indications

CS may be performed for the benefit of the mother, the fetus or both (Table 31.2), although in practice maternal indications will ultimately affect the fetus adversely if not relieved, and vice versa. For elective CS, 39 weeks is commonly chosen as the optimum gestation, reflecting a balance between the benefit to the neonate of a longer gestation and the greater risk of spontaneous labour and emergency surgery.

Procedure

For lower segment CS, skin incision is usually low transverse (i.e. in the L1 dermatome) but may be midline. Once exposed, the rectus sheath is split longitudinally and stretched laterally and the peritoneum incised. The uterus is incised transversely in its thin lower segment. A 'classical' CS involves a midline incision, and the uterus is incised longitudinally in its upper segment. Classical CS is associated with a greater risk of haemorrhage, infection and ileus but is quicker to perform and easier than lower segment CS. It may be indicated if the lower segment is poorly formed, e.g. in premature delivery, and in placenta praevia, transverse/unstable lie or uterine fibroids.

Uterine incision is accompanied by removal by suction of amniotic fluid if the membranes have not ruptured (mothers and partners may find the noise alarming if unexpected). Delivery of the baby may be difficult if the head has descended well into the pelvis, and may require forceps. If the placenta has already started to separate, the uterus may contract around the baby's head, especially if CS is in the second stage of labour; increased inspired concentration of volatile agent has been used to relax the uterus during general anaesthesia; glyceryl trinitrate 50–100 µg intravenously or sublingually, repeated as necessary, has also been used to good effect and is suitable during regional anaesthesia.

The time between induction of general anaesthesia and delivery (I–D interval) may affect fetal wellbeing since if very short, the induction agent may be present in the fetus at high levels; if the interval is very long, fetal accumulation of inhalational agents may occur. The time from uterine incision to delivery (U–D interval) is thought to be more important, since placental disruption may occur once the uterus is incised; fetal acidosis is unlikely if the U–D interval is less than 3 minutes.

Following delivery of the baby, oxytocin (Syntocinon) is given (typically 5 U slowly intravenously, though there is some evidence that even smaller doses may be effective). Rapid injection of larger doses may cause severe tachycardia and may be no more effective than smaller doses. Uterine contraction may be aided by vigorous rubbing of the uterus; an oxytocin infusion may be required (e.g. 40 U in 500 ml saline at ~125 ml/h), especially after prolonged augmented labour, multiple delivery, in the presence of polyhydramnios and with a previous history of postpartum haemorrhage or multiple deliveries. Increasingly, this infusion is requested as routine for all cases by the obstetricians. An analogue of oxytocin, carbetocin, is longer acting and may be a suitable alternative.

Once the baby and placenta have been delivered, the uterus is checked for tears and then sutured. Many obstetricians prefer the ease of access conferred by exteriorising the uterus, although this may be accompanied by discomfort and nausea/vomiting during regional anaesthesia, bradycardia and an increased incidence of air embolism. The obstetrician should always check with the anaesthetists before performing this manoeuvre.

Problems/special considerations

- Surgical problems relating to the procedure itself include difficulty caused by adhesions (especially following previous CS or other abdominal surgery), haemorrhage, surgical trauma to the baby, difficulty delivering the baby with the risk of fetal hypoxia or physical trauma, difficulty delivering the placenta and damage to neighbouring structures. There may be large veins on the anterior wall of the uterus and wide transverse incisions may extend to the uterine angles when the baby is delivered, leading to severe bleeding. Usual blood loss is ~400–700 ml (increased with general anaesthesia) but is notoriously difficult to estimate accurately. There is an increased risk of placenta accreta in women who have had previous CS, especially if the placenta overlies the previous scar. Overall the risk of further surgery is increased from ~3 per 10 000 after CS to ~50 per 10 000 after vaginal delivery, with the risk of hysterectomy increased from 1–2 per 10 000 to up to 80 per 10 000 (though it isn't clear how much the reason for CS may also influence the need for further surgery).
- Anaesthetic problems include those of general or regional anaesthesia generally. Pain during CS under regional anaesthesia has replaced awareness under general anaesthesia as the main reason for litigation associated with CS. Chest pain and/or electrocardiographic changes may occur; their cause is unknown (although small air emboli or coronary artery/oesophageal spasm have been suggested) and they may occur independently of each other. Elevations of maternal troponin I levels have also been

reported. Shoulder-tip pain may occasionally occur, probably related to blood irritating the diaphragm. Other possible problems related to the procedure include air or amniotic fluid embolism and allergic phenomena.

- Postoperative problems are as for any surgery and include infection (prophylactic antibiotics have been shown to reduce infection; although traditionally often given after delivery to avoid exposing the fetus to the drug, and in case a severe maternal allergic reaction should occur, recent National Institute for Health and Clinical Excellence (NICE) guidelines suggest administration before skin incision) and thromboembolism (heparin is given prophylactically to women at high risk in some units and to all women in others. If the former, the Royal College of Obstetricians and Gynaecologists' guidelines should be followed). NICE guidelines suggest that observations (including assessment of pain and sedation) should be half hourly for 2 hours after CS, then hourly, up to 12 hours after intrathecal diamorphine. Many units cannot manage such an intensive observation regimen. Postoperative analgesia is discussed in Chapter 39, Postoperative analgesia.

Management options

The choice of anaesthetic technique depends on the degree of urgency, whether an epidural catheter is already in place, specific obstetric factors (e.g. complicated surgery anticipated) or anaesthetic (e.g. known difficult intubation, previous back surgery), the personal preference of the anaesthetist and the wishes of the mother (see Chapters 32–34). Absolute figures are unavailable, but it is thought that two thirds to three quarters of CS are performed under regional anaesthesia in the UK, reflecting the above preferences and the widely perceived greater safety of regional over general anaesthesia for CS. Particular concerns are the possibly inadequate exposure of anaesthetic trainees to general anaesthesia for CS, the greater tendency of trainees to use general anaesthesia (especially for emergency CS) than more experienced consultants, and the anxiety caused when this occurs. There is also concern that the incidence of failed intubation in obstetrics is increasing and that this may be related to the above factors.

Key points

- Caesarean section rate in the UK is ~25–30%.
- Indications may be maternal, fetal or both.
- Complications include shoulder-tip, abdominal or chest pain, air or amniotic fluid embolism, haemorrhage, surgical trauma and awareness.

Further reading

Lucas DN, Yentis SM, Kinsella SM, *et al.* Urgency of Caesarean section: a new classification. *JRSM* 2000; **93**: 346–50.

National Institute for Health and Clinical Excellence. Caesarean section. *Clinical Guideline 132.* London: NICE 2004, http://guidance.nice.org.uk/CG132.

Royal College of Obstetricians and Gynaecologists/ Royal College of Anaesthetists. Classification of urgency of caesarean section – a continuum of risk. *Good Practice No. 11.* London: RCOG 2010, http://www.rcog.org.uk/classification-of-urgency-of-caesarean-section-good-practice-11.

Yentis SM. Whose distress is it anyway? 'Fetal distress' and the 30-minute rule. *Anaesthesia* 2003; **58**: 732–3.

Chapter 32

Spinal anaesthesia for caesarean section

Continuous audit by the Obstetric Anaesthetists' Association suggests that half to two thirds of caesarean sections are currently done under single-shot spinal anaesthesia in the UK.

Problems/special considerations

- Rapid onset of widespread vasodilatation coupled with the effect of aortocaval compression means that hypotension is an almost inevitable accompaniment to spinal anaesthesia unless specific precautions are taken. Avoidance of the supine position, frequent blood pressure measurement and instant availability of intravenous fluid and vasopressors are prerequisites for the safe use of this technique.
- Careful assessment of the level of block is essential before starting the operation. Despite an apparently adequate block, pain may still occur, although this is less likely than if an epidural anaesthetic has been used. Mothers should be warned of this possibility in advance, and adequate treatment, even to the extent of inducing general anaesthesia, must be offered. Pain during caesarean section under regional anaesthesia is currently the most common successful cause of litigation against obstetric anaesthetists in the UK.
- The incidence of postdural puncture headache (PDPH) is related to the size and type of needle used. 'Pencil-point' and conical tip needles, such as the Sprotte and Whitacre, are associated with a much lower rate of headache than Quincke needles with a cutting tip, so much so that a 24 G pencil-point needle is probably better than a 27 G Quincke needle.
- Meningitis and encephalitis are extremely rare. However, once the dura mater has been penetrated, the cerebrospinal fluid (CSF) is particularly susceptible to contamination, and it is considered good practice to use a completely aseptic technique, including the wearing of mask, gown and gloves.

Management options

Suitability of the technique

In experienced hands, spinal anaesthesia can be almost as fast as general anaesthesia, and there are few occasions when the urgency of the situation means that there is no time for this technique. If the mother already has an effective epidural *in situ* then time permitting, this should be topped-up in preference to establishing a new block. If time is short, a single-shot spinal has been suggested as an alternative to general anaesthesia in a mother with an epidural *in situ*. If spinal supplementation of an existing epidural block is thought appropriate, it may be necessary to use a reduced dose, as there have been case reports of very high blocks in these circumstances. Spinal anaesthesia is contraindicated in patients with hypovolaemia, coagulation disorders (whether iatrogenic or pathological) and systemic sepsis. Although regional anaesthesia was traditionally avoided previously if massive blood loss was expected, such as in placenta praevia, many anaesthetists would now use a spinal block in this situation. There is some evidence to suggest that blood loss and the need for blood transfusion is reduced if regional anaesthesia is used in these circumstances.

Although traditionally favoured as being better for the baby than general anaesthesia, there is evidence that spinal anaesthesia may be associated with greater neonatal acidosis than after epidural or general anaesthesia, possibly related to the rapidity of onset and cardiovascular changes. However, the rapid onset and more profound block compared with epidural anaesthesia, and the greater maternal safety profile compared with general anaesthesia, make spinal anaesthesia the technique preferred by most obstetric anaesthetists for caesarean section

Preoperative preparation

Preoperative assessment may be compromised by the urgency of the case, but should include assessment for difficult intubation, since general anaesthesia may be needed if the block is unsatisfactory. An explanation of the technique should be given, and the mother should be warned about the risks of hypotension with associated nausea and vomiting. The possibility of pain during the operation must be mentioned, although she should be reassured that this is unusual and will be treated if necessary with intravenous opioids, inhaled nitrous oxide or even general anaesthesia. Most mothers prefer their partners to be present for the delivery, and it is good practice to involve them in these discussions so that they are aware of what may happen.

Preparation

Standard monitoring is mandatory. Most anaesthetists prefer to perform spinal anaesthesia with the patient on the operating table, since this minimises the need for movement after the local anaesthetic has been administered. Sitting and lateral positions are both acceptable, although there is evidence that the former may be easier if the bony landmarks are difficult to palpate. The block tends to develop more rapidly in the lateral position, probably owing to the slope of the vertebral canal in this position in women (the hips are wider than the shoulders, causing a downward slope towards the head, unlike in men, in which the opposite tends to occur).

Intravenous access

Good intravenous access is essential, and a preload of 1000–2000 ml was traditionally used before the spinal dose was given. However, 'co-loading' (giving 400–800 ml fluid together with a prophylactic vasopressor) is now widely used, and this avoids excessive fluid administration. Colloid solutions have been shown to be more efficacious than crystalloids at preventing hypotension, but are more expensive and there is a small risk of allergy. A vasopressor must be to hand and phenylephrine is now the vasopressor of choice as it has been shown to cause less fetal acid–base disturbance compared with ephedrine. Phenylephrine may be given as intermittent boluses or as an infusion; infusions may be associated with more cardiovascular stability but the doses given greatly exceed those when bolus injections are used.

Administration of the spinal anaesthetic

Full asepsis should be used, and an interspace below L3 should be chosen to ensure that the needle tip is well below the termination of the cord. A pencil-point or conical tip needle is standard practice in obstetrics nowadays. Once free-flowing CSF has been identified, the chosen dose of local anaesthetic should be administered over 10–20 seconds. 'Dry tap' or pain during insertion or injection should be a signal to withdraw the needle and try again.

Drugs

Hyperbaric bupivacaine 0.5% is the most commonly used local anaesthetic for spinal anaesthesia in the UK. A dose of 10–15 mg (2–3 ml) is typically used, although low-dose techniques (< 10 mg) have been used in an attempt to reduce hypotension and nausea/vomiting – though at the expense of less reliable anaesthesia. Fentanyl 15–20 μg, preservative-free morphine 75–100 μg, or morphine/diamorphine 0.3–0.4 mg is usually added for postoperative analgesia. However, caution must be observed when using intrathecal morphine as there have been case reports associated with delayed respiratory depression; this is thought to be less likely with intrathecal diamorphine and there have been no case reports to date of delayed respiratory depression in the obstetric population with diamorphine. The mother should be moved quickly but carefully into a left-wedged supine position, ensuring that there is no head-down tilt, and the blood pressure checked at 1–2 minute intervals. Some practitioners prefer to turn the mother into a full lateral posture, avoiding the wedged supine position until just before draping and incision.

Testing the block

To minimise the risk of pain, the block should extend up to T5 on both sides when testing to touch, and this is now considered the 'gold standard'. A block to light touch extending to T5 has been shown to be associated with a low incidence of intraoperative pain and a reduced need for intraoperative supplementation, compared with the same extent of block to pinprick or cold sensation. Although a complete block below the upper level is fairly certain when spinal anaesthesia is used, it is good practice to check that the sacral segments are covered and that the mother cannot straight leg raise against gravity. A recalcitrant block can be extended by using a variety of techniques such as turning from side to side, coughing, a Valsalva manoeuvre or judicious head-down tilt. The extent of the block and the modality used for testing must always be recorded.

During the operation

The patient should be watched for premonitory signs of hypotension, such as pallor, yawning or nausea. Bradycardia may indicate a high block affecting the sympathetic cardiac accelerator fibres, or be related to the use of phenylephrine. The mother may complain that her chest 'feels heavy'; this sensation is common when the intercostal muscles are affected, and reassurance should be offered. Complaints of discomfort or pain may be treated with inhaled nitrous oxide or intravenous boluses of fentanyl (12.5–25 μg) or alfentanil (125–250 μg) at first; intravenous ketamine (5–10 mg) has also been used. Pain is more likely during peritoneal traction, swabbing of the paracolic gutters or exteriorisation of the uterus. If the patient still complains of breakthrough pain, then a general anaesthetic must be offered.

After the operation

Positional changes may cause sudden cranial spread of the block even at this late stage. A fully-staffed recovery area is mandatory, and the sitting position may be carefully adopted if the blood pressure is stable. The mother should not be moved to the ward until cardiovascular stability is certain and the block is receding. Postoperative monitoring is discussed in Chapter 31, Caesarean section. Anaesthetic follow-up for symptoms of PDPH or persistent block should continue for 48 hours.

Key points

- Pencil-point or conical tip needles should be used to minimise the risk of postdural puncture headache.
- Hypotension is almost invariable unless actively prevented with vasopressors.
- The extent of the block must be tested and recorded, and the patient should be warned of the risk of pain.

Further reading

Arzola C, Wieczorek PM. Efficacy of low-dose bupivacaine in spinal anaesthesia for Caesarean delivery: systematic review and meta-analysis. *Br J Anaesth* 2011; **107**: 308–18.

Dahl V, Spreng UJ. Anaesthesia for urgent (grade 1) caesarean section. *Curr Opin Anesthesiol* 2009; **22**: 352–6.

Langesæter E, Dyer RA. Maternal haemodynamic changes during spinal anaesthesia for caesarean section. *Curr Opin Anesthesiol* 2011; **24**: 242–8.

Sia AT, Fun WL, Tan TU. The ongoing challenges of regional and general anaesthesia in obstetrics. *Best Pract Res Clin Obstet Gynaecol* 2010; **24**: 303–12.

Chapter

33 Epidural anaesthesia for caesarean section

Although no longer the technique of choice for elective caesarean section, the popularity of epidural analgesia for pain relief in labour means that many women presenting for emergency caesarean section have an epidural *in situ*. A greater understanding of methods to enhance the speed of onset and quality of epidural block has reduced the need for general anaesthesia in this group of mothers; extension of the block is the technique of choice, unless epidural analgesia during labour has been of poor quality or there is a very urgent indication for delivery within 5–10 minutes.

Problems/special considerations

- Poor block with breakthrough pain is more common with epidural anaesthesia than with spinal anaesthesia, and a careful assessment of block is therefore particularly important in this group. The block should be 'mapped out' to ensure that there are no missed segments or patchy areas and the extent of block carefully recorded. The mother must be warned of the risk of pain before starting the procedure, and the anaesthetist should be prepared to supplement the block with further top-ups, intravenous analgesia or even general anaesthesia. Pain during caesarean section is the commonest failure cited in negligence suits against obstetric anaesthetists in the UK.

- Hypotension is slower in onset and normally less severe than with spinal anaesthesia, but vasoconstrictors may still be required, and great care should be taken to avoid aortocaval compression.

- The possibility of migration of the epidural catheter, whether into the subdural, intrathecal or intravenous compartments, must be borne in mind, especially when large, concentrated doses of local anaesthetic are being used. Doses should be fractionated or given by slow injection and the level of block regularly checked. It is unacceptable to leave a mother for any reason once the process of establishing the block has started. (See also Chapter 23, Epidural test doses.)

Management options

Suitability of the technique

Extending a pre-existing epidural block for anaesthesia for caesarean section is not as fast as general anaesthesia. Thus, for very urgent caesarean sections, spinal or general anaesthesia remains the techniques of choice. However, with appropriate top-up solutions given over 2–3 minutes (see below), surgical anaesthesia may be produced within 5–10 minutes – though there is considerable variation in onset times between patients. Further, slow injection of a bolus conflicts with the precautions mentioned above about fractionating doses. The risks and benefits to the mother and fetus of epidural versus general anaesthesia in these circumstances must be carefully considered, and these can be among the most difficult clinical decisions taken by anaesthetists.

A 'fresh' spinal anaesthetic is preferable to attempting to top up a poorly functioning epidural catheter, since the chance of inadequate anaesthesia during surgery is greater if analgesia has been poor during labour. Also, if extension of the epidural proves to be inadequate and a spinal anaesthetic is then chosen, the spread of the spinal dose may be more unpredictable after large volumes of solution have already been injected epidurally.

Contraindications to epidural anaesthesia are discussed in Chapter 22, Epidural analgesia for labour.

Preoperative preparation

This is as discussed in Chapter 32, Spinal anaesthesia for caesarean section. It is particularly important in women having an epidural top-up to mention the risk of intraoperative pain and to have a plan to deal with this should it occur. The reported need for general anaesthesia after an epidural top-up is ~2–4%; therefore an intravenous H_2-antagonist should be given if the mother has not received it during the last 6–8 hours. Many anaesthetists do not routinely give the mother oral sodium citrate (though it should be immediately available) since it has an unpleasant taste, it only lasts ~30 minutes, and the likelihood of general anaesthesia is small. Prophylactic vasopressors are rarely needed, but should be available, and a large-bore intravenous cannula must be inserted to allow rapid fluid infusion. Before giving an epidural top-up, it is important to test the block that is already present; whilst the top-up required does not need modifying as a result in most cases, failure to do so will allow an unexpectedly extensive block, that might indicate subdural or subarachnoid migration of the catheter, to go undetected.

Choice of drugs

Bupivacaine 0.5% was the mainstay for many years for epidural caesarean section, but large doses (often in excess of the recommended upper limits) are frequently required, and resuscitation from systemic toxicity is less likely to succeed than with other local anaesthetics. Lidocaine 2% has a faster onset for elective cases, especially if pH-adjusted, but adrenaline must be added to minimise systemic absorption; this also enhances its efficacy. Slow bolus injection (including through the needle) has been shown to produce more rapid and reliable block (with lower final volumes) than boluses of 5 ml repeated every 5–10 minutes, but with attendant risks if the injection is misplaced.

For emergency caesarean section, the use of a bolus dose of 15–20 ml concentrated local anaesthetic solution (e.g. (levo)bupivacaine 0.5% or ropivacaine 0.75%), given over 2–3 minutes, can convert labour epidural analgesia to a block suitable for surgery within about 15–20 minutes in most cases. Lidocaine with adrenaline and bicarbonate (e.g. 20 ml lidocaine 2%, 0.1 ml 1:1000 adrenaline and 2 ml 8.4% bicarbonate) has been shown to produce surgical anaesthesia in approximately half this time, though approximately one minute may be 'lost' by mixing the drugs, and care must be taken to avoid drug errors (although lidocaine and bicarbonate are stable when mixed, the adrenaline degrades within a few hours of addition).

The use of 2-chloroprocaine 3% has been reported as having a very short onset time but reports of back pain and neurological damage, shortly after its introduction several decades ago, have led to a very restricted availability (e.g. the USA and a handful of countries in continental Europe), though the modern preparation is free of the preservatives that have since been implicated in causing these complications. Another potential problem with chloroprocaine is that its effects wear off rapidly and so supplementation with further epidural local anaesthetic is required to avoid intraoperative pain.

Opioids (e.g. fentanyl 50–100 μg, diamorphine 2–3 mg, morphine 3–4 mg) are commonly added, either during the initial topping up or towards the end of the case. The evidence that addition of fentanyl might speed the onset of block and/or improve analgesia is weak, especially if the mother has been receiving regular epidural fentanyl in labour and the epidural has been working well.

Administration of the epidural anaesthetic

If a catheter is being sited *de novo*, it is often best done on labour ward or in a suitable area outside the operating theatre, since the slower onset of epidural anaesthesia would otherwise mean that the mother would have to lie on the operating table for some time while waiting for the block to take effect. In most cases, the epidural catheter is already *in situ*; if this is the case, then it has been argued that the epidural may be topped up in the delivery room before transfer, thus saving what may be important time. This practice is controversial, however, since the delivery room is not an ideal place for dealing with extensive block, severe hypotension or local anaesthetic toxicity. The anaesthetist must, of course, remain with the mother from the point of topping up an epidural with concentrated solutions, wherever this is done, and ensure adequate monitoring. If he/she is 'trapped' in the delivery room then he/she is unable to check and prepare the required drugs and equipment in the operating theatre.

Testing the block

The principles should be as for spinal anaesthesia, though an epidural block is more likely to have missed segments or be unilateral than a spinal block, so the extent of sensory loss should be mapped with great care. The epidural catheter allows further doses to be given, and appropriate positioning of the patient, although not as effective as with spinal anaesthesia, may encourage spread into recalcitrant areas. In emergency cases when the epidural has been topped up, it may be more difficult to determine sensory block resulting from the top-up if the mother already has a sensory block from the labour epidural. In such circumstances, the development of a profound motor block in the legs is very reassuring that the top-up is becoming effective.

During the operation

Hypotension is less common than with spinal anaesthesia, but blood pressure should be carefully monitored and treated expeditiously. Inadequate block may become apparent during peritoneal incision, and exteriorisation of the uterus, a manoeuvre much favoured by certain obstetricians, may be poorly tolerated. A delicate surgeon can make all the difference if the block is borderline, and good communication between medical staff is rarely more important. Nausea and vomiting, if associated with vagal stimuli such as exteriorisation of the uterus or peritoneal manipulation, may be treated with glycopyrronium 200–600 μg.

After the operation

If opioids have not been given, an epidural dose of e.g. diamorphine may be given in combination with rectal non-steroidal analgesics, if not contraindicated, at the end of surgery. The same precautions regarding discharge from recovery and monitoring should be followed as for spinal anaesthesia. The epidural catheter lends itself to further low-dose local anaesthetic/opioid top-ups or infusion, but this can only be done if there are facilities and staff to care for the patient safely. Postoperative monitoring is discussed in Chapter 31, Caesarean section, and postoperative analgesia is discussed in Chapter 39.

Key points

- The full extent of the block must be tested before giving an epidural top-up for caesarean section.
- Pain during the operation is more common than with spinal anaesthesia, and the patient must be warned.
- Slow-bolus epidural injection may produce a faster block of good quality, but may be more hazardous than fractionated injection.

Further reading

Allam J, Malhotra S, Hemingway C, Yentis SM. Epidural lidocaine–bicarbonate–adrenaline vs. levobupivacaine for emergency Caesarean section: a randomised controlled trial. *Anaesthesia* 2008; **63**: 243–9.

Lam DT, Ngan Kee WD, Khaw KS. Extension of epidural blockade in labour for emergency Caesarean section using 2% lidocaine with epinephrine and fentanyl, with or without alkalinisation. *Anaesthesia* 2001; **56**: 790–4.

Lucas DN, Ciccone GK, Yentis SM. Extending low-dose epidural analgesia for emergency Caesarean section – a comparison of three solutions. *Anaesthesia* 1999; **54**: 1173–7.

Malhotra S, Yentis SM. Extending low-dose epidural analgesia in labour for emergency Caesarean section – a comparison of levobupivacaine with or without fentanyl. *Anaesthesia* 2007; **62**: 667–71.

Sanders SD, Mallory S, Lucas DN, *et al.* Extending low-dose epidural analgesia for emergency caesarean section using ropivacaine 0.75%. *Anaesthesia* 2004; **59**: 988–92.

Chapter

34 General anaesthesia for caesarean section

There has been a general trend away from general anaesthesia in many countries over the past few decades because of the associate potential morbidity and mortality, with about 80–90% of caesarean sections in the UK now performed under regional anaesthesia.

General anaesthesia is usually reserved for those women who adamantly refuse a regional technique, for those in whom such a technique is contraindicated e.g. by medical disease, or if there is lack of time.

Problems/special considerations

- *Airway difficulty* (see Chapter 36, Failed and difficult intubation): The incidence of failure to intubate the trachea is approximately 1 in 300–500 in the obstetric population, compared with a ten-fold lower incidence in the general surgical population. Reasons for this are not completely clear but are thought to include the following:
  - The pregnant woman has a tendency to fluid retention and generally increased vascularity. Attempts at laryngoscopy, tracheal intubation or passage of oro/nasogastric tubes are more likely to encounter swollen tissues and result in soft tissue trauma and bleeding.

- Full dentition is the norm; dental hazards may be increased by expensive restorative dentistry. Increased breast mass and the application of cricoid pressure may make insertion of the laryngoscope difficult. Positioning of the patient on the operating table to avoid aortocaval compression may increase the likelihood of incorrectly applied cricoid pressure.
- Psychological pressure on the anaesthetist, especially in the emergency situation, may increase the chances of failed intubation.
- Current anaesthetic teaching is that anaesthetists must declare failure early and wake the patient; thus cases in which intubation might be successful with the aid of other staff/equipment in non-obstetric settings are being counted as failed intubations in the delivery suite.

Pressure to achieve tracheal intubation may lead to prolonged attempts during which hypoxia occurs. Fatalities typically arise from failure of oxygenation rather than failure of tracheal intubation.

- *Pulmonary aspiration of gastric contents* (see Chapter 54, Aspiration of gastric contents; Chapter 14, Gastric function and feeding in labour).
- *Hypovolaemia* (see Chapter 72, Major obstetric haemorrhage): The extent of blood loss in fit young people is usually underestimated. Induction of general anaesthesia in an unresuscitated hypovolaemic mother may precipitate catastrophic cardiovascular collapse. Tachycardia should alert the anaesthetist to the possibility of hypovolaemia, although the significance of tachycardia may be difficult to assess in an extremely anxious mother.
- *Awareness:* The risks of awareness during general anaesthesia for caesarean section are thought to be minimal if modern techniques are used (see Chapter 55, Awareness). Suitable opioid analgesia should be administered to the mother after delivery of the baby. Meticulous anaesthetic record keeping is vital. Most cases of supposed intraoperative awareness are in fact episodes occurring during recovery from anaesthesia, but claims of intraoperative awareness are difficult to refute if the anaesthetic record is inadequate. Some authorities recommend that all mothers are warned preoperatively of an extremely small risk of intraoperative awareness, and that this warning is recorded in the preoperative assessment.
- *So-called 'minor' problems:* General anaesthesia is associated with a tendency towards longer immediate recovery, more pain (see Chapter 39, Postoperative analgesia), more postoperative nausea and vomiting, and more neonatal depression than regional anaesthesia. In addition, the parents do not experience the moment of birth as with spinal or epidural anaesthesia.

Management options

Preoperative assessment

The time available for preoperative anaesthetic assessment may be brief but vital aspects should not be omitted, especially any previous anaesthesia, drug allergy, recent oral intake, indication (and urgency) for caesarean section, and the mother's airway.

Therapy to raise intragastric pH and minimise intragastric volume is given. It is usual to administer ranitidine (or cimetidine) or omeprazole preoperatively, either orally or parenterally, depending on timing. Metoclopramide is also given in many units. Some obstetric units advocate the administration of antacid prophylaxis routinely to every woman in labour, but this is controversial. 0.3 M sodium citrate (30 ml) is administered immediately before preoxygenation and induction of anaesthesia to neutralise any gastric contents.

Induction of anaesthesia

- It is customary to induce anaesthesia for caesarean section in the operating theatre. The obstetric anaesthetist should check the anaesthetic machine in the obstetric theatre at least once a day. A suitably trained anaesthetic assistant must be present before induction of general anaesthesia. There should be an airway trolley equipped with a range of differently sized tracheal tubes, intubation aids, laryngoscopes and equipment for dealing with failed intubation. The uterus must be displaced off the aorta and vena cava either manually (uncommon in the UK), by a wedge placed under the woman's right hip, or by laterally tilting the operating table.
- A large-bore intravenous cannula (14 G or 16 G) that is connected to a freely running infusion must be in place before induction of anaesthesia.
- Adequate preoxygenation must always precede induction of anaesthesia, regardless of urgency for delivery. It is crucial to ensure a tight fit of the facepiece and if a circle system is being used, at least 12 l/min of oxygen. The standard recommendation is preoxygenation for 3 minutes or 4–5 vital capacity breaths, although a better guide is the difference between the inspired and expired oxygen content, indicated on the gas monitor (in ideal conditions with no leak, both should exceed 90% when de-nitrogenation is complete).
- Monitoring of the mother should include blood pressure, capnography, electrocardiography, pulse oximetry and end-tidal volatile concentration.
- Rapid sequence induction of anaesthesia with an intravenous induction agent and suxamethonium 1–1.5 mg/kg is standard practice in the UK. Although use of all induction agents has been described in the literature, most UK obstetric anaesthetists still prefer thiopental, which should be given in an adequate dose (350–500 mg unless there is hypovolaemia or a fixed cardiac output). Propofol has been associated with a less favourable neonatal acid–base profile, though the clinical significance of this is disputed; in addition, it has been claimed that propofol's short duration of action might increase the risk of awareness before adequate brain levels of volatile agent are reached, especially if intubation is difficult. The induction agent may be supplemented with hypotensive agents and/or opioid analgesics in mothers with pre-eclampsia or cardiac disease. Cricoid pressure is applied before consciousness is lost and maintained until the airway is secured and tracheal intubation confirmed (see Chapter 35, Cricoid pressure).
- Use of non-depolarising neuromuscular blocking drugs, e.g. rocuronium, has been advocated instead of suxamethonium on the basis that intubation conditions will be maintained for long enough to achieve intubation if the latter is unsuccessful on the first attempt. The traditional counter-argument has always been that the intubation conditions suxamethonium produces are the best, within the shortest time, and if intubation fails, the return of muscle power favours earlier self-ventilation. However, with the introduction of sugammadex, rocuronium may become the drug of choice,

since sugammadex has been shown to reverse the effects of rocuronium within 2–3 minutes (compared with the offset of suxamethonium of up to 10 minutes). As sugammadex is still a relatively new drug, familiarity with its use is still limited, especially in obstetrics; furthermore its cost is high and the incidence of anaphylaxis associated with its use is still not known.

- Every obstetric anaesthetist should be familiar with both failed intubation and failed ventilation drills and should mentally rehearse these before every induction of general anaesthesia in the obstetric patient. Every obstetric theatre should have monitoring equipment that includes measurement of end-tidal carbon dioxide, and there should be access to specialised airway equipment, e.g. cricothyroid cannulae and a fibreoptic endoscope.

Perioperative and postoperative management

- Common practice is to use 50% nitrous oxide in oxygen plus a volatile anaesthetic agent (e.g. isoflurane) to ventilate the lungs, reverting to conventional mixtures of 70% nitrous oxide in 30% oxygen after delivery of the baby. The volatile agent should be continued throughout anaesthesia. In severe fetal compromise, 100% oxygen with a corresponding increase in the inspired concentration of volatile agent may be chosen.

- A short-acting non-depolarising neuromuscular blocking drug should be used when the suxamethonium has worn off, and if the surgeon is fast it may not be necessary to use further neuromuscular blockers after the initial dose of suxamethonium. Deaths have occurred from inadequate reversal of neuromuscular blockade following the use of long-acting drugs.

- Oxytocin (Syntocinon) is usually given as a slow intravenous bolus of 5 U at delivery of the baby, often followed by an intravenous infusion of 40 U in 500 ml saline at ~125 ml/h.

- Adequate analgesia should be given following delivery of the baby; the combination of a long-acting opioid such as morphine and a non-steroidal anti-inflammatory drug (NSAID) such as diclofenac is used in many units. It is important to obtain pre-operative consent to rectal administration of drugs. Intravenous paracetamol is now widely available in the UK and may also be given intraoperatively.

- At the end of surgery, residual neuromuscular blockade is reversed and the mother is turned into the left lateral position before the trachea is extubated. It is important to remember that the risk of aspiration is present at extubation and possibly during the initial phase of recovery from anaesthesia, as well as during induction of anaesthesia. Extubation of the trachea should not be performed until there is evidence of return of protective reflexes.

- The mother must be nursed in a properly equipped recovery room by trained staff before returning to the postnatal wards. Deaths have occurred due to inadequately staffed and equipped recovery facilities.

- Postoperative analgesia must be provided; patient-controlled opioids are popular, and NSAIDs appear to be particularly effective in combating 'afterpains' of uterine involution. NSAIDs should not be used in severe pre-eclamptics and severe asthmatics. Bilateral ilio-inguinal block has been suggested as a simple, safe and effective way to provide postoperative analgesia. More recently, transversus abdominis plane blocks have been used to provide postoperative pain relief. Further aspects are discussed in Chapter 39, Postoperative analgesia.

- Heparin should be given preoperatively if it is known that general anaesthesia will be given, as for any operation; if general anaesthesia is unexpected the first dose may be given during surgery or shortly afterwards.

Key points
- All obstetric patients requiring general anaesthesia should be considered high-risk.
- Emergency general anaesthesia is associated with increased morbidity and mortality.
- Failure to intubate the trachea is ten times more common in the obstetric population than in the general surgical population.

Further reading

Dahl V, Spreng UJ. Anaesthesia for urgent (grade 1) caesarean section. *Curr Opin Anesthesiol* 2009; **22**: 352–6.

Sia AT, Fun WL, Tan TU. The ongoing challenges of regional and general anaesthesia in obstetrics. *Best Pract Res Clin Obstet Gynaecol* 2010; **24**: 303–12.

Chapter

35 Cricoid pressure

The cricoid cartilage is the only cartilaginous part of the upper airway to be a complete ring, and so pressure on its anterior aspect results in compression of the upper oesophagus/ hypopharynx against the vertebral body of C6 posteriorly. First described by Sellick in 1961 (hence 'Sellick's manoeuvre'), cricoid pressure is widely used as a means of preventing passive regurgitation (and thus aspiration) of gastric contents during induction of general anaesthesia in at-risk patients. It is thus a standard technique in obstetric anaesthesia, although precisely when the period of risk begins and ends is controversial. In addition, whether cricoid pressure is actually necessary has also been questioned, since it is not routinely practised in many continental European countries without apparent increases in morbidity and mortality, and there is some evidence that it does not completely occlude the oesophagus when applied.

Method

As originally described by Sellick, the assistant's forefinger is placed over the cricoid cartilage and firm pressure exerted posteriorly, with the thumb and middle finger supporting on either side. In the two-handed technique, the assistant's second hand is placed behind the patient's neck, resisting any flexion of the cervical spine as cricoid pressure is applied. However, it is unclear whether the two-handed technique has any consistent advantage and it does mean that the assistant has both of his/her hands occupied should the anaesthetist need any more equipment.

The optimal time to start exerting pressure is somewhat controversial since cricoid pressure is uncomfortable when the patient is awake, whereas regurgitation may occur if it is applied too late. As a compromise, many advocate gentle pressure until consciousness is lost, with firmer pressure thereafter (as Sellick originally described), although there is evidence that gentle pressure itself may cause relaxation of the lower oesophageal sphincter. Estimates of the force required to prevent regurgitation range from 10 N to over 40 N.

Although the use of cricoid pressure is standard practice, it may hinder tracheal intubation, first because the assistant's hand may obstruct insertion of the laryngoscope blade into the mouth and second because if incorrectly applied (it has been suggested that this is more likely in obstetrics because of lateral tilt) it may distort the laryngeal anatomy. If pressure is excessive, it may also flex the neck (or hyperextend it if two-handed cricoid pressure is used). It is therefore important that anaesthetic assistants are properly trained in its application; studies have demonstrated considerable variation in assistants' ability but also considerable improvement following training.

In cases of failed intubation, release of cricoid pressure should be considered, especially if mask ventilation or placement of a laryngeal mask airway is considered, as these may be hindered by cricoid pressure. Release is also advocated if there is active vomiting since oesophageal rupture has been reported; however, cricoid pressure should only be released on the anaesthetist's instruction.

Key points

- Cricoid pressure should be applied as consciousness is lost.
- A force of 10–40 N is required.
- Incorrect application may impede intubation.
- Assistants should be properly trained in its application.

Further reading

El-Obarney M, Connolly L. Rapid sequence induction and intubation: current controversy. *Anesth Analg* 2010; **110**: 1318–25.

Benhamou D, Vanner R. Controversies in obstetric anaesthesia: cricoid pressure is unnecessary in obstetric general anaesthesia. *Int J Obstet Anesth* 1995; **4**: 30–3.

Brimacombe JR, Berry AM. Cricoid pressure. *Can J Anaesth* 1997; **44**: 414–25.

Lerman J. On cricoid pressure: 'may the force be with you'. *Anesth Analg* 2009; **109**: 1363–6.

Chapter 36

Failed and difficult intubation

Over the last 30 years the number of deaths associated with failed intubation has declined, though more recently there has been concern that the incidence of failed intubation may be increasing. It is important to remember that patients do not die from failed intubation; they die from hypoxia or acid aspiration if the failed intubation is unrecognised or the corrective measures are inadequate.

Problems/special considerations

Tracheal intubation is more difficult in obstetric anaesthesia and the incidence of failed or difficult intubation is usually quoted as between 1 in 250 and 1 in 500 obstetric general anaesthetics, compared with 1 in 2000 to 1 in 3000 for non-obstetric general anaesthetics. There are many reasons for difficulties with intubation and the increased risk of developing hypoxia (Table 36.1). Laryngoscopy and placement of a tracheal tube may thus be more difficult whilst hypoxaemia develops more rapidly than in general surgical patients. This is compounded by the anaesthetist's being under considerable stress during induction of anaesthesia.

The consequences of failed intubation in obstetrics are serious for both maternal and fetal health. Obstetric anaesthetists have been encouraging regional anaesthesia to reduce the numbers of general anaesthetics administered. There is a decreased percentage of general anaesthetics administered although the absolute numbers of general anaesthetics may not have fallen dramatically. However, there are now many obstetric units where very few general anaesthetics are given and this, although a commendable trend, has led to a reduction in training opportunities, not only for trainees but also for trainers. It has been suggested that simulation courses may help address the issue of reduced training in general anaesthesia for obstetrics, but although simulation has been shown to improve practical skills, it is yet to be validated as a training tool.

Management options

If general anaesthesia is to be administered then it is important to do the following:
- Attempt to predict difficult intubation
- Use an anaesthetic technique that will minimise the risk of failing
- Have a failed intubation drill.

Table 36.1 Causes of increased incidence of problems relating to tracheal intubation in obstetric anaesthesia

Anatomical	Difficulty inserting laryngoscope	Large breasts Weight gain/increased fatty tissue Oedema (especially pre-eclampsia) Complete dentition Cricoid pressure
	Poor laryngoscopic view	Weight gain/increased fatty tissue Laryngeal oedema Cricoid pressure causing distortion Swollen mucosa
Physiological	Increased risk of aspiration Increased oxygen demand Reduced lung capacity	
Iatrogenic	Incorrectly applied cricoid pressure Urgency leading to haste Inexperience of staff	

Prediction of difficult intubation

Prediction of difficult intubation is attempted using the same clinical examination as in the non-pregnant patient:

- Mallampati score
- Co-existing neck pathology
- State of dentition
- Mouth opening
- Thyromental distance.

Unfortunately, even in combination these tests have low predictive value (i.e. relatively few of the cases predicted as being difficult will actually be difficult), partly because of the poor function of the tests and partly because difficult intubation is uncommon, even in obstetric cases. Mallampati scores have been shown to change during pregnancy and even during labour.

Anaesthetic technique

The delivery suite theatre should be well equipped for a difficult intubation, and the equipment should include a variety of aids to intubation as well as equipment to aid oxygenation if a problem arises. Skilled assistance for the anaesthetist is essential.

The anaesthetist should ensure that the patient is well positioned and that adequate doses of induction agent and neuromuscular blocking drug are given after a full 3 minutes' preoxygenation or 3–5 vital capacity breaths. Proper fitting of the facemask is important to ensure efficient preoxygenation. The correct application of cricoid pressure by a trained assistant is important, since badly applied cricoid pressure can make laryngoscopy difficult.

Although suxamethonium is still the standard neuromuscular blocking drug used, there is a suggestion that with the introduction of sugammadex, rocuronium may be more

- A retained placenta prevents the uterus from contracting effectively so there may be excessive bleeding from any areas of separation. Occasionally, retained placenta is complicated by uterine inversion (either partial or complete). Unless the uterus is rapidly replaced manually the mother will become severely hypotensive and may become bradycardic. A similar clinical picture may be seen with so-called 'cervical shock' in which there is increased vagal tone caused by trapping of the placenta in the cervix.
- Severe perineal tears may require lengthy repair and can be associated with significant blood loss that may go relatively unrecognised.

Management options

For retained placenta, early conservative management is appropriate if bleeding is not excessive and vital signs are stable. An intravenous infusion of oxytocics may be started, and putting the baby to the breast for suckling sometimes stimulates delivery of the placenta. Turning the woman into the left lateral position is anecdotally reported to assist spontaneous placental delivery, and emptying the bladder may also be helpful. If the uterus is very bulky, there is still a risk of aortocaval compression in the supine position.

Choice of anaesthetic technique in both situations should be based on assessment of the relative risks of general and regional anaesthesia. Intravenous access via a large cannula (at least 16 G) with a freely flowing infusion is mandatory before starting any anaesthetic technique. If epidural analgesia has been used for labour it is usually possible to extend this for surgery. There is usually no reason to separate mother and baby if regional anaesthesia is used, and there should be no delay in initiating breastfeeding. Adequate fluid replacement is essential, particularly as the sympathetically induced vasodilatation accompanying regional blockade will aggravate any existing hypovolaemia. Suitable solutions for topping up the epidural catheter are similar to those used for instrumental delivery. An upper extent of block to T8 is required for retained placenta since uterine manipulation may be considerable; lower blocks may be suitable for perineal repair.

In the absence of epidural analgesia, spinal anaesthesia should be instituted, unless the mother is significantly hypovolaemic (see below). It is often more comfortable for the mother to have spinal anaesthesia induced in the lateral rather than sitting position. A dose of 1.5–2 ml 0.5% heavy bupivacaine with 15–20 µg fentanyl is usually adequate.

If there is evidence of hypovolaemia and continuing bleeding despite adequate resuscitation, general anaesthesia should be used. The mother is assumed to have a full stomach and the same technique as for caesarean section should be used, including antacid prophylaxis and rapid-sequence induction of anaesthesia. Blood should be cross-matched and preferably two large (14 G) intravenous cannulae inserted, and the case managed as for any obstetric haemorrhage. If there is uterine inversion, general anaesthesia may be required to aid replacement of the uterus, unless the mother is stable and regional analgesia is already present.

Postoperative analgesia should be considered, especially for women with extensive perineal repairs. Intrathecal or epidural opioids, together with regular paracetamol and non-steroidal anti-inflammatory drugs, may be required.

Key points

- There is a risk of massive bleeding from retained placenta. Repair of perineal tears may be lengthy and associated with significant blood loss.
- Resuscitation should take place before induction of anaesthesia.
- Spinal or epidural anaesthesia is appropriate in haemodynamically stable patients.
- General anaesthesia (with cricoid pressure and tracheal intubation) is indicated in hypovolaemic patients.

Further reading

Royal College of Obstetricians and Gynaecologists. The management of third- and fourth-degree perineal tears. *Green-top 29*. London: RCOG 2007, http://www.rcog.org.uk/womens-health/clinical-guidance/management-third-and-fourth-degree-perineal-tears-green-top-29.

Chapter

39 Postoperative analgesia

Adequate pain relief following caesarean section is particularly important because the mother needs to be sufficiently comfortable to care for her baby; she is also at increased risk of thromboembolism, and effective analgesia facilitates early mobilisation.

It is also important to remember that women having other procedures (e.g. repair of perineal tears) may be in considerable discomfort or pain afterwards.

Problems/special considerations

- Psychological considerations are important. The mother who has been delivered by elective caesarean section under regional anaesthesia, with preoperative preparation and discussion about postoperative analgesia, cannot be directly compared with the mother who has been delivered by emergency caesarean section under general anaesthesia after many hours of labour and a failed trial of forceps delivery. (In the worst scenario she may also have received an episiotomy.)
- Most published studies of post-caesarean section analgesia are, for logistical reasons, performed in women having elective section, and the results should therefore be interpreted cautiously.
- The ideal analgesic should of course be extremely effective, universally applicable, cheap to use and free from unwanted side effects. The ideal analgesic does not exist, and the demand for freedom from unwanted effects is particularly important in obstetric patients.

It is important to remember that unwanted effects include the need for intravenous cannulae and infusions, urinary catheters and additional monitoring equipment. Safety is vital in a patient population that is young and fit with newly born dependants. Other side effects that may be acceptable to an elderly general surgical population (e.g. pruritus, nausea and sedation), are unacceptable to women wishing to care for babies.

The use of various opioids by the subarachnoid or epidural routes has become routine, but the level of nursing care required by women who have received this method of analgesia remains controversial. The relative risk and timing of respiratory depression associated with different opioids varies, but none can be considered completely safe in this respect. Equally, all centrally administered opioids cause nausea, vomiting and pruritus, although to differing degrees. Although there can be no doubt that high-dependency care, either in a high-dependency unit, or given in a normal postnatal ward by one-to-one or one-to-two patient supervision, is ideal, many obstetric units are unable to provide this. Protagonists of spinal opioids point out that all opioids, given by any route, have the capacity to cause respiratory depression, and that no special precautions are taken after the administration of intramuscular opioids. Various compromises are made at a local level.

Women undergoing non-caesarean procedures can experience considerable postoperative pain (e.g. perineal) but may find that this is not always appreciated by the medical and midwifery staff, who may focus on mothers who had caesarean section.

Management options

A combination of paracetamol, opioids and non-steroidal anti-inflammatory drugs (NSAIDs) is used in the majority of women to provide analgesia following caesarean section. Analgesics prescribed regularly are more likely to be given than those prescribed 'as required', but midwives should be educated about assessment and management of postoperative pain and encouraged to give analgesics as prescribed. Published research has failed to demonstrate clearly the superiority of any one route or of any one drug or drug combination.

Caesarean section under general anaesthesia

The most commonly used drugs in this situation are intraoperative intravenous opioids (e.g. morphine 10–20 mg or diamorphine 5–10 mg), an NSAID (e.g. diclofenac 100 mg given rectally at the end of surgery) and either intramuscular or patient-controlled intravenous opioids postoperatively. Regular paracetamol and NSAIDs act synergistically with both strong and weak opioids.

NSAIDs are contraindicated in women with severe pre-eclampsia because of their effect on platelet function and should also be used with caution in asthmatics. The potentially adverse effect of NSAIDs on renal function should be considered in women who are hypovolaemic and in those who have compromised renal function.

Bilateral ilioinguinal blocks have been shown to improve postoperative pain control, and should be considered for all cases under general anaesthesia. Rectus sheath blocks may also be used although they are more difficult immediately after caesarean section than in elective gynaecological surgery. Increasingly popular are transversus abdominis plane (TAP) blocks, which may be performed under ultrasounded guidance at the end of the surgery. Although TAP blocks have been described as easy to perform, the efficacy of the block is variable and very operator-dependent, and there have been case reports of bowel injury, and intraperitoneal and intravascular injection of local anaesthetic.

In the emergency situation there may be an epidural catheter in place but insufficient time to extend a block for anaesthesia, but this does not preclude use of the catheter for postoperative analgesia using epidural opioids.

Caesarean section under regional analgesia

It is common anecdotal evidence that women experience less pain following caesarean section under regional anaesthesia than under general anaesthesia, although this is difficult to substantiate. The pre-emptive action of epidural or spinal anaesthesia remains unproven. Subarachnoid fentanyl (10–20 µg) is used to improve the quality of intra-operative anaesthesia, but its action does not extend significantly into the postoperative period. This had led to many North American anaesthetists using a combination of subarachnoid fentanyl and morphine (0.1–0.2 mg), which provides very effective analgesia for up to 24 hours, but is considered by some anaesthetists to be associated with the highest risks of nausea, vomiting, pruritus and respiratory depression. In the UK, subarachnoid diamorphine (200–400 µg) is commonly used, providing analgesia both during surgery and extending 6–8 hours postoperatively.

Epidural or combined spinal–epidural anaesthesia allows greater flexibility for post-operative analgesia. Epidural local anaesthetic alone is unsuitable since women are unable to mobilise and dislike the sensation of being numb. Fentanyl (e.g. 50–100 µg) is relatively short acting (3–4 hours) but is reported to have the lowest incidence of side effects; morphine (e.g. 2–4 mg) has delayed onset of action but long duration (18–24 hours) and a higher incidence of side effects, including delayed respiratory depression. Diamorphine (e.g. 2–3 mg) is available in the UK although in few other countries in the world and has an intermediate duration of action and incidence of side effects. Sufentanil is widely used in North America and Europe but is not available in the UK.

Patient-controlled administration of epidural opioids (e.g. fentanyl or pethidine) has been described but this is uncommon in the UK.

Regardless of choice of opioid, analgesia is improved by the addition of an NSAID (subject to the same precautions outlined above) and by the regular administration of simple analgesics such as paracetamol.

Other procedures

Women having perineal repairs and other procedures should be told that adequate analgesia will be made available should they need it, and the staff looking after them encouraged to take their pain seriously. Neuraxial opioids and regular analgesics may be required, and it may be easiest and kindest to prescribe the same postoperative analgesics as for caesarean section.

Key points

- The mother needs to be alert and comfortable in order to feed, care for and bond with her baby.
- Paracetamol, opioids and non-steroidal anti-inflammatory drugs are the mainstay of postoperative analgesia.

- Opioids are associated with respiratory depression, nausea and vomiting with all routes of administration.
- The epidural and subarachnoid routes are also associated with pruritus and possible delayed respiratory depression.

Further reading

Gadsden J, Hart S, Santos AC. Post-Cesarean delivery analgesia. *Anesth Analg* 2005; **101**: S62–9.

Lavand'homme P. Postcaesarean analgesia: effective strategies and association with chronic pain. *Curr Opin Anesthesiol* 2006; **19**: 244–8.

McDonnell NJ, Keating ML, Muchatuta NA, Pavy TJ, Paech MJ. Analgesia after caesarean delivery. *Anaesth Intensive Care* 2009; **37**: 539–51.

Petersen PL, Mathiesen O, Torup H, Dahl JB. The transversus abdominis plane block: a valuable option for postoperative analgesia? A topical review. *Acta Anaesthesiol Scand* 2010; **54**: 529–35.

Chapter 40

Bloody tap

Cannulation of an epidural vessel may occur with either the needle or the catheter during siting of an epidural. Its incidence is uncertain since widely varying figures have been quoted (e.g. 5–45%), possibly related to different methods of locating the epidural space, different needles or different definitions. It is thought to be less likely when the paramedian approach is used, when 5–10 ml fluid is injected before threading the catheter and when smaller needles are used.

Bloody tap is important because if unrecognised, injection of local anaesthetic solution intravenously instead of epidurally may result in systemic toxicity (depending on the drug and dose) as well as not producing a block; and continued bleeding from a punctured vessel (e.g. after the epidural has been re-sited) may theoretically lead to an epidural haematoma if coagulation is impaired.

Problems/special considerations

Diagnosis is not usually a problem, especially if the needle has punctured a vessel. Puncture of a vessel by the catheter may be marked by discomfort as the vessel wall is pierced. Blood may then be aspirated from the catheter – although this is not always the case, hence the use of a test dose. Similarly, the absence of a bloody tap does not guarantee correct placement of the catheter. Therefore, it is important to aspirate all epidural catheters before administering any top-up solution.

Management options

If blood flows from the needle there is no option other than to remove the needle and re-insert it at a different interspace. If blood is obtained again, it may represent a new vascular puncture or blood from the original puncture. If blood is aspirated from the catheter, withdrawing the catheter in 0.5 cm increments, and flushing it with saline after each increment until aspiration is no longer possible, may remove the catheter from the vessel whilst still leaving enough length in the epidural space for effective anaesthesia. If this is not possible, then it should be re-sited in another interspace.

Key points

- In cases of bloody tap, flushing and incremental withdrawal of the catheter may avoid having to re-site the epidural.
- Bloody tap may not always be present when the catheter is placed intravascularly.

Dural puncture

Dural puncture usually refers to puncture of the dura and the underlying arachnoid mater. It may be deliberate during subarachnoid anaesthesia or accidental during epidural analgesia. The incidence in the latter case is traditionally said to be around 1% in teaching centres but many authorities consider this to be unacceptably high, with an incidence of 0.5–1% being more realistic and < 0.5% attainable in experienced hands. Most would routinely include dural puncture in their discussion with patients of the risks associated with regional analgesia.

Most accidental dural punctures are caused by the epidural needle, although it is possible for an epidural catheter to migrate through the dura. In vitro studies suggest that this can only occur if there has been prior (unrecognised) dural puncture or partial tear of the dura by the needle. Rotating the Tuohy needle once its tip is within the epidural space has been implicated in this and is now generally considered undesirable. Reduced incidence of accidental dural puncture has been associated with use of saline rather than air for loss-of-resistance (LOR), and possibly use of the paramedian rather than midline approach.

Problems/special considerations

Dural puncture poses three main problems if it occurs:

- *Diagnosis:* Dural puncture is usually heralded by a 'give' as the needle passes through the dura, and passage of cerebrospinal fluid (CSF) through the needle. For subarachnoid block, these two signs may be influenced by the design of the needle. In a combined spinal–epidural technique, it is usually easier to identify the dura by feel, especially in less experienced hands, since the starting position of the spinal needle in relation to the dura is more precisely known.

  When a 16–18 G Tuohy needle is accidentally passed into the subarachnoid space, there is usually free flow of CSF, which poses no diagnostic difficulty. However, studies during deliberate dural puncture when placing lumbar drains before neurosurgery have revealed that occasionally, free flow is not obtained. Thus, the appearance of slowly dripping clear fluid at the hub of the needle may represent CSF from a dural puncture or backflow of saline injected into the epidural space during an LOR technique and may cause confusion, especially during a difficult procedure. In this situation, testing for temperature, glucose and protein content and pH (the last three by using urinary testing strips) will reliably distinguish CSF from saline (even saline that has been injected into the epidural space).

  Occasionally, typical postdural puncture headache (PDPH) may be the first evidence that dural puncture has occurred, although this more often reflects either inexperience on the part of the operator in not recognising accidental dural puncture or the operator not wishing to 'own up' in the hope that PDPH will not occur.

- *Management:* The aims of management of accidental dural puncture during establishment of epidural analgesia should include provision of adequate analgesia, safety of the patient and, if possible, reduction of risk from the adverse consequences of the dural puncture, as discussed below.
- *Adverse consequences:* Adverse consequences of dural puncture are PDPH (which occurs in 60–90% of cases of accidental dural puncture in parturients) and its sequelae such as cranial nerve palsies, convulsions and subdural or intracranial haemorrhage.

Management options

Traditional management of accidental dural puncture comprises removing the needle and placing an epidural catheter at the adjacent (cranial) interspace. Most units advocate that all subsequent top-ups during labour should be administered by an anaesthetist. The woman, her partner and the attending midwives/obstetricians should be informed that accidental dural puncture has occurred.

Other management options include converting the initial block to subarachnoid ± inserting the catheter into the subarachnoid space for a continuous subarachnoid block, e.g. by using 1–2 ml of standard low-dose epidural solution as top-ups or 1–2 ml/h by infusion. Some observational studies suggest that inserting the catheter has been associated with a reduced incidence of PDPH, and it has been suggested that a possible mechanism is via initiating an inflammatory reaction around the catheter. However, other studies have not found this to be the case. If the catheter is placed intrathecally, it must be clearly labelled and the whole team informed since there is a risk that it might be mistaken for an epidural catheter.

Traditionally, women who have had an accidental dural puncture have been advised to accept instrumental delivery to avoid pushing, but this is now generally considered unnecessary.

Prophylactic epidural blood patch (via the catheter after delivery) is not thought to be useful, and problems include the difficulty it might cause with analgesia (e.g. postoperatively), the fact that some women will receive an intervention they may not need, the possible risk of infection if the catheter is left in place throughout a prolonged labour, and the reduced efficacy of prophylactic, compared with therapeutic, blood patch. Epidural infusion of crystalloid after delivery (e.g. a litre of saline over 24 hours) has also been advocated, though this is rarely done nowadays.

The use of epidural or spinal opioids has also been claimed to reduce the incidence of PDPH, although most of the evidence for this is weak apart from one randomised control study that has shown a reduction in the incidence of PDPH with epidural morphine. A recent randomised controlled trial has suggested that intravenous administration of cosyntropin, an ACTH analogue, after delivery may be useful in reducing the incidence of PDPH.

After delivery, there is no benefit in restricting the mother to bed since this does not prevent PDPH. Similarly, although dehydration can exacerbate PDPH there is no evidence that overhydration has any beneficial effect. The mother should be visited regularly and given full support, and if PDPH occurs she should be offered the various management options available. She should also be informed about the possible serious sequelae of dural puncture, but reassured that they are rare. It is equally important that the anaesthetist is honest with his/her colleagues, since attempting to conceal accidental dural puncture may only serve to delay appropriate management. Each unit should have a clear protocol for managing accidental dural puncture, and there should be a system in place for recording and monitoring such cases, usually involving a senior anaesthetist. Postpartum follow-up at 6–10 weeks is recommended in order to check that symptoms have resolved and to advise about future pregnancies.

Key points
- Incidence of accidental dural puncture should be less than 1%.
- Immediate management includes re-siting the epidural or inserting the catheter into the subarachnoid space.
- All top-ups should be administered by an anaesthetist.
- The mother should be allowed to mobilise freely and advised to avoid dehydration.
- Mothers should be followed up regularly and any headache managed promptly.

Further reading

Apfel CC, Saxena A, Cakmakkaya OS, *et al.* Prevention of postdural puncture headache after accidental dural puncture: a quantitative systematic review. *Br J Anaesth* 2010; **105**: 255–63.

Hakim S. Cosyntropin for prophylaxis against postdural puncture headache after accidental dural puncture. *Anesthesiology* 2010; **113**: 413–20.

Sprigge JS, Harper SJ. Accidental dural puncture and post dural puncture headache in obstetric anaesthesia: presentation and management: a 23-year survey in a district general hospital. *Anaesthesia* 2008; **63**: 36–43.

Van de Velde M, Schepers R, Berends N, Vandermeersch E, De Buck F. Ten years of experience with accidental dural puncture and post-dural puncture headache in a tertiary obstetric anaesthesia department. *Int J Obstet Anesth* 2008; **17**: 329–35.

Chapter

42

Postdural puncture headache

Postdural puncture headache (PDPH) is typified by severe headache, usually frontal and bilateral, which is worsened by standing and relieved by lying. There may be associated neck stiffness, nausea, tinnitus, visual disturbances and photophobia. It is thought to arise from intracranial hypotension resulting from leakage of cerebrospinal fluid (CSF) through the dural hole, with stretching of the cranial nerve roots and meninges in the upright position. Thus, the incidence and severity of PDPH are greatest following dural puncture with large cutting needles that leave large holes in the dura (60–90% in parturients after accidental

Table 42.1 Causes of postpartum headache

Tension, stress, fatigue, depression
Intracranial hypotension, e.g. postdural puncture headache
Intracranial hypertension, e.g. tumour, haematoma, cortical vein thrombosis, benign intracranial hypertension
Migraine
Infection, e.g. meningitis, sinusitis, encephalitis
Pre-eclampsia (including posterior reversible encephalopathy syndrome)
Electrolyte imbalance, hypoglycaemia
Drugs, e.g. ondansetron

dural puncture with a 16 G Tuohy needle), whereas small non-cutting needles are associated with a low incidence (under 1% with 25–27 G pencil-point needles). Parturients are more susceptible to PDPH than any other patient group.

There may be associated cerebral vasodilatation, leading to similarities being made between PDPH and migraine.

Symptoms usually begin within 1–2 days of dural puncture and last less than 1–2 weeks, although PDPH may occasionally persist for many months or even years.

Problems/special considerations

- Symptoms may be severe enough to prevent the mother mobilising and caring for her baby; this is particularly unwelcome in the early postpartum period. Discharge from hospital may be delayed, increasing costs and the risks of hospital-acquired infection and thromboembolism.
- Rarely, more sinister sequelae may occur. These include cranial nerve palsies, convulsions and subdural or intracranial haemorrhage.

Management options

It is important that a full history is taken and neurological examination performed, since there are many causes of postpartum headache (Table 42.1). Neurological referral may be wise in difficult cases. PDPH is suggested by a history of dural puncture and typical symptoms, especially the postural element. However, it may follow apparently unremarkable epidural analgesia; the incidence is unknown, although it may involve a number of factors including: lack of recognition at the time of dural puncture; lack of reporting dural puncture for fear of retribution; a possible tear of the dura but not arachnoid at the time of epidural insertion, with rupture of the arachnoid subsequently; and migration of the epidural catheter intrathecally during labour. It has been suggested that an otherwise typical PDPH that only becomes severe hours after getting up is caused by a very small dural hole with slow leak of CSF, e.g. after spinal anaesthesia with a very fine needle. A useful confirmatory sign is the lessening of headache produced by gradually compressing the upright patient's upper abdomen. This is thought to displace spinal CSF into the cranium by causing venous engorgement in the extradural space. Magnetic resonance imaging and computerised tomography scanning have been used to diagnose intracranial hypotension and to demonstrate cerebrospinal fluid leaks (in the latter case involving further diagnostic dural puncture), but are not widely used.

Initial management includes simple analgesics such as paracetamol and non-steroidal anti-inflammatory drugs. Although dehydration can exacerbate the headache, there is no evidence that overhydration has a beneficial effect. Other medical management includes oral caffeine 150–300 mg 6–8 hourly, which has been shown to improve the symptoms. Caffeine may cause nausea and vomiting in overdosage and has been implicated in convulsions occurring after dural puncture. Use of sumatriptan and ACTH analogue has been described, but the evidence supporting their use is weak.

Invasive procedures involve infusion or injection of various substances into the extra-dural space, firstly to shift CSF from the spine into the skull and secondly to tamponade leakage of CSF through the dural hole and even to seal the hole. Saline infusions have been used both diagnostically and therapeutically, and dextran has been used in an attempt to provide longer-lasting relief. However, epidural blood patch (EBP) is now generally accepted as the definitive treatment in persistent PDPH, with an initial reported success rate of 70–100%, although the headache may recur. Many anaesthetists would now proceed to EBP early (e.g. within 24–48 hours of symptoms) if there is a good history rather than delay for several days as was common previously.

Full discussion with, and support of, the patient is of prime importance, since she may be more distressed by apparent indifference to the severity of her symptoms than by the complication itself. She should be regularly visited and the various options discussed, preferably by a senior anaesthetist. If she decides against an EBP, she should be reassured that she may come back at any time should her symptoms persist. She should also be told about the rare possibility of serious sequelae. It is not known whether EBP prevents these, although this is generally assumed if symptoms resolve. Postpartum follow-up at 6–10 weeks is recommended in order to check that symptoms have resolved and to advise about future pregnancies.

Key points

- Postdural puncture headache occurs in 60–90% of parturients after accidental dural tap with a 16 G Tuohy needle.
- The postural element is the most important confirmatory feature.
- Initial management includes paracetamol, non-steroidal anti-inflammatory drugs, avoidance of dehydration; ± caffeine.
- Definitive treatment is with epidural blood patch.

Further reading

Basurto Ona X, Martínez García L, Solà I, Bonfill Cosp X. Drug therapy for treating post-dural puncture headache. *Cochrane Database Syst Rev* 2011; (8): CD007887.

Klein AM, Loder E. Postpartum headache. *Int J Obstet Anesth* 2010; **19**: 422–30.

Sprigge JS, Harper SJ. Accidental dural puncture and post dural puncture headache in obstetric anaesthesia: presentation and management: a 23-year survey in a district general hospital. *Anaesthesia* 2008; **63**: 36–43.

Thew M, Paech MJ. Management of postdural puncture headache in the obstetric patient. *Curr Opin Anesthesiol* 2008; **21**: 288–92.

Van de Velde M, Schepers R, Berends N, Vandermeersch E, De Buck F. Ten years of experience with accidental dural puncture and post-dural puncture headache in a tertiary obstetric anaesthesia department. *Int J Obstet Anesth* 2008; **17**: 329–35.

Chapter 43

Epidural blood patch

Injection of blood into the epidural space as a treatment for postdural puncture headache (PDPH) was first suggested in the 1960s, following the observation that the incidence of PDPH was lower when dural tap followed a bloody tap. In fact, this relationship was later found not to be so, but epidural blood patch (EBP) has became widely accepted as the gold standard treatment for PDPH, despite early fears about adverse effects.

The mechanism of action of EBP is uncertain; traditional teaching is that the blood seals the dural hole, preventing further leakage of cerebrospinal fluid. However, an alteration of cerebrospinal haemodynamics by EBP has been suggested, accounting for EBP's immediate effect and the observation that lumbar EBP is effective even following cervical dural puncture.

Problems/special considerations

- Current opinion favours early use of EBP for PDPH (e.g. within 1–2 days if headache is severe). Prophylactic EBP (via the catheter after delivery) is not thought to be useful (see Chapter 41, Dural puncture).
- Contraindications are those of epidural analgesia generally; in particular the risk of epidural abscess is often quoted if the mother is pyrexial. In that situation, other methods of treating PDPH may be tried; alternatively, prophylactic use of antibiotics has been suggested. Some authorities advocate routine sending of blood for microbiological culture in case bacteraemia is present, although this practice is not universal.
- Adverse effects of EBP include those of epidural analgesia (including failure or another dural puncture), back pain, transient nerve root pain and pyrexia. Transient bradycardia has been reported but its significance is uncertain.

Management options

Other causes of postpartum headache should be excluded (see Table 42.1). Two operators are required. Whilst one locates the epidural space in the usual way, the other prepares to draw 20 ml of blood under aseptic conditions. The blood is injected slowly and the patient is asked to report any unpleasant effects. The interspace at or below the level of the original dural puncture is usually recommended, since injected blood has been shown to track mainly upwards after injection. One of the controversial issues regarding EBP is the volume of blood to inject. It was thought that the more blood that was injected, the greater the chance of success. A recent multicentre randomised controlled trial has shown that the likelihood of success is limited if only 15 ml of blood is injected, whilst there is no advantage in terms of efficacy if > 20 ml of blood is injected.

The patient is usually kept lying for 2–4 hours after EBP (reduced efficacy has been suggested if mobilisation is immediate). The success rate of EBP has been reported as 70–100%; typically, there is complete relief of headache, although some degree of headache may return in up to 30–50% of women. Repeat EBP is sometimes required, rarely more than once. The procedure is performed on an outpatient basis in some units.

The mother should be fully informed of the benefits and risks of EBP (including the fact that proper randomised trials are few, as concluded by a recent Cochrane review). A senior anaesthetist should perform the EBP for two reasons: first, the original epidural may have been difficult, and a second dural puncture occurring during EBP would be at best embarrassing; second, the mother has suffered considerable distress and deserves the reassurance of knowing that a senior anaesthetist is handling her case. Since the headache may return after EBP, she should be invited to contact the anaesthetist if this occurs.

Key points

- Epidural blood patch should be performed by a senior anaesthetist.
- Strict asepsis is required.
- 15–20 ml of blood is injected if tolerated.
- The mother is kept supine for 2–4 hours after patching.
- Epidural blood patch is thought to affect cerebrospinal haemodynamics ± plug the dural hole.
- Treatment is effective in 70–100% of cases but headache may recur in 30–50%.

Further reading

Boonmak P, Boonmak S. Epidural blood patching for preventing and treating post-dural puncture headache. *Cochrane Database Syst Rev* 2010; (1): CD001791.

Paech MJ, Doherty DA, Christmas T, Wong CA; Epidural Blood Patch Trial Group. The volume of blood for epidural blood patch in obstetrics: a randomized, blinded clinical trial. *Anesth Analg* 2011; **113**: 126–33.

Thew M, Paech MJ. Management of postdural puncture headache in the obstetric patient. *Curr Opin Anesthesiol* 2008; **21**: 288–92.

Van de Velde M, Schepers R, Berends N, Vandermeersch E, De Buck F. Ten years of experience with accidental dural puncture and post-dural puncture headache in a tertiary obstetric anaesthesia department. *Int J Obstet Anesth* 2008; **17**: 329–35.

Extensive regional blocks

Obstetric anaesthetists, in routinely extending neuraxial analgesia up to the level of T4, are accustomed to dealing with regional anaesthetic blocks that other practitioners would regard as excessively high. It is inevitable that occasionally the block will extend beyond the anticipated area, either because of accidental subarachnoid or subdural administration or merely because of the unpredictability of spread in some individuals. Although many such blocks may be quite benign and not cause any cardiovascular or respiratory embarrassment, it is important that they are detected in order to pick up misplacement of the local anaesthetic, which may cause more serious problems later.

'Total spinal block' is strictly defined as a spinal block that results in unconsciousness and central depression of respiratory and myocardial activity, accompanied by massive vasodilatation. Since the same may also result from epidural and subdural blocks, and one should not wait until unconsciousness before acting, the terms 'high regional block' or 'extensive regional block' are preferred. A practical definition of these terms would be a regional block that results in the need for tracheal intubation or other airway intervention. The reported incidence of such blocks is between 1 in ~2000 and 1 in ~13 000, probably reflecting differences in definitions used in the studies from which these figures arise.

Problems/special considerations

- The effect and spread of local anaesthetic drugs is enhanced in pregnancy and this should be borne in mind when planning doses for a spinal or epidural block.
- An apparently fixed spinal block may extend further if the patient is moved, even 30 minutes or more after the local anaesthetic has been administered. This particularly applies to rotation through the fully supine position from one side to the other and may be due to dural compression resulting from dilatation of the epidural veins, which act as a collateral circulation during aortocaval compression.
- Early features of extensive block include weakness/tingling of the upper arms and shoulders, breathing difficulties, slurred speech and sedation. Symptoms and signs may develop late and insidiously.
- Hypotension may be severe and may be associated with reduced placental perfusion and fetal hypoxia/ischaemia. Urgent delivery may be necessary both to relieve maternal hypotension and to protect the fetus.
- Airway management following total spinal block is made more difficult in pregnancy because of the increased risk of aspiration and the difficulty in maintaining a clear airway without tracheal intubation.

Epidural analgesia/anaesthesia

Relatively large doses of local anaesthetic drugs are used which, if they find their way into the wrong compartment, can cause a dangerously extensive block.

Prevention is the key, and this is achieved by maintaining a high index of suspicion and regarding every dose of local anaesthetic as subarachnoid until proven otherwise. The potential problems are best discussed under the following headings:

- *Epidural analgesia:* A test dose suitable for distinguishing subarachnoid placement should be used after the epidural catheter is inserted, and the effect should be assessed before further local anaesthetic is given. Each epidural dose should be given sufficiently slowly to allow detection of a spinal block before it spreads to a dangerously high level; doses should be administered at intervals of 5 minutes or longer, with the mother moving between increments. These precautions should be used with every dose in labour, since catheter migration has been known to occur between doses. The use of low-dose local anaesthetic/opioid mixtures reduces the risk to the mother if accidentally given intrathecally; the local anaesthetic concentration should be the lowest for the effect required.

- *Epidural top-up for instrumental or caesarean delivery:* Volumes of up to 20 ml concentrated solution may be injected over 3 minutes, the risk of extensive block being weighed against the need for rapid extension for surgery. Alternatively, 3–4 ml of the top-up solution can be given as a test dose, 3–5 minutes before the main dose. It has been suggested that the top-up can safely be given in the labour room and the patient transferred to theatre while the block is extending although this is controversial, since the ability to monitor and/or resuscitate may not be ideal before/during transit. It is essential that the anaesthetist is by the patient at all times and ensures adequate monitoring and lateral tilt. Regular testing of the block is mandatory.

- *Epidural after dural puncture with the Tuohy needle:* If an epidural catheter has been re-sited following accidental dural puncture, the risk of high block is increased, both because the local anaesthetic can leak through the puncture and because the catheter can migrate. Epidural doses/infusions should be reduced and given by an anaesthetist.

- *Subdural block:* This is thought to occur in up to 1% of 'epidurals'. It may occur when the epidural catheter is passed into the potential space between the dura mater and the arachnoid, probably after the needle has torn the dura. The block is characteristically slow (20–30 minutes) in onset and spreads cranially much higher than expected, often involving the lower cervical dermatomes. Extensive motor block is, however, uncommon, and hypotension is usually mild. The block tends to spare the lumbar and sacral segments and may be patchy; consequently, pain relief is often poor. If analgesia is acceptable, it is tempting to leave the catheter *in situ* and to continue to use smaller doses. This technique is not recommended, because of the risk of a top-up rupturing the arachnoid, with subsequent development of an extensive subarachnoid block.

- *Accidental subarachnoid block:* This is rarer than subdural block, largely because the anaesthetist is usually alerted by the free flow of cerebrospinal fluid from the hub of the catheter. The consequences are far more hazardous, however, since the resulting block is very rapid in onset, has a considerable motor component and is normally associated with severe hypotension.

Spinal anaesthesia

High blocks associated with spinal anaesthesia are related to greater spread rather than deposition of local anaesthetic into the wrong space. This may result from use of hypobaric solutions, or compression of the dural sac from the outside as a result either of recent epidural top-up or of aortocaval compression, or it may represent an extreme of normal variation as anaesthetists have sought higher and higher blocks in order to avoid pain during surgery. The continuous presence of the anaesthetist and the immediate availability in the operating theatre of the necessary equipment and assistance ensure that further supportive measures are readily available if needed.

Prevention of excessive block is achieved by using the minimum necessary dose of local anaesthetic. Excessive barbotage should also be avoided. Maintenance of the natural kyphosis of the thoracic spine if in lateral tilt, or the use of pillows under the shoulders and head if in the full lateral position, will help prevent hyperbaric local anaesthetic spreading higher than the T4 dermatomes. Head-down tilt is very occasionally needed to encourage a recalcitrant block to spread high enough for surgery, but this should be used with great care and reversed as soon as the desired effect has been achieved. The same precautions apply if the mother is rolled through the full supine position as part of the positioning or if she is coughing or otherwise performing a Valsalva manoeuvre; these can result in sudden cranial spread of the block, and this can even happen at the end of a procedure when the block has been established for some time.

The ideal dose of spinal solution to use after a recent (failed) epidural top-up is uncertain. There have been reports of extensive blocks if normal spinal doses are used, presumably as a result of dural compression, but there have also been reports of normal responses or even inadequate anaesthesia if smaller doses are used.

Management options

- The basics (ABC) of resuscitation should be remembered. Aortocaval compression should be prevented and the full lateral position is best if cardiopulmonary resuscitation is not needed.
- Oxygen should be given by facemask and tracheal intubation performed early if a raising block progresses; waiting until the patient is unconscious may risk airway obstruction and/or aspiration of gastric contents.
- Cardiovascular support includes intravenous fluids, vasopressors such as phenylephrine (adrenaline may be needed if hypotension is resistant) and cardiopulmonary resuscitation if cardiac arrest or severe myocardial depression is compromising cerebral oxygenation.
- Delivering the fetus should be considered to protect it from hypotension and to relieve aortocaval compression.

Key points

- All epidural doses should be divided into safe aliquots, if time permits.
- Subdural catheter placement is common and may progress to subarachnoid block.
- Spinal blocks can spread cranially even 30 minutes after administration.

- Careful and regular monitoring of the height of block is required after institution of spinal or epidural anaesthesia.
- Delivery of the fetus may protect it from ischaemia and may also benefit the mother.

Further reading

Jenkins JG. Some immediate serious complications of obstetric epidural analgesia and anaesthesia: a prospective study of 145,550 epidurals. *Int J Obstet Anesth* 2005; **14**: 37–42.

Yentis SM, Dob DP. High regional blockade – the failed intubation of the new millennium? *Int J Obstet Anesth* 2001; **10**: 159–61.

Chapter

45

Inadequate regional analgesia in labour

Although epidural analgesia has an excellent track record for relieving the pain of labour, a proportion of epidurals fail to deliver adequate pain relief. Approximately 10% of women will have initially unsatisfactory blocks, and around 2% of these will be persistently inadequate. Poor blocks may be divided into those involving inadequate spread, and those where spread is apparently adequate but the degree of block is insufficient.

Problems/special considerations

- *Inadequate spread:* This may be one of several types:
  - A very limited block involving only one or two dermatomes, thought to be caused by the tip of the catheter 'escaping' from the epidural space via an intervertebral foramen when excessive length of catheter is left in the epidural space.
  - Satisfactory cranial and caudal spread, but limited to one side of the body only. Contrast studies of this type of block have shown that it is associated with distribution of fluid to one side of the epidural space only. The most likely explanation is the existence of a dorsal midline septum arising from the posterior aspect of the dura mater, which acts as a barrier to the free spread of local anaesthetic. Unilateral block has also been shown to be more common in cases of scoliosis and this is also presumed to be due to anatomical barriers to spread of local anaesthetic in the epidural space.

- Missed segment, whereby one or more segments remain unblocked despite normal analgesia above and below; this was more commonly seen when low volumes of concentrated local anaesthetic solution were routinely used during labour, but is relatively uncommon with the higher-volume, low concentrations used in modern techniques. Missed segments were thought to arise from isolation of some nerve roots from the local anaesthetic by longitudinal septa or air used in loss of resistance techniques, or from larger nerve roots' (typically lumbar) relative resistance to penetration by local anaesthetic.

- Limited cranial or caudal spread despite attempts to extend it with further doses, e.g. because of a horizontal septum preventing flow or presumed scarring in patients who have undergone spinal surgery.

  Catheters with single terminal eyes are commonly used in the USA, whereas most UK practitioners prefer multi-holed, blind-ending catheters. Studies have demonstrated a higher incidence of unsatisfactory blocks with the former, mostly due to unilateral blocks and missed segments. This is probably due to a 'streaming' effect, whereby all the solution is directed along a single track, encouraging longitudinal spread at the expense of lateral flow.

- *Inadequate density of block despite apparently adequate spread:* This may occur when excessively dilute mixtures of local anaesthetic are used, when the intensity of pain is increased (e.g. occipito-posterior position, or placental abruption or impending uterine rupture), or in some women who just seem to have lower pain thresholds.

Management options

The key to managing poor blocks is early detection. All mothers who have had an epidural block in labour should be checked by the anaesthetist within 30 minutes of the first dose and the level of analgesia tested with a suitable stimulus. Continued review of the patient and the efficacy of epidural analgesia is mandatory throughout subsequent labour. Any complaint of persistent pain at any time during the labour should prompt further testing and review.

A limited unilateral block is usually due to an excessive amount of catheter having been inserted into the epidural space. Anything greater than 5 cm is generally regarded as likely to lead to transforaminal escape of the catheter tip. Even multi-holed catheters can be freely pulled back to leave 3–5 cm in the space in an attempt to overcome this problem. Unfortunately, once a 'track' has been established for the local anaesthetic solution, it may persist despite the catheter being pulled back, and the only solution may be to remove the catheter and re-site it in a different space. Even if the catheter was originally inserted to the optimum distance, the possibility of it being drawn further into the epidural space should not be discounted; this has been shown to happen as a result of traction imposed by movements of the vertebrae and activity of the spinal muscles.

Unilateral block can occasionally be overcome by laying the patient on the affected side and administering large volumes of local anaesthetic, with or without opioid. It is presumed that this encourages spread of the solution up and down the epidural space and thus beyond the boundaries of any midline septum or allows any breaches in the septum to be exploited. These manoeuvres may be effective but there will often be a marked tendency for the block to affect the 'good' side more than the other. In the more recalcitrant unilateral block, the catheter may need to be re-sited in another interspace. In general, when the above manipulations have been unsuccessful, a paramedian approach may help, since the catheter has been shown to travel a straighter course in the epidural space when inserted via this route. A combined spinal–epidural technique may be used to overcome poor spread or missed segments, and for some anaesthetists this is the technique of choice following a failed epidural, as it allows rapid onset of analgesia and it has been suggested that the epidural catheter is less likely to fail if a CSE technique has been used compared with a plain epidural technique. Other causes for poor block should not be overlooked.

Continuous infusion techniques may fail if the syringe pump is not functioning properly, has been incorrectly set up or has become occluded. The commonest reason for a previously satisfactory block failing is the epidural catheter falling out – another good reason for checking the catheter first.

Finally, it should be remembered that an inadequate epidural for labour is likely to be inadequate for caesarean section should one be required in an emergency; in such situations it might be appropriate to consider spinal anaesthesia instead. Furthermore, in women with a high risk of caesarean section the anaesthetist should have a low threshold for re-siting an epidural if the latter is less than perfect during labour.

Key points

- Blocks should be checked regularly to allow early detection of failure.
- In the event of a poor block, especially when previously satisfactory, the catheter should be checked.
- Poor spread is often caused by an excessive length of catheter in the epidural space. A length of 3–5 cm is usually considered optimum.
- Re-siting the catheter early is often a better option than repeated 'fiddling'.

Further reading

Agaram R, Douglas MJ, McTaggart RA, Gunka V. Inadequate pain relief with labor epidurals: a multivariate analysis of associated factors. *Int J Obstet Anesth* 2009; **18**: 10–14.

Pan PH, Bogard TD, Owen MD. Incidence and characteristics of failures in obstetric neuraxial analgesia and anesthesia: a retrospective analysis of 19, 259 deliveries. *Int J Obstet Anesth* 2004; **13**: 227–33.

Backache

Backache is not a trivial symptom. It is one of the commonest causes of time off work in the UK, and can be particularly debilitating for the nursing mother.

Backache is very common, and a high proportion of women have significant backache before pregnancy, with surveys putting this figure at around 15%. During pregnancy, the prevalence of backache rises to ~50%.

Long-term backache after childbirth (defined as backache lasting longer than 3 months) occurs in about a third of women and this increases to half if there is a history of backache before or during the pregnancy. The incidence of new, long-term backache in women with no symptoms of backache before or during pregnancy is much lower, at around 5–10%.

Problems/special considerations

Prospective studies have found no significant increase in the risk of backache when epidural analgesia is used in labour, nor an association with motor block. Despite this, there is a popular belief among parturients, midwives and even obstetricians that there is a causative link between epidural analgesia in labour and subsequent backache, largely arising from retrospective surveys of mothers in the late 1980s. Many women who develop intractable backache shortly after an anaesthetist has inserted a needle into their back will, not surprisingly, believe that the two are connected, and commonly refer to their backache as starting 'after the epidural' instead of 'after the baby'.

This is not to say, of course, that a poorly administered epidural cannot cause trauma that might lead to backache or that backache should be ignored after an epidural. In particular, acute tenderness over the epidural site should always raise the suspicion of an epidural abscess or haematoma, especially when accompanied by pyrexia and signs of nerve root irritation or cauda equina syndrome. Finally, rare coincidental causes such as a tumour should not be overlooked.

Management options

Women with backache often present to the anaesthetist in the antenatal period. Referral to the obstetric physiotherapist, lumbar support, simple analgesia and transcutaneous electrical nerve stimulation (TENS) may all be of help.

Whilst the evidence does not support a causal link between epidural/spinal analgesia/ anaesthesia and long-term backache, many women ask about this complication, especially at antenatal classes, and the best approach is to inform them of the high risk of backache associated with pregnancy and childbirth, and to reassure them that these techniques do not appear to increase this risk.

The woman who presents with severe backache or a long history of back trouble in the antenatal clinic should be warned that it is very likely that this will continue after childbirth. Epidural analgesia should not be contraindicated in these cases but it may sometimes be more painful having an epidural sited in a sensitive back. Care should be taken to avoid unnatural postures that will unduly stress the ligaments and the patient should be allowed to move freely in labour. Support of lumbar lordosis and prevention of hyperextension at the hips are helpful.

Midwives should be alerted to refer severe, acute, localised backache after epidural insertion to the anaesthetist. Management should include a full neurological examination, and a low threshold for early referral to a neurologist and imaging to exclude haematoma or abscess formation.

Localised tenderness and limitation of movement may be due to a small haematoma in the interspinous ligament or paraspinous muscles and these will often respond to physiotherapy.

Key points

- Backache is very common after childbirth.
- There is no apparent link between epidural/spinal analgesia and long-term postpartum backache.
- Tenderness associated with pyrexia should raise the suspicion of abscess.

Further reading

Anim-Somuah M, Smyth RM, Jones L. Epidural versus non-epidural or no analgesia in labour. *Cochrane Database Syst Rev* 2011; (12): CD000331.

Han IH. Pregnancy and spinal problems. *Curr Opin Obstet Gynecol* 2010; **22**: 477–81.

Orlikowski CE, Dickinson JE, Paech MJ, McDonald SJ, Nathan E. Intrapartum analgesia and its association with post-partum back pain and headache in nulliparous women. *Aust N Z J Obstet Gynaecol* 2006; **46**: 395–401.

Chapter 47

Horner's syndrome and cranial nerve palsy

Horner's syndrome is the combination of partial ptosis, myosis (small pupil), enophthalmos and hypohydrosis, and represents interruption of the ipsilateral sympathetic supply to the head anywhere along its length. There may also be associated nasal stuffiness and reduced taste sensation on the ipsilateral side (Gustav's sign). Horner's syndrome may occasionally occur during an otherwise unremarkable epidural block.

Palsies of cranial nerves V and VI have been reported following uncomplicated obstetric epidural anaesthesia, although much less commonly than Horner's syndrome. In addition, cranial nerve palsies are well known to occur (albeit uncommonly) following dural puncture, and cases (including cranial nerve VII palsy) have been reported after accidental dural tap during childbirth. An idiopathic lower motor neurone lesion of cranial nerve VII (Bell's palsy) may occur rarely in pregnancy but there is no evidence that it is related to regional anaesthesia.

Problems/special considerations

The mechanism for Horner's syndrome occurring during apparently normal and non-extensive epidural analgesia and anaesthesia is uncertain; partial subdural cranial extension of local anaesthetic solution has been suggested, although there may be no other features of atypical block. The sympathetic innervation of the iris is variable and may arise from C8 to T5; in addition sympathetic fibres are thought to be more sensitive to local anaesthetics than somatic fibres. Increased incidence in pregnancy has been suggested and may be related to the greater susceptibility of pregnant women to local anaesthetics generally or to more extensive central neural blocks in particular. Cranial nerve palsy is also thought to be related to excessively high blockade; palsy of cranial nerve V is commonly associated with Horner's syndrome. Cranial nerve palsy following dural puncture is thought to be related to stretching of the nerve caused by traction of intracranial contents and is usually associated with postdural puncture headache.

Lesions may go unnoticed or may cause alarm to the patient, her partner or labour ward staff. In addition, if another possibly unrelated complication or event were to occur or if general anaesthesia was administered subsequently, the pupillary signs especially may cause confusion.

Management options

For cases occurring during uncomplicated epidural analgesia and anaesthesia, no specific treatment is required other than reassurance, since the signs themselves are harmless and disappear when the epidural block wears off. Although there are other more sinister causes of Horner's syndrome and cranial nerve palsies, they are rare and would not be expected to cause signs to appear so acutely in the absence of other symptoms or signs, and last such a short time. Palsies associated with dural puncture should be managed as for the headache; it has been suggested that resolution of the palsy is less likely if epidural blood patch is delayed.

There is no evidence that the occurrence of Horner's syndrome or cranial nerve palsy during one labour epidural predisposes the patient to the same thing during subsequent epidurals.

It must not be forgotten that some individuals naturally have unequal pupils or an asymmetrical face; it is therefore worth asking the patient and her partner whether the signs are new. Once diagnosed, simple observation is all that is required, bearing in mind that the intense interest of medical and midwifery staff may cause more anxiety than the syndrome itself.

Key points

- Horner's syndrome:
  - Comprises partial ptosis, myosis, enophthalmos and hypohydrosis.
  - May occur during an otherwise unremarkable epidural.
  - Is harmless and requires no treatment if related to epidural anaesthesia.

- Cranial nerve palsy:
  - Most commonly involves nerves V or VI although the incidence is lower than that of Horner's syndrome.
  - Requires no treatment if of short duration and associated only with regional anaesthesia.

Further reading

Barbara R, Tome R, Barua A, *et al.* Transient Horner syndrome following epidural anesthesia for labor: case report and review of the literature. *Obstet Gynecol Surv* 2011; **66**: 114–19.

Day CJE, Shutt LE. Auditory, ocular, and facial complications of central neural block. *Reg Anesth* 1996; **21**: 197–201.

Loo CC, Dahlgren G, Irestedt L. Neurological complications in obstetric regional anaesthesia. *Int J Obstet Anesth* 2000; **9**: 99–124.

Chapter

48

Peripheral nerve lesions following regional anaesthesia

Although spinal and epidural needles and catheters must, by virtue of their mode of action, pass close to nerve roots, the incidence of neurological damage appears to be very low. Surveys have suggested that around 1 in 2000 obstetric epidurals/spinals is complicated by numbness, paraesthesia or weakness in the distribution of a single nerve root that may take several days to a few months to resolve. The incidence of permanent symptoms is approximately 1 in 15 000.

Problems/special considerations

- *Other causes of nerve damage:* While it is perhaps natural to blame any lower limb neurological deficit on the neuraxial block that preceded it, nerve palsy is more likely to arise as a result of obstetric factors, as witnessed by patients with demonstrable permanent lesions despite not having had epidural or spinal procedures. The overall incidence of these complications is estimated to be around 1 in 2000 deliveries, and the causes and features are listed in Table 48.1. The potential for nerve damage during childbirth is apparent when one considers the anatomy of the nerves arising in the pelvis (Fig. 10.6).

Table 48.1 Nerve lesions with non-anaesthetic, obstetric causes

Lesion	Presentation	Cause
Lumbosacral trunk	Foot drop Loss of sensation, esp. L4–5, S1	Pressure in pelvis from fetal head or forceps
Peroneal nerve	Foot drop	Pressure from lithotomy poles or prolonged squatting
Femoral nerve	Loss of sensation front of thigh Quadriceps weakness Reduced knee jerk	Hyperflexion of thighs, esp. squatting or lithotomy position
Lateral cutaneous nerve of thigh	Meralgia paraesthetica – altered sensation over anterolateral aspect of thigh	Antenatal weight gain ± lumbar lordosis
Conus of spinal cord	Anterior spinal artery syndrome – cauda equina/paraplegia	Obstruction of aberrant blood supply to conus by fetal head during prolonged labour

Table 48.2 Neurological deficit following nerve root trauma

Root	Sensory loss	Motor weakness
L2	Upper anterior thigh	Hip flexion
L3	Lower anterior & medial thigh	Thigh adduction
L4	Lateral thigh, knee & medial leg	Leg extension
L5	Lateral leg & dorsum of foot	Ankle dorsiflexion
S1	Lateral foot	Ankle plantar flexion

- *Aetiology of nerve root damage:* A needle or catheter touching a nerve root is almost certain to cause paraesthesia in the awake patient, usually of a severe, lancinating quality and characteristically described as being like an electric shock in the distribution of the nerve root. Unless transient and mild, paraesthesia should always prompt the anaesthetist to remove the needle or catheter and to reorientate it. Presence or absence of paraesthesia should always be recorded. If damage has occurred, symptoms are usually experienced in the same distribution (Table 48.2).
- *Central neurological lesions:* Single nerve damage should be distinguished from the more serious central lesions that occur extremely rarely (see Chapter 49, Spinal cord lesions following regional anaesthesia; Chapter 50, Arachnoiditis; Chapter 51, Cauda equina syndrome).

Management options

Prevention is the most important aspect of management. Blocks should be performed with the patient awake (not normally an issue in obstetric practice), and care should be taken to ensure that the interspace chosen is below the level of termination of the spinal cord. Patients should be asked to indicate if they feel paraesthesia, and this should be a signal to the anaesthetist to remove the needle or catheter and start again. Spinal injections should only be given if there is free flow of cerebrospinal fluid, to ensure that the needle tip is not obstructed by nerve tissue. A note should always be made as to the presence or absence of paraesthesia during the procedure, as this information can be invaluable later.

Routine follow-up should be carried out assiduously, and midwives should be alerted to notify the anaesthetist if any mother shows signs of slow recovery of sensory or motor function. Careful mapping of the deficit should be carried out at the earliest opportunity to establish a baseline from which improvement can be measured. Other, non-anaesthetic, causes should be considered; the aetiology may be suggested by the distribution of the deficit and by other precipitating factors (see Table 48.1). The benign course of the vast majority of these lesions means that an explanation to the patient can include a reassuring prognosis. Generally neuropraxias recover in 3–4 months though occasionally chronic pain may ensue so postpartum follow-up should always be offered.

Except for minor and resolving lesions, further management should generally involve referral to a neurologist or neurophysiologist. Imaging of the lumbar region is rarely helpful but may be used to exclude coincidental causes such as a prolapsed intervertebral disc. Nerve conduction studies are often invaluable as they allow the site of the lesion to be identified and may help in estimating prognosis.

Key points

- Paraesthesia should always be documented and is a sign to withdraw the needle, reorientate it and start again.
- Delayed recovery needs assiduous follow-up to detect neuraxial haematoma/abscess.
- Nerve palsy is usually a result of pregnancy/childbirth and unrelated to regional anaesthesia.

Further reading

Cook TM, Counsell D, Wildsmith JAW, on behalf of the Royal College of Anaesthetists Third National Audit Project. Major complications of central neuraxial block: report on the 3rd National Audit Project of the Royal College of Anaesthetists. *Br J Anaesth* 2009; **102**: 179–90.

Moen V, Irestedt L. Neurological complications following central neuraxial blockades in obstetrics. *Curr Opin Anesthesiol* 2008; **21**: 275–80.

Russell R. Neurological complications in obstetric regional anaesthesia. *Anaesth Intensive Care Med* 2007; **8**: 323–5.

Wong CA. Nerve injuries after neuraxial anaesthesia and their medicolegal implications. *Best Pract Res Clin Obstet Gynaecol* 2010; **24**: 367–81.

Chapter 49

Spinal cord lesions following regional anaesthesia

Postpartum neurological lesions are often blamed on peripartum anaesthetic interventions, even though non-anaesthetic causes are much more likely. Obstetric anaesthetists may therefore find themselves involved in the assessment and management of these problems. There are many causes of spinal cord lesions (Table 49.1).

Problems/special considerations

The initial problem is one of diagnosis. Different lesions may present in different ways that may overlap with each other and with other conditions (Table 49.1). Spinal cord lesions are more commonly associated with spinals and combined spinal–epidurals, and it should be remembered that peripheral neuropathies may arise as a result of obstetric interventions especially involving the lithotomy position. Although cord lesions generally present with upper motor neurone signs and sensory impairment below the level of injury, and peripheral nerve injuries

Table 49.1 Causes of postpartum spinal cord lesions

Mechanism	Condition	Comment
Compression	Epidural haematoma	Not associated with back pain
	Epidural abscess	Associated with back pain plus evidence of local and/or systemic infection; typically presents several days postpartum
	Prolapsed disc	Associated with back pain; may present *de novo* intra- or postpartum
	Tumour	May be associated with back pain
Ischaemia*	Severe hypotension	Not associated with back pain
	Anomalous arterial blood supply plus prolonged labour or hypotension	Includes arteriovenous malformations or a predominantly pelvic blood supply to the conus medullaris and cauda equina
	Normal vascular supply and normotension	Has been reported in spinal stenosis following rapid injection of a large epidural bolus
Neurotoxicity	Injection of wrong solution	May be associated with back pain
Trauma	Back injury	Associated with back pain
	Direct damage during regional anaesthesia	May be associated with back pain although paraesthesia is more common

*N.B. Compression results in local ischaemia.

present with lower motor neurone signs, it may be surprisingly difficult to distinguish them clinically (see Chapter 48, Peripheral nerve lesions following regional anaesthesia). Sinister signs such as pyrexia, severe back pain, bilateral distribution, or loss of bladder or bowel function are suggestive of a compressive lesion such as epidural or spinal haematoma abscess. These conditions are very rare (less than 1 in 100 000) but may cause major, irreversible damage unless relieved within hours of presentation. Any suspicion should prompt immediate referral for a neurosurgical opinion. In the case of early lesions, some effects of spinal or epidural blockade may persist for several hours, occasionally over 12 hours (up to 48 hours has been observed, with no apparent cause), obscuring the underlying pathology. Since regression of a block often occurs under observation by non-anaesthetic staff, there may be delay in appropriate medical input being requested. In the case of acute potentially reversible spinal cord damage, e.g. cord compression caused by haematoma, delay of more than 6–8 hours is associated with an increasing chance of permanent impairment.

Similarly, problems that present later, such as epidural abscess, may be missed if associated back pain is dismissed as trivial.

Management options

Anaesthetic-related problems may be reduced by attention to details such as:

- Assessing the coagulation status and pre-existing neurological status before performing regional techniques
- Aseptic technique
- Determining appropriate anatomical landmarks during the procedure and awareness of the risk of and from inserting the needle too high
- Removal of the needle if severe paraesthesia or pain is experienced during a regional block
- Prevention and management of hypotension after anaesthesia.

Any unexpectedly dense or prolonged block should always be observed carefully, especially if other risk factors (e.g. heparin therapy) are present. A careful history and examination, and knowledge of the relevant anatomy, are vital to distinguish the various lesions from less severe conditions, and neurological referral is always advisable if there is any suspicion.

Individual conditions are managed as for non-pregnant patients, e.g. surgical decompression for cord compression, plus antibiotics for abscess.

Key points

- Anaesthetists may be involved in the assessment and management of postpartum spinal cord lesions.
- Knowledge of the appropriate anatomy is crucial.
- In acute spinal cord compression, delay in decompression beyond 6–8 hours may result in permanent disability.

Further reading

Cook TM, Counsell D, Wildsmith JAW, on behalf of the Royal College of Anaesthetists Third National Audit Project. Major complications of central neuraxial block: report on the 3rd National Audit Project of the Royal College of Anaesthetists. *Br J Anaesth* 2009; **102**: 179–90.

Moen V, Irestedt L. Neurological complications following central neuraxial blockades in obstetrics. *Curr Opin Anesthesiol* 2008; **21**: 275–80.

Porter JR, Christie LE, Yentis SM, Durbridge J, Dob DP. Prolonged neurological deficit following neuraxial blockade for caesarean section. *Int J Obstet Anesth* 2011; **20**: 271.

Russell R. Neurological complications in obstetric regional anaesthesia. *Anaesth Intensive Care Med* 2007; **8**: 323–5.

Wong CA. Nerve injuries after neuraxial anaesthesia and their medicolegal implications. *Best Pract Res Clin Obstet Gynaecol* 2010; **24**: 367–81.

Chapter

50

Arachnoiditis

Arachnoiditis is a rare condition comprising chronic radicular pain associated with radiologically diagnosed abnormalities, classically filling defects in the subarachnoid space, absence of spinal nerve root sleeves, arachnoid cysts and obstruction to flow of radio-opaque contrast medium. It is important to realise that radiological abnormalities may be present in asymptomatic patients, and a diagnosis of arachnoiditis should not be made on radiological criteria alone. It may occur spontaneously, although it has followed radiation and perispinal injection of irritant substances, e.g. oil-based contrast medium that used to be employed for myelography. Antiseptic solutions, powder from surgical gloves and preservatives in drug solutions (e.g. sodium metabisulphite) have been implicated, as have infection and traumatic bleeding.

Arachnoiditis may occasionally be confused with cauda equina syndrome; typical features of the two conditions are shown in Table 50.1.

Problems/special considerations

Chronic adhesive arachnoiditis may develop several months or even years after the trigger, so it may be difficult to establish a causal link. Typically arachnoiditis presents with back pain, with or without leg pain, paraesthesia or weakness. It is usually steadily progressive and may follow neurological complications of regional anaesthesia.

Management options

Although obstetric regional analgesia and anaesthesia is considered to be extremely safe, it is important to maintain scrupulous attention to aseptic and atraumatic technique and to minimise the use of novel drugs and multiple combinations of drugs. Thus all solutions

Table 50.1 Typical features of arachnoiditis and cauda equina syndrome

	Aetiology	Features
Arachnoiditis	Inflammation of the arachnoid meningeal layer and subarachnoid space. Progressive fibrosis may cause spinal canal narrowing, ischaemia and permanent nerve damage	Meningeal irritation may occur early, although usually presents months or years later. May involve the cauda equina, presenting with similar features. Rarely extends cranially
Cauda equina syndrome	Damage to the lumbosacral nerve roots	Presents soon after regional anaesthesia, with numbness in corresponding dermatomes, weakness of corresponding myotomes, sphincter dysfunction

injected epidurally or spinally should be carefully checked first. Once the diagnosis is suspected, early involvement of a neurologist is mandatory with confirmation of the diagnosis by MRI scan. Detailed follow-up and possibly long-term support will be required. There is no specific treatment for arachnoiditis; steroids may have been tried although they are thought to be effective only in the very acute stage of the inflammatory process. Psychological support is important since the consequences of the condition may be catastrophic.

Key points

- Arachnoiditis is inflammation of the arachnoid and subarachnoid space; it typically occurs months or more after injury.
- Although rare, it may cause permanent neurological damage.

Further reading

Aldrete JA. Neurologic deficits and arachnoiditis following neuroaxial anesthesia. *Acta Anaesthesiol Scand* 2003; **47**: 3–12.

Moen V, Irestedt L. Neurological complications following central neuraxial blockades in obstetrics. *Curr Opin Anesthesiol* 2008; **21**: 275–80.

Rice I, Wee MYK, Thompson K. Obstetric epidurals and chronic adhesive arachnoiditis. *Br J Anaesth* 2004; **92**: 109–20.

Cauda equina syndrome

Cauda equina syndrome is a rare condition that has been associated with ultra-fine spinal catheters, especially when hyperbaric lidocaine has been injected. It is thought that poor mixing of local anaesthetic in the cerebrospinal fluid results in pooling of anaesthetic in the terminal dural sac, especially if large doses are used to extend an inadequate block. Local anaesthetics are known to be directly neurotoxic in high concentrations, lidocaine more than bupivacaine. The cauda equina nerve fibres may be more vulnerable to damage than other structures because they lack protective sheaths.

Cauda equina syndrome may occasionally be confused with arachnoiditis (for typical features of the two conditions, see Chapter 50, Arachnoiditis).

Problems/special considerations

Isolated areas of numbness on the leg and disturbances of perineal sensation are relatively common after delivery, making diagnosis difficult. Cauda equina syndrome may cause permanent neurological impairment.

Management options

Scrupulous attention to technique should be used when performing regional analgesia and anaesthesia. Special precautions should be taken when using continuous spinal blockade (e.g. avoiding lidocaine, especially in high concentrations, and not injecting large volumes of hyperbaric solutions). Once the diagnosis is suspected, early involvement of a neurologist is mandatory since detailed follow-up and possibly long-term support will be required. There is no specific treatment for cauda equina syndrome, although steroids may be tried. Psychological support is important since the consequences of the condition may be catastrophic.

Key points

- Cauda equina syndrome results from damage to the lumbosacral nerve roots; the condition occurs soon after the insult.
- Although rare, it may cause permanent neurological damage.

Further reading

Cook TM, Counsell D, Wildsmith JAW, on behalf of the Royal College of Anaesthetists Third National Audit Project. Major complications of central neuraxial block: report on the 3rd National Audit Project of the Royal College of Anaesthetists. *Br J Anaesth* 2009; **102**: 179–90.

Moen V, Irestedt L. Neurological complications following central neuraxial blockades in obstetrics. *Curr Opin Anesthesiol* 2008; **21**: 275–80.

Opioid-induced pruritus

Itching can result from the administration of opioids by any route but is much more common following epidural and intrathecal opioids than with systemically administered opioids. The reported incidence of itching varies from 0 to 100% and it is sometimes only discovered as a result of observing the patient or asking direct questions. Severe itching is only a problem in a very small number of cases (possibly as low as 1%). The incidence of itching associated with opioids is higher in the obstetric population, probably due to an oestrogenic influence at the opioid receptors.

Facial itching predominates after epidural and intrathecal opioids. This is possibly due to migration of opioid in the cerebrospinal fluid to the trigeminal nucleus and the trigeminal nerve roots. More generalised itching occurs with systemically administered opioids and may be due to activation of peripheral opioid receptors and partly due to histamine release (especially with morphine). The mechanism of opioid-induced itching is still not completely understood.

Problems/special considerations

The incidence of pruritus varies considerably between different opioids, being highest with morphine and lowest with the most lipophilic drugs such as fentanyl and sufentanil. Mixed agonist–antagonist drugs such as buprenorphine and butorphanol have been used via the epidural route to reduce the incidence of itching without decreasing analgesia.

Itching following administration of intrathecal fentanyl for caesarean section does not appear to predict that itching will also occur after epidural administration of diamorphine for postoperative analgesia.

Management options

No treatment is necessary for opioid-induced itching unless the mother is distressed. Simple antihistamines may be effective. Naloxone is an effective treatment for pruritus, but reduces the duration of analgesia obtained with neuraxial opioids, although a low-dose continuous infusion (0.4–0.6 mg/h) of naloxone is said to treat itching whilst maintaining analgesia from intrathecal morphine.

A variety of other treatments have been proposed, including intravenous droperidol, subhypnotic doses of propofol, ondansetron, nalbuphine and intramuscular promethazine. There is little evidence that any are effective.

Key points

- Itching can occur following the administration of any opioid drug by any route, but is most common following the epidural or intrathecal administration of morphine.
- Although the incidence of pruritus may exceed 90%, it is not often distressing for the mother and may not require any treatment other than reassurance.

Further reading

Bonnet MP, Marret E, Josserand J, *et al*. Effect of prophylactic 5-HT3 receptor antagonists on pruritus induced by neuraxial opioids: a quantitative systematic review. *Br J Anaesth* 2008; **101**: 311–19.

Szarvas S, Harmon D, Murphy D. Neuraxial opioid-induced pruritus: a review. *J Clin Anesth* 2003; **15**: 234–9.

Waxler B, Dadabhoy Z, Stojiljkovic L, Rabito S. Primer of postoperative pruritus for anes- thesiologists. *Anesthesiology* 2005; **103**: 168–78.

Chapter

53

Shivering

Although shivering may occur in about 10% of normal labours and following general anaesthesia, it is particularly associated with regional (especially epidural) anaesthesia and analgesia, during which it has been reported to occur in up to two thirds of cases. The cause is uncertain, but evidence suggests the tremor is at least partly thermoregulatory and may be accompanied by vasoconstriction in the arms. It also appears that epidural blockade may inhibit the subjective feeling of being cold, even when the core temperature has fallen. Other postulated mechanisms include altered control of peripheral muscles and a central effect resulting from systemic absorption of local anaesthetic or its transport via the cerebrospinal fluid to the brain. In labour, the high levels of circulating catecholamines and general arousal may also be important. Finally, the tendency for maternal temperature to increase after prolonged epidural analgesia may contribute to shivering, although it has also been suggested that shivering may contribute to the increase in temperature.

Shivering is also commonly seen after misprostol, with reported incidences of 50–70%.

Problems/special considerations

In most cases, shivering is mild and benign, although if severe it may increase maternal catecholamine concentrations and metabolic rate, interfere with fetal and maternal monitoring and be alarming to the mother. It also increases maternal oxygen consumption and carbon dioxide production, although this is rarely a problem in practice. Rarely, the mother may be unable to cooperate with medical and midwifery staff during examinations, etc.

Management options

If shivering is mild, simple reassurance is often all that is required. Measures that have been studied include warming of epidural and intravenous solutions and administration of intravenous opioids (pethidine 10–30 mg has been shown to be especially effective in the non-pregnant population). Epidural opioids may also reduce the incidence and severity of shivering. Other drugs shown to be effective after general anaesthesia outside of obstetrics include clonidine and doxapram, although these are infrequently used in the maternity suite.

Key points

- Shivering is common during epidural analgesia and anaesthesia.
- Simple reassurance is adequate treatment in most cases.

Further reading

Crowley LJ, Buggy DJ. Shivering and neuraxial anesthesia. *Reg Anesth Pain Med* 2008; **33**: 241–52.

Witte J, Sessler DI. Perioperative shivering: physiology and pharmacology. *Anesthesiology* 2002; **96**: 467–84.

Chapter 54

Aspiration of gastric contents

Aspiration is one of the three factors consistently associated with maternal deaths related to obstetric general anaesthesia, the others being emergency operation and difficult tracheal intubation. Often, these three factors occur together.

Problems/special considerations

Several risk factors make the pregnant woman more prone to aspiration:

- Reduced efficacy of the lower oesophageal sphincter caused by progesterone
- Reduced gastric emptying if opioids have been given

- The physical effect of the gravid uterus on the stomach
- The presence of gastric contents if the mother has eaten (see Chapter 14, Gastric function and feeding in labour).

Every mother in the third trimester should be considered at risk of aspiration, although the point during pregnancy at which increased risk occurs, and the point postpartum at which the risk returns to normal, are controversial. Many obstetric anaesthetists would consider 16–18 weeks of pregnancy as representing the onset of the 'at-risk' period, although an earlier cut-off point has also been suggested, especially if there are symptoms of gastro-esophageal reflux, the mother is obese, or the procedure requires her to be positioned head-down. Similarly, although hormonal profiles alter dramatically within a few hours of delivery, studies of gastric emptying have not produced consistent results, although some have suggested as little as 4–8 hours postpartum as the time required for the risk to return to normal (longer if opioids have been administered). However, other general physiological changes of pregnancy may take several weeks to disappear.

Finally, it should not be forgotten that any pregnant woman with an obtunded level of consciousness may be at risk from aspiration, e.g. during or after convulsions, drug overdose, anaphylaxis, etc. Thus, women identified as high risk may not only be those in whom surgical intervention is planned or expected.

Mortality or morbidity may be related to:

- Impairment of the view at laryngoscopy causing difficulty with intubation
- Obstruction of the upper airway by solid or semi-solid matter causing complete or partial airway obstruction and hypoventilation
- Chemical pneumonitis (Mendelson's syndrome), related to the pH and volume of the aspirated material. Extrapolation from animal work suggested an increased risk of pneumonitis if the pH is less than 2.5 and the volume is more than 25 ml, although it is now generally accepted that there is a continuum of risk, such that smaller volumes are required if the pH is lower. The alveolar inflammatory reaction may be intense, with oedema, cellular infiltration and the features of acute lung injury. There may be associated hypotension and poor peripheral perfusion if large amounts of fluid have been transferred from the intravascular space into the alveoli. Aspiration pneumonitis may also be caused by particulate antacids, e.g. magnesium trisilicate.

Management options
Prevention

- *Reduction of the volume and acidity of gastric contents:* This may be achieved by:
  - Withholding oral intake during labour
  - Administration of metoclopramide or other prokinetic drugs
  - Use of antacids or acid-reducing drugs such as H_2-antagonists and omeprazole
  - Emptying the stomach with a stomach tube before general anaesthesia or by inducing vomiting (rarely used although it has been suggested that a stomach tube should be routinely passed during general anaesthesia for emergency caesarean section in order to reduce the risk of aspiration after extubation).

  The first three measures are used to differing extents in different situations and countries. Thus, for example, all women in a particular unit might be given regular oral antacids and ranitidine throughout labour, whereas only women identified as being at high risk of intervention might be treated in another unit. Similarly, feeding in labour occurs to different degrees on different labour wards (see Chapter 14, Gastric function and feeding in labour). Proponents of all-inclusive treatment point to the potentially devastating effect of aspiration, the relative cheapness of therapy and the difficulty of identifying women truly at risk of a general anaesthetic. Supporters of selective treatment cite the low incidence of aspiration overall, the relatively low incidence of general anaesthesia in modern obstetric practice, the cost of therapy compared with no therapy, and resistance from many women and midwives to the 'medicalisation' of normal labour.

A practical breakdown of commonly used pharmacological preventative measures might be as follows (although as already mentioned, the protocol in use may vary widely between units):

- Normal (i.e. low risk) labour: nil
- High-risk labour (e.g. obstetric complications, multiple pregnancy, etc.): regular oral ranitidine 150 mg 6-hourly in active labour; following administration of pethidine: ranitidine 50 mg intramuscularly 8-hourly
- Emergency caesarean section: ranitidine 50 mg ± metoclopramide 10 mg slowly intramuscularly or intravenously when the decision for surgery is made, 30 ml sodium citrate 0.3 M orally immediately before induction of general anaesthesia
- Elective caesarean section: oral ranitidine 150 mg the night before and repeated the morning of surgery, metoclopramide/sodium citrate as above.

- *Preventing regurgitation during general anaesthesia:* Standard general anaesthetic practice includes a rapid sequence induction with application of cricoid pressure, although the method of its application and the possibility that cricoid pressure might make laryngoscopy more difficult are controversial areas (see Chapter 35, Cricoid pressure). Tracheal extubation should be in the lateral position with the patient awake, following return of full protective reflexes.
- *Avoidance of general anaesthesia altogether by using regional anaesthesia for operative procedures:* This is generally thought to be a major factor in the reduction in maternal mortality associated with anaesthesia that occurred over the 1970s–1990s, although there is no doubt that improvements in training in, and assistance and facilities for, general anaesthesia also occurred during this period.

Diagnosis

Regurgitation may be obvious, either during induction of anaesthesia or intra-/postoperatively. It may or may not be associated with aspiration. It is also possible for aspiration to occur without obvious, massive regurgitation, e.g. during induction or intraoperatively past the cuff of the tracheal tube. Features include bronchospasm, raised airway pressure, hypoxaemia, tachypnoea, tachycardia and pyrexia; these may present for the first time postoperatively following otherwise uneventful anaesthesia. A high index of suspicion is therefore required. If fluid is aspirated from the pharynx, larynx or tracheal tube, simple litmus paper is useful for identifying its acidity, although this may not always be reliable if antacid therapy has been used.

Treatment

Initial management comprises removing the regurgitated material from the airway by using pharyngeal, laryngeal and tracheal suction and maintaining oxygenation; tracheal intubation has the advantage of securing the airway and protecting it against further aspiration, as well as allowing ready access to the tracheobronchial tree for suction. Cricoid pressure may prevent further regurgitation during intubation. The head-down lateral position may be appropriate depending on the particular circumstances of the case, in order to encourage drainage of fluid from the upper airway and discourage further aspiration should regurgitation recur. Although popular in the past, the use of prophylactic steroid and antibiotic therapy in cases where aspiration is suspected is no longer advocated, since this approach has not been shown to reduce mortality and may even increase it. Solid particles may be removable via bronchoscopy; bronchoalveolar lavage may also be used to dilute the acidic fluid aspirated.

A chest x-ray may be useful to show the presence of large amounts of aspirated material (usually in the right lower lobe) and as a baseline, although a normal appearance does not exclude aspiration. In 25% of cases, there are no visible changes seen on x-ray. Patients suspected of having aspirated should be observed and monitored carefully for at least 12–24 hours since their condition may worsen considerably during this time.

Key points

- Aspiration of gastric contents is a major factor in maternal death associated with general anaesthesia, especially related to emergency caesarean section and difficult tracheal intubation.
- Prevention includes sensible policies on feeding in labour, use of pH-raising drugs and antacids, emptying the stomach, rapid-sequence induction when general anaesthesia is used and avoidance of general anaesthesia by encouraging regional anaesthetic techniques.
- Diagnosis may not always be obvious.
- Treatment includes general supportive measures; antibiotics and steroid therapy are no longer advocated.

Further reading

Gyte GM, Richens Y. Routine prophylactic drugs in normal labour for reducing gastric aspiration and its effects. *Cochrane Database Syst Rev* 2006; (3): CD005298.

Ng A, Smith G. Aspiration of gastric contents in anaesthesia. *Anesth Analg* 2001; **93**: 494–513.

Mendelson CL. The aspiration of stomach contents into the lungs during obstetric anaesthesia. *Am J Obstet Gynecol* 1946; **52**: 191.

Awareness

Awareness is a shorthand term referring to a state of inadequate general anaesthesia, resulting in the patient's remembering all or part of a surgical procedure. It is almost exclusively associated with techniques involving the use of neuromuscular blocking drugs, when the patient is unable to move or otherwise attract attention to her plight. Awareness is not an all-or-nothing phenomenon and may range from unpleasant 'dreams' via vague memories of painful stimuli to the extreme situation where the patient is fully conscious and alert but unable to move.

Problems/special considerations

Awareness is particularly associated with anaesthesia for caesarean section and is thought to have a higher incidence in the obstetric population. This probably results from the perceived need to protect the fetus from the sedative effects of the anaesthetic agent, coupled with an exaggerated fear of the adverse effects of volatile agents upon uterine contractility. Fortunately, pregnancy reduces anaesthetic requirements by as much as 40%, or complaints of awareness would probably be more common.

The incidence of awareness is dependent upon the anaesthetic technique being used. Before the early 1970s it was common practice to avoid volatile agents altogether and use a 50:50 mixture of nitrous oxide and oxygen; not surprisingly this led to maternal awareness in 12–26% of cases. The addition of a low concentration of a volatile agent (e.g. isoflurane 1%) reduces this to less than 1%. The effect of these concentrations upon uterine contractility is minimal and, even at 1.5 minimum alveolar concentration (MAC) the uterus will respond normally to oxytocic drugs.

The need for adequate fetal oxygenation during caesarean section has led to the use of higher inspired concentrations of oxygen (and therefore less nitrous oxide) than for other surgical procedures and this also has an impact on the depth of anaesthesia. There is little evidence to support the use of more than 30% oxygen for delivery of the unstressed fetus, but when fetal distress is present, 50% or even 100% oxygen has been advocated. The loss of the anaesthetic contribution of nitrous oxide and the second-gas effect mean that higher concentrations of volatile agent should be used throughout these cases, and the initial concentration should be higher still (overpressure) to drive up the alveolar concentration quickly.

The contribution of opioid drugs to the anaesthetic should not be ignored, and part of the explanation for the high incidence of awareness during obstetric anaesthesia lies in the common practice of withholding these drugs until after the baby is delivered. This also has adverse consequences for cardiovascular stability during tracheal intubation, and there is an increasing tendency to use a modest dose of short-acting drugs such as fentanyl and alfentanil to obviate both of these problems.

Even minor degrees of awareness can lead to significant long-term psychological morbidity, typified by 'waking dreams', difficulty in sleeping, depression, and fear of hospitals and doctors. Full-blown post-traumatic stress disorder may also occur.

In addition to awareness, inadequate anaesthesia may result in release of catechol- . amines, which further decrease placental perfusion and promote fetal hypoxia.

Management options

It has been recommended by some authorities that patients undergoing general anaesthesia for a caesarean section should be warned about the risk of awareness, but this is not widely practised. It is advisable to warn women that they may wake up with a 'tube in their throat' so that their memory of this is less likely to be confused with intraoperative awareness.

Some incidents of awareness may be clearly traced back to a technical problem with the anaesthetic apparatus, vaporiser faults being the most common. When checking the anaesthetic machine, correct seating of the chosen vaporiser on its mount and adequate filling should be ensured. The anaesthetist should be familiar with the breathing system and ventilator and understand how air or oxygen can be entrained into the system and how the inspired concentration of volatile agent can be lower than that set on the vaporiser (e.g. a circle system). A volatile agent monitor is now considered mandatory.

There is no guaranteed 'sleep' dose of an induction agent, and the drug must be titrated against the patient's response, bearing in mind that it will be responsible for maintaining anaesthesia throughout the onset of neuromuscular blockade and tracheal intubation. Factors such as obesity will influence the induction dose that is used. Thiopental is probably still considered the drug of choice for induction, and the anaesthetist should have 6 mg/kg available in the syringe. It has been suggested that propofol is more likely to be associated with awareness than thiopental because of its shorter duration of action (for example during prolonged attempts at tracheal intubation). One particular risk associated with thiopental is that it is easily mistaken for antibiotic, and vice versa; concern has been raised that recent guidelines advocating administration of prophylactic antibiotics before skin incision could lead to the preparation of two very similar-looking syringes at a time of potential stress, increasing the chance of a drug error.

Volatile agents with a low lipid solubility will achieve alveolar-inspired equilibrium most quickly. Isoflurane is the best of the 'established' agents, but desflurane and sevoflurane are commonly used now as a result of their more rapid onset times. Concentrations representing at least 0.5 MAC should be used during the procedure and this should be higher if the inspired nitrous oxide concentration is less than 60%. An overpressure of 1.5–2 MAC should be employed in the first 2–3 minutes if a more soluble agent is being used.

The patient should be closely watched for signs of lightening anaesthesia (tears, sweating), and the monitors should be observed frequently for evidence of sympathetic overactivity (tachycardia, hypertension). Some practitioners advocate the use of specific monitors of anaesthetic depth, but these have not been evaluated yet in obstetrics and none has so far been shown to be any more effective than simply watching vital signs (Table 55.1). A meticulous record should be kept, which should include vaporiser settings and end-tidal volatile concentrations, if available.

A generous dose of a suitable opioid drug should be given directly after cord clamping and the volatile agent left on until the skin is being sutured. It is better to wait a few minutes at the end of the operation rather than risk awareness.

Table 55.1 Methods for monitoring depth of anaesthesia

Clinical signs – PRST score (pressure, rate, sweating, tears)
Isolated forearm technique
Lower oesophageal contractility
Skin resistance
Evoked auditory/somatosensory potentials
Electroencephalogram/cerebral function analysing monitor and derivations thereof (e.g. bispectral
index, entropy)

All mothers undergoing general anaesthesia for caesarean section should be followed up within 24 hours of delivery and questioned about dreaming or sensation during the operation. The psychological sequelae of awareness can be minimised by a sympathetic approach. Many such patients complain that medical staff do not believe them when they first report that they have memories of the operation; this can exacerbate the degree of trauma, so all such complaints should be taken seriously and handled at a senior level. Midwives should be alert to the possibility of awareness and ensure early referral to an anaesthetist. Early referral to a psychologist with experience of post-traumatic stress disorder is desirable.

Some patients will mistake their memory of awake extubation for true intraoperative awareness. This risk can be minimised by careful preoperative explanation, but any markers as to the timing of such memory should be sought in order to reassure the patient if possible. Just because true awareness did not occur does not mean that the patient will not be traumatised.

Key points

- Clinical signs are still the best indicator of awareness.
- A clinically effective concentration of volatile agent, suitably monitored, should be used at all times.
- Patients should be warned about awake extubation.
- Complaints of awareness should be treated seriously and sympathetically.

Further reading

Paech MJ, Scott KL, Clavisi O, *et al.* A prospective study of awareness and recall associated with general anaesthesia for caesarean section. *Int J Obstet Anesth* 2008; **17**: 298–303.

Robins K, Lyons G. Intraoperative awareness during general anesthesia for cesarean delivery. *Anesth Analg* 2009; **109**: 886–90.

Air embolism

Subclinical entry of air into the circulation has been shown with Doppler techniques to occur in up to 60% of caesarean sections (possibly more if the head-down position is used or if the uterus is exteriorised), although the significance of circulating microscopic bubbles is uncertain. It has been suggested that chest pain or ST segment depression occurring during caesarean section under regional anaesthesia may be related to air in the coronary circulation, although both are frequently unaccompanied by Doppler demonstration of bubbles. Large amounts of air may cause cardiovascular impairment, although this is less common (up to 2%); the mechanism is obstruction of right ventricular output by the presence of compressible gas within the contracting ventricle. In addition, bubbles may lodge in the pulmonary circulation, increasing dead space, whilst paradoxical embolism may occur there is a patent foramen ovale (a probe-patent foramen is found in about 30% of 'normal' hearts on routine autopsy) or other right-to-left shunt.

Although most cases are related to caesarean section, it should not be forgotten that air embolism may occur whenever open veins are above the level of the heart, e.g. when central venous lines are manipulated with the patient in the sitting position or when the arm in which a peripheral venous cannula has just been placed is held aloft to prevent spillage of blood; both are more likely to occur when staff are inexperienced in the management of intravenous lines, as may (unfortunately) occur on the labour ward. Finally, the danger of accidental intravenous injection of air, e.g. when pressurising devices are used with air-containing bags of intravenous fluid or when bubbles are allowed into intravenous infusion lines, must not be forgotten. In patients with right-to-left shunts, even small bubbles may have disastrous systemic effects.

Problems/special considerations
- The diagnosis may not be clear, especially at first. Clinical features are fairly non-specific and include hypotension, tachycardia, reduced arterial saturation and reduced end-expiratory carbon dioxide concentration (during general anaesthesia), the last firstly because of reduced cardiac output and hence return of carbon dioxide from the tissues and secondly because of increased pulmonary dead space. There may be an audible churning sound on cardiac auscultation, although this is usually only present in massive air embolism. Paradoxical embolism may result in systemic infarction of vital organs, especially heart and brain.
- The differential diagnosis of air embolism therefore includes any cause of cardiovascular impairment or collapse, at least initially; a high level of awareness is thus required. In particular, amniotic fluid embolism or thromboembolism may cause the same initial right ventricular outflow obstruction. If it occurs during regional anaesthesia, it may mimic hypotension produced by anaesthesia-induced sympathetic blockade. Doppler or

ultrasound detection is the gold standard in diagnosing air embolism, but most units do not have the necessary equipment to hand. It may be possible to aspirate bubbles from the right ventricle or atrium via a central venous catheter, but inability to do so does not exclude the diagnosis.

- Manoeuvres for preventing further embolism and managing the current embolism (as described below) may be difficult to carry out midway through a caesarean section, especially if the patient is awake and distressed. In addition, some of the traditional advice concerning positioning of the patient is self-contradictory (head-up for prevention of further embolism; head-down for its management).

Management options

- Prevention of further embolism is important as soon as the diagnosis is considered. This includes immediately informing the obstetrician, who should return the uterus to the abdomen if possible, flood the surgical field with saline and look for open veins (the ability to do this will obviously depend to some extent on the stage of surgery). Positioning the patient head-up is generally suggested to raise the level of the heart and increase venous pressure in the pelvis and abdomen.

- Damage limitation is generally achieved by reducing the size of the bubble(s); this is done firstly by stopping any nitrous oxide that is being administered and secondly by attempting to remove air from the circulation, or more specifically from the right side of the heart. It may be possible to aspirate air from a routine central venous cannula or catheter; special wide-bore multi-perforated cannulae are manufactured specifically for this task but are not generally available on many labour wards. The head-down position is traditionally required for central venous cannulation, and the left lateral head-down position is advised for isolation of the bubbles away from the right ventricular outflow tract and easier aspiration of air. Both of these positions may compromise the advice given above, and moving to the left lateral position is at best awkward in the middle of surgery.

- Further management consists of general supportive treatment (increased concentration of inspired oxygen, vasopressor/inotropic drugs, intravenous fluids) and basic resuscitative measures as appropriate. If the baby has not yet been delivered, the cardiovascular effects of air embolism will be exacerbated by aortocaval compression; thus lateral displacement of the uterus is especially important and delivery should be expedited.

It has been suggested that caesarean section should always be performed in the head-up position to reduce the incidence of air embolism; however, this has implications for the incidence and effects of hypotension following regional anaesthesia and for the spread of spinal blockade. It has also been suggested that Doppler or ultrasound monitoring (trans-thoracic or oesophageal) should always be available during caesarean section, but this is hampered by the lack of equipment and expertise in its use.

Key points

- Air embolism occurs in up to 60% of caesarean sections as detected by Doppler studies.
- Air embolism may cause cardiovascular collapse if large.
- Management includes general resuscitation, preventing further embolism and removal of air already in the circulation.

Chapter

57

Induction and augmentation of labour

Induction of labour (IOL) is the artificial commencement and stimulation of labour and involves the ripening of the cervix, artificial rupture of the membranes (ARM) and stimulation of uterine contractions. It is indicated when delivery of the baby before spontaneous labour occurs is in the best interests of the mother or fetus, or both.

Augmentation of labour is used where the normal progression of labour is too slow.

Induction of labour

The indications for IOL are shown in Table 57.1.

Once the decision to induce labour has been made, the ease of induction is usually assessed by using the Bishop score, based on the result of pelvic examination. A low Bishop score indicates that the cervix is unfavourable and will need to be ripened. This is usually achieved by vaginal dinoprostone (PGE_2), which may be repeated at intervals of 12–24 hours depending on the change in the Bishop score. This process may take more than 48 hours. Misoprostol has also been used to induce labour, but is currently only used in women who have an intrauterine fetal death.

Surgical induction of labour (ARM) is performed if the cervix is favourable or following cervical ripening with prostaglandins. This stimulates labour and allows the colour of the liquor to be assessed and a fetal scalp clip electrode to be applied to monitor the fetal heart, both of which give information about the wellbeing of the fetus.

Table 57.1 Indications for induction of labour

Fetal reasons	Prolonged pregnancy
	Intrauterine growth retardation
	Multiple pregnancy
	Unstable lie
	Infection
	Rhesus disease
	Lethal fetal abnormality
	Intrauterine death
Maternal reasons	Pregnancy-induced hypertension
	Essential hypertension
	Other maternal disease, e.g. renal, malignant
	Antepartum haemorrhage
	Poor obstetric history, e.g. previous stillbirth

Oxytocics (Syntocinon) are usually an integral part of the management of IOL, and therapy is normally commenced after ARM has been performed.

Augmentation of labour

Augmentation of labour is used when labour is not proceeding at the standard rate (see Chapter 19, Normal labour) or when there has been premature rupture of membranes without signs of labour after 12–24 hours. It is usually done by ARM (if intact) and/or oxytocics.

Problems/special considerations

- The most common complications of IOL are:
  (i) Prolapse of the cord
  (ii) Abruption of the placenta
  (iii) Acute fetal distress – particularly when ARM is performed in the presence of polyhydramnios
  (iv) Hyperstimulation of uterine contractions – tetanic contraction may cause acute fetal distress
  (v) Postpartum haemorrhage associated with uterine atony.
- Complications of augmentation are as above; in addition there is an increased risk of infection if the membranes have been ruptured for some time.
- Induction of labour is often prolonged and may be particularly tiring and painful; therefore epidural analgesia should be discussed as part of the labour management, as well as the above complications. Contractions augmented by oxytocic drugs are more painful. There may also be maternal or fetal reasons for the advisability of epidural analgesia, e.g. pregnancy-induced hypertension.
- Induction of labour may not be successful and since there has been a commitment to deliver the baby these women may need to be delivered by caesarean section.
- Induction of labour is often associated with a high-risk pregnancy.
- Induction of labour increases the strengths of the contractions, which are therefore more painful.
- There is an increased risk of precipitous labour and instrumental delivery.

Further reading

Mozurkewich EL, Chilimigras JL, Berman DR, et al. Methods of induction of labour: a systematic review. BMC Pregnancy Childbirth 2011; 11: 84.

Mozurkewich E, Chilimigras J, Koepke E, Keeton K, King VJ. Indications for induction of labour: a best-evidence review. BJOG 2009; 116: 626–36.

National Institute for Health and Clinical Excellence. Induction of labour. Clinical Guideline 70. London: NICE 2007, http://guidance.nice.org.uk/CG70.

Oxytocic and tocolytic drugs

Oxytocic drugs are used to promote uterine contractions whereas tocolytic drugs relax the uterus. Both groups of drugs are widely used in obstetric practice.

Oxytocic drugs

These drugs may be given during labour to augment progress, at delivery and in the puerperium to reduce postpartum haemorrhage and aid expulsion of the placenta and at earlier stages of pregnancy to help empty the uterus, e.g. following evacuation of retained products of conception or termination of pregnancy.

Although the third stage of labour can be managed without oxytocic drugs ('physiological management of the third stage'), it is common practice to give an oxytocic to all women at childbirth, usually on delivery of the anterior shoulder (vaginal delivery) or following delivery of the baby (caesarean section). In most units, the drug used is either a mixture of oxytocin analogue and ergometrine (vaginal delivery) or oxytocin analogue alone (caesarean section), although local practice varies.

- *Oxytocin analogues:* The most widely used is Syntocinon; its effects resemble those of natural oxytocin, released from the posterior pituitary gland. Oxytocin causes milk ejection from the lactating breast and acts directly on specific oxytocin receptors in the uterine myometrium, increasing the force and frequency of contractions. In early pregnancy, the uterine receptors are present in small numbers and their sensitivity is low; thus there is little value in giving the drug for operative procedures in early pregnancy, although this is commonly done. Syntocinon may cause vasodilatation and tachycardia; the latter is especially likely if the intravenous route is used, if large doses are given (> 5 U) by bolus injection and if other drugs causing tachycardia (e.g. ephedrine) are given concurrently. These effects can be disastrous in patients with fixed cardiac output states, e.g. aortic stenosis. A potential problem with prolonged Syntocinon therapy during labour is related to its antidiuretic effect, which may result in excessive water retention, compounded by excessive fluid administration if infused in weak solution over a long period of time. This has resulted in hyponatraemia and convulsions, hence the recommendation that Syntocinon should be diluted in physiological saline rather than dextrose solutions. The half-life of Syntocinon is approximately 10 minutes, another reason for giving it by infusion at caesarean section.

  Carbetocin is a longer-acting oxytocin analogue, otherwise similar to Syntocinon. It is more expensive than Syntocinon and not routinely used in most units.

- *Ergometrine:* This acts on smooth muscle generally; thus it may cause vasoconstriction and hypertension (both systemic and pulmonary) and increased central venous pressure. It may also cause severe vomiting, and bronchospasm has been reported. It is therefore avoided in women with hypertensive disease. It is commonly given intramuscularly together with oxytocin analogue (Syntometrine; 5 U Syntocinon and 500 μg ergometrine) at vaginal delivery. Intravenous administration (125–250 μg, repeated if necessary) may be useful in severe postpartum haemorrhage and has now been recommended by the Confidential Enquiries into Maternal Deaths to be the second-line agent in these situations. It increases the force, frequency and duration of uterine contractions.

- *Prostaglandins:* Gemeprost (PGE$_1$) is given vaginally to soften and ripen the cervix before termination of pregnancy or to induce abortion. Dinoprostone (PGE$_2$) has also been used for this purpose but is more commonly used to induce labour. Both may cause nausea, vomiting, pyrexia, diarrhoea, bronchospasm and hypertension (especially dinoprostone, which may also cause uterine hypertonus and fetal distress. The occurrence of bronchospasm and hypertension is despite PGE$_2$'s traditionally ascribed broncho- and vasodilator effects).

    Misoprostol has been used for medical termination of pregnancy, induction of labour and prevention/treatment of postpartum haemorrhage. The main side effects seen are shivering and pyrexia, although uterine hyperstimulation has been reported when used for induction.

    Carboprost (PGF$_2$α) is used in postpartum haemorrhage associated with uterine atony if standard oxytocics are ineffective. It is given intramuscularly (250 μg) and has been injected directly into the myometrium (off-licence); following reports of myometrial ischaemia, this mode of administration has now become obsolete. Carboprost is associated with the same side effects listed above.

    All the prostaglandins are more effective in late pregnancy, although this is thought to be related to increased sensitivity rather than increased number of receptors.

Tocolytic drugs

There are several different groups of drugs that have been used or studied as tocolytics. As with many areas of obstetric practice, their value (and even efficacy in some cases) is controversial.

- *β$_2$-adrenergic agonists:* These act on uterine β$_2$-receptors causing relaxation of myometrium. Although the most commonly prescribed tocolytics for premature labour, improvement in outcome has not been conclusively proven. The emphasis of therapy has shifted away from long-term prolongation of pregnancy towards allowing enough time for steroids to promote fetal lung maturity before delivery. The most commonly used drugs are terbutaline, salbutamol and ritodrine and these may be given orally, subcutaneously or by intravenous infusion. They may cause tremor, restlessness, hypotension, tachycardia and pulmonary oedema. The last is thought to arise from fluid overload during the infusion, together with increased pulmonary blood flow resulting from β$_2$-receptor mediated pulmonary vasodilatation, often compounded by maternal steroid administration. Careful monitoring of blood pressure, pulse and arterial oxygen saturation is required during therapy. Metabolic effects include hypokalaemia and hyperglycaemia (thus they should be used with caution in diabetics).

    Both regional and general anaesthesia may be used following β$_2$-agonist therapy; excessive fluid administration (e.g. during regional anaesthesia) should be avoided and drugs that may cause tachycardia (e.g. ephedrine) used with caution.

The drugs may also be given by intravenous bolus (salbutamol or terbutaline 100–250 μg) as part of intrauterine resuscitation of the fetus, e.g. in severe fetal distress.

- *Oxytocin antagonists (e.g. atosiban):* These bind competitively to uterine oxytocin receptors, causing dose-dependent reduction in contractions. Atosiban has been shown to be comparable with β_2-agonists in preterm labour and to have fewer side effects (although it may cause nausea, vomiting, tachycardia and hypotension), though more expensive.
- *Calcium channel antagonists:* Calcium antagonists (e.g. nifedipine) are commonly used as tocolytics as they are associated with superior efficacy and fewer side effects than other drugs. However, the safety of calcium channel antagonists has not been rigorously tested and nifedipine is still unlicensed for use as a tocolytic.
- *Glyceryl trinitrate (GTN):* This acts directly on uterine smooth muscle and has been given intravenously (50 μg boluses) or sublingually (200–400 μg) to produce acute but relatively brief uterine relaxation, e.g. in cases of uterine hypertonicity, retained placenta and uterine inversion and for external cephalic version. Similar doses have been used in severe fetal distress as above. Hypotension and headache are the main side effects. The use of GTN delivered by dermal patch has been studied as a means of preventing premature labour following premature rupture of membranes.
- *Magnesium sulphate:* This acts directly on smooth muscle via calcium ion antagonism; it is rarely used as a tocolytic in the UK although it is more commonly given for this purpose elsewhere, e.g. the US. (Anaesthetic considerations of magnesium therapy are discussed in Chapter 81, Magnesium sulphate.)

Key points

- Oxytocic drugs are used routinely during labour, following delivery, in early pregnancy and in the emergency management of postpartum haemorrhage.
- Tocolytic drugs are used in premature labour and for intrauterine resuscitation of the fetus.
- Drugs of both groups may have implications for the anaesthetist because of their side effects.

Further reading

Dyer RA, Butwick AJ, Carvalho B. Oxytocin for labour and caesarean delivery: implications for the anaesthesiologist. *Curr Opin Anesthesiol* 2011; **24:** 255–61.

Royal College of Obstetricians and Gynaecologists. Tocolytic drugs for women in preterm labour. *Green-top 1B*. London: RCOG 2011, http://www.rcog.org.uk/womens-health/clinical-guidance/tocolytic-drugs-women-preterm-labour-green-top-1b.

Vercauteren M, Palit S, Soetens F, Jacquemyn Y, Alahuhta S. Anaesthesiological considerations on tocolytic and uterotonic therapy in obstetrics. *Acta Anaesthesiol Scand* 2009; **53:** 701–9.

Chapter 59

Premature labour, delivery and rupture of membranes

Labour or rupture of membranes are defined as preterm if they occur at less than 37 completed weeks' gestation. Rupture of membranes is defined as premature if it occurs without being followed by spontaneous uterine contractions – the period of latency required before the diagnosis is made varies but is usually up to 8 hours. The term premature labour is often used interchangeably with preterm labour.

About 5–10% of deliveries are preterm in the UK, in about a third of cases without premature rupture of membranes (PROM) as the initiating event. Prematurity is a major cause of fetal and neonatal morbidity and accounts for the majority of infant deaths in the developed world. Many epidemiological studies have investigated neonatal morbidity and mortality according to birth weight instead of gestation, although there is evidence that the interplay of these two factors is more important than either one alone. For example, at a given gestation, heavier babies have less morbidity and mortality than lighter ones; similarly, at a given birth weight, mature babies do better than immature ones.

Although several risk factors for preterm delivery are recognised, about half of preterm deliveries have no obvious precipitating cause. Known risk factors include: a previous history of prematurity; young maternal age; maternal disease (especially infection), surgery or trauma; uterine abnormality; stress; smoking and use of recreational drugs; multiple gestation; placenta abnormality; and fetal disease.

Problems/special considerations

- *Diagnosis:* Careful obstetric assessment is required to establish the diagnosis of PROM since it is not always obvious. Amniotic fluid can be tested for by using special reagent sticks (nitrazine). The diagnosis of preterm labour is made according to gestation, the frequency of uterine contractions and changes in cervical dilatation or effacement. In some countries (not routinely in the UK) fetal maturity is assessed by the lecithin–sphingomyelin (LS) ratio, which increases as surfactant production increases and may indicate the likelihood of respiratory distress syndrome.

- *Maternal problems:* Prolonged rupture of membranes may lead to chorioamnionitis with or without systemic features of infection. Thus there may be theoretical risks from regional anaesthesia (see Chapter 135, Pyrexia during labour, and Chapter 130, Sepsis).

  Administration of tocolytic drugs may result in tachycardia, fluid overload and pulmonary oedema (see Chapter 58, Oxytocic and tocolytic drugs). Tachycardia may also be related to maternal sepsis and anxiety; the latter may be considerable because of the mother's fears for her baby.

  Any underlying cause of preterm labour or PROM (such as maternal disease) may have implications for the anaesthetic management.

The best method of delivery is controversial, but operative delivery rate is higher than for term deliveries. Breech presentation is more common. Classical caesarean section may be required if the lower uterine segment is poorly formed (uncommon after 26 weeks' gestation), with a greater risk of haemorrhage and other complications.

- *Neonatal problems:* These can be short- or long-term. The immediate problems for the neonate are respiratory distress (occurring in approximately 50–60% of babies at 26–28 weeks, 20–40% at 30–32 weeks and 5–10% at 34–36 weeks), hypoglycaemia and intracranial haemorrhage. The last may be related to trauma during delivery although it may also occur postpartum in severe respiratory distress. The neonate is more likely to require resuscitation. Necrotising enterocolitis and patent ductus arteriosus are also more common in premature neonates. Long-term problems include cerebral palsy (in around 20% of babies born at 22–26 weeks, with 7% severe), neurodevelopmental delay and chronic lung disease. If maternal infection is suspected, neonatal screening is performed since infection may also be present in the baby. Survival rates are approximately 40–45% for babies born at 24 weeks, and 80% for babies born at 26 weeks. It should be remembered that even with modern neonatal intensive care, the neonate has a greater risk of morbidity when born at 35–36 weeks than at 37–38 weeks.

Management options

Management includes finding the cause and ensuring that the timing of delivery is optimised. Steroids are given to the mother to aid maturation of the fetal lungs. Since steroids require 24 hours to become optimally effective, delivery is usually delayed for this period if possible. Tocolytic drugs are commonly used in an attempt to prevent or stop labour, but their use is controversial since the evidence suggests that although they may delay labour, they do not improve perinatal outcome. Antibiotics have been shown to reduce the incidence of preterm labour in women with PROM. Delivery is required in the presence of chorioamnionitis or fetal distress, although the precise mode of delivery is controversial. Since the preterm infant is more susceptible to intracranial haemorrhage, the need to prevent trauma during delivery often leads to caesarean section although the benefit of this is unproven.

Anaesthetic options are discussed more fully under the relevant related topics. In general, regional analgesia is often preferable in labour and is considered safe in the absence of systemic features of infection and if antibiotic cover has been provided, since it provides good conditions for a controlled delivery and can be readily extended for instrumental delivery. If caesarean section is required, regional anaesthesia may offer the parents their only chance to see and hear their baby free of tubes, etc. if the chance of neonatal survival is poor. In addition, neurobehavioural and physiological outcome is better in premature neonates when regional anaesthesia is used than with general anaesthesia. It is important to appreciate the dangers of concurrent tocolytic therapy with any anaesthetic technique. The preterm fetus is especially vulnerable to the adverse effects of maternal hypotension.

Key points

- 5–10% of deliveries in the UK are preterm.
- Potential maternal problems are those of fever and sepsis, use of tocolytic drugs and the increased requirement for instrumental delivery and anaesthetic intervention.
- Fetal and neonatal problems are those of prematurity, infection and the increased need for neonatal resuscitation.

Further reading

Royal College of Obstetricians and Gynaecologists. Antenatal corticosteroids to reduce neonatal morbidity. *Green-top 7*. London: RCOG 2010, http://www.rcog.org.uk/womens-health/clinical-guidance/antenatal-corticosteroids-prevent-respiratory-distress-syndrome-gree.

Royal College of Obstetricians and Gynaecologists. Preterm prelabour rupture of membranes. *Green-top 44*. London: RCOG 2010, http://www.rcog.org.uk/womens-health/clinical-guidance/preterm-prelabour-rupture-membranes-green-top-44.

Simhan HN, Canavan TP. Preterm premature rupture of membranes: diagnosis, evaluation and management strategies. *BJOG* 2005; **112** (Suppl 1): 32–7.

Simhan HN, Caritis SN. Prevention of preterm delivery. *N Engl J Med* 2007; **357**: 477–87.

Chapter

60

Malpresentations and malpositions

Definitions

Lie – the relationship of the long axis of the fetus to that of the mother, e.g. longitudinal, transverse, oblique.

Presentation – the part of the fetus that is foremost in the birth canal, e.g. cephalic, breech or compound.

Position – the relationship of the presenting part of the fetus, using a reference point such as the occiput or sacrum, to the maternal pelvis, e.g. left occipito-anterior (LOA) or right sacral transverse (RST).

Approximately 85% of fetuses at term lie longitudinally, with a cephalic presentation in an occipito-anterior position. A malpresentation is anything that does not fulfil these criteria.

Problems/special considerations

The malpresenting fetus is less likely to deliver spontaneously, and instrumental or operative intervention is often required. Labour is often prolonged and particularly painful. Although it has been suggested that epidural analgesia may increase the likelihood of malpresentation, there is little, if any, evidence to support this view.

- *Occipito-posterior:* This is the commonest malpresentation, occurring in 10% of term pregnancies. Progress of labour may be slow, and the mother often experiences particularly severe pain in the back, which may be resistant to treatment by regional blockade. Manual or instrumental rotation may be attempted to bring the head into a more favourable occipito-anterior position

- *Breech presentation:* This occurs in 3–4% of term pregnancies and can be subdivided into frank (hips flexed and legs extended over abdominal wall), complete (hips and legs flexed) and footling (foot or knee presenting). The mother with a breech presentation may get the urge to 'push' before the cervix is fully dilated, thus running the risk of trapping the fetal head; this is a particular risk if the labour is preterm. It is becoming increasingly common for women with breech presentation to be delivered by elective caesarean section, especially if primiparous as this reduces neonatal morbidity by two thirds and mortality by three quarters. External cephalic version (ECV) is routinely offered to women with breech presentation; in this manoeuvre, the obstetrician applies external pressure to rotate the fetus to a vertex presentation (see Chapter 61, External cephalic version).

- *Transverse lie:* This occurs in 0.3% of term pregnancies and may be associated with placenta praevia, polyhydramnios and grand multiparity. Spontaneous delivery is impossible unless the lie is converted to longitudinal, which may be achieved by external version provided that placenta praevia has been excluded. Caesarean section is usually necessary, and a vertical uterine incision may be needed to aid delivery.

- *Face and brow presentations:* These are rare presentations, where the head is hyperextended. A face presentation may deliver vaginally, but caesarean section is often needed.

- *Prolapsed cord:* Cord prolapse occurs in 0.4% of cases when the vertex is presenting, but this incidence rises to 0.5% in frank breech, 4–6% in complete breech and 15–18% in footling presentations. It is generally more common when the fetus does not fully occlude the pelvic inlet, as in preterm labour, and may follow artificial rupture of the membranes with a high presenting part. If immediate vaginal delivery is not feasible, the presenting part is pushed and held out of the pelvis to prevent cord compression, often aided by steep head-down tilt, while the mother is transferred to theatre for immediate caesarean section.

Management options

Good regional analgesia is desirable at an early stage since intervention is more likely to be required. If there is breakthrough pain, e.g. with an occipito-posterior position, addition of an epidural opioid such as fentanyl may improve pain relief, although more concentrated solutions of local anaesthetic than those used in 'low-dose' techniques may be required.

If vaginal delivery of a breech presentation is planned, epidural analgesia will help prevent premature 'pushing' and will enable controlled manipulation, extensive episiotomy and application of forceps to the aftercoming head.

For cord prolapse requiring caesarean section, general anaesthesia is usually the quickest option, although extension of a pre-existing epidural block or institution of spinal anaesthesia is also possible (see Chapter 67, Prolapsed cord).

Key points

- Regional analgesia is particularly indicated in malpresentation.
- Prolapsed cord is often associated with breech and transverse presentations and preterm delivery.
- Early multidisciplinary communication will help optimise management.

Further reading

Hannah ME, Hannah WJ, Hewson SA, *et al.* Planned caesarean section versus planned vaginal birth for breech presentation at term: a randomised multicentre trial. *Lancet* 2000; **356**: 1375–83.

Royal College of Obstetricians and Gynaecologists. Management of breech presentation. *Green-top 20b.* London: RCOG 2006, http://www.rcog.org.uk/womens-health/clinical-guidance/management-breech-presentation-green-top-20b.

Chapter

61

External cephalic version

External cephalic version (ECV) is a procedure performed to convert a breech or shoulder presentation into a cephalic one by manipulating the fetus through the mother's abdominal wall and anterior wall of the uterus. Its reported success rate is 30–80%, and Royal College of Obstetricians and Gynaecologists guidance suggests that overall success rates of 40% for nulliparous women and 60% for multiparous women should be possible.

Problems/special considerations

ECV is usually attempted at 36–37 weeks' gestation; a fetus at earlier gestation is more likely to revert to a breech presentation subsequently since there is more room available to it, and since the procedure carries a risk of premature delivery a more mature gestation is preferable. On the other hand, the larger the fetus the more difficult it may be to achieve successful version, especially if the presenting part is engaged.

Contraindications include multiple pregnancy (although ECV is occasionally used to turn the second twin), antepartum haemorrhage, placenta praevia, ruptured membranes, fetal abnormalities and factors that indicate caesarean section. Previous caesarean section, intrauterine growth retardation, pre-eclampsia and obesity are controversial relative contraindications. The mother should be nil-by-mouth in case a complication occurs. The fetus is monitored continuously, and with the mother in the tilted supine position, talcum powder is applied to the abdominal wall and rotationary pressure applied to the fetus whilst attempting to lift the presenting part out of the pelvis. Tocolytic drugs, e.g. β_2-agonists, may be given. There may be considerable discomfort, particularly if the mother is especially tense, which reduces the chance of success. Various maneouvres have been used in an attempt to improve the success and tolerability of ECV, including sedation (e.g. with benzodiazepines) and regional analgesia, although many obstetricians consider the degree of discomfort a useful indicator of when to stop the attempted procedure and prefer to avoid the use of adjuncts. In the UK, anaesthetists are rarely involved, although meta-analysis suggests that the success rate can be significantly improved with regional analgesia. A maximum of 10 minutes is usually allowed before considering the attempt at version unsuccessful.

Apart from discomfort, complications of ECV include maternal or fetal bradycardia, onset of labour and placental abruption, with about 0.5% of cases requiring immediate caesarean section. It should also be remembered that breech presentation is more common in fetuses with other congenital abnormalities and in placenta praevia or uterine abnormalities.

Management options

From the anaesthetic viewpoint, awareness that ECV is being planned is usually the main issue, since anaesthetic input may be required at short notice. However, anecdotal experience suggests that many obstetricians perform ECV in clinics, wards or the delivery suite without routinely informing anaesthetists.

Key points

- External cephalic version has a reported success rate of 30–80%.
- Analgesia or sedation may occasionally be required.
- Regional analgesia improves the success rate but is uncommonly used in the UK.
- Complications include fetal distress, onset of labour and haemorrhage.

Further reading

Goetzinger KR, Harper LM, Tuuli MG, Macones GA, Colditz GA. Effect of regional anesthesia on the success rate of external cephalic version: a systematic review and meta-analysis. *Obstet Gynecol* 2011; **118**: 1137–44.

Hutton EK, Hofmeyr GJ. External cephalic version for breech presentation before term. *Cochrane Database Syst Rev* 2006; (1): CD000084.

Royal College of Obstetricians and Gynaecologists. External cephalic version (ECV) and reducing the incidence of breech presentation. *Green-top 20a*. London: RCOG 2006, http://www.rcog.org.uk/womens-health/clinical-guidance/external-cephalic-version-and-reducing-incidence-breech-presentation.

Sultan P, Carvalho B. Neuraxial blockade for external cephalic version: a systematic review. *Int J Obstet Anesth* 2011; **4**: 299–306.

Multiple pregnancy

The incidence of multiple pregnancy has increased owing to an increase in assisted conception programmes, although twins, triplets and quadruplets also occur naturally. The natural incidence of twins is 1:80 pregnancies, triplets 1:8000 and quadruplets 1:800 000. The obstetric anaesthetist has an important part to play in the management of these deliveries.

Problems/special considerations

The mother carrying a multiple pregnancy experiences all the minor pregnancy complaints in excess. She will be more likely to be very uncomfortable and to suffer from backache, heartburn and varicose veins. Often she will be dyspnoeic at rest or on minor exertion and she may be unable to lie on her back because of supine hypotension; it is often difficult to relieve aortocaval compression except in the full lateral position. She is also more prone to the following complications:

- Anaemia (real and dilutional)
- Pregnancy-induced hypertension
- Intrauterine growth retardation
- Malpresentations
- Premature labour
- Prolonged labour
- Malpresentation of the second twin after delivery of the first twin
- Postpartum haemorrhage (because of uterine atony and the large placental site)
- Intrauterine death.

Management options

Twins may be delivered vaginally although the labour and delivery may not be straightforward and the above factors should be considered. Epidural analgesia is recommended; firstly it will provide excellent analgesia for what may be a long labour requiring oxytocic drugs, and secondly – and most importantly – the epidural can be used if there are problems with the second twin. Malpresentation of the second twin may require external or internal version and/or operative delivery, including caesarean section (which may be required in approximately 10%). The anaesthetist should be present for the delivery of twins to ensure that the epidural block is adequate for these manipulations. The second stage is usually conducted in the operating theatre. If caesarean section is indicated for the second twin, the anaesthetist must be able to extend the epidural block for the operation. Some anaesthetists advocate extending the epidural to produce a block suitable for caesarean section in all cases of twins, in case surgery is required. In rare instances, general anaesthesia may be required for the delivery of the second twin.

Many twins and nearly all triplets and quadruplets are booked for delivery by elective caesarean section, although because premature labour is more common, caesarean section is often performed as a non-elective procedure. The indications for twins to be delivered by elective caesarean section include malpresentation of the first twin, previous caesarean section, poor obstetric history (which may include assisted conception) and maternal request.

Regional anaesthesia is considered preferable for caesarean section in multiple pregnancy. Great care must be taken when performing regional anaesthesia in these women to ensure that supine hypotension is avoided. A Syntocinon infusion is usually set up post-delivery.

Key points

- Women with multiple pregnancies are an 'at-risk' group.
- The anaesthetist should be actively involved with the care of these women whether they are in labour or not.
- Special care is required to avoid aortocaval compression.
- There is increased likelihood of premature or prolonged labour, instrumental delivery and postpartum haemorrhage.

Further reading

National Institute for Health and Clinical Excellence. Multiple pregnancy: the management of twin and triplet pregnancies in the antenatal period. *Clinical Guideline 129.* London: NICE 2011, http://www.nice.org.uk/CG129.

Royal College of Obstetricians and Gynaecologists. Management of monochorionic twin pregnancy. *Green-top 51.* London: RCOG 2008, http://www.rcog.org.uk/womens-health/clinical-guidance/management-monochorionic-twin-pregnancy.

Chapter

63

Trial of scar

Trial of scar is the term used for the trial of labour in a woman who has a scar on her uterus. The scar has usually resulted from a lower segment caesarean section, but may also be from a hysterotomy or myomectomy. Traditionally, a previous classical caesarean section has been considered a contraindication to a trial of scar, but there are many reports of this being done successfully. In the USA and increasingly in the UK, vaginal delivery after a lower segment caesarean section is commonly called VBAC (vaginal birth after caesarean).

Problems/special considerations

- Risk factors for unsuccessful trial of scar are induction of labour, high BMI and no previous vaginal delivery. A previous vaginal delivery is the single biggest predictor of success.
- A trial of scar would be considered if the reason for the scar was not a recurrent obstetric problem, such as cephalopelvic disproportion. The major anxiety is rupture of the uterine scar, particularly during strong uterine contractions. The incidence of uterine rupture is ~3–4 per 1000 cases. The risk is thought to be increased if prostaglandins are used for the induction of labour although Syntocinon, which is more controllable, is not usually considered contraindicated.

    Features of uterine rupture are:

    (i) Fetal compromise
    (ii) Hypotension
    (iii) Tachycardia
    (iv) Intrapartum bleeding
    (v) Cessation of labour.

    If uterine rupture occurs, urgent delivery is required.
- There is a 25–30% likelihood of a repeat caesarean section if the reason for the previous caesarean section is non-recurrent.
- There have been anxieties that epidural analgesia may mask the pain of uterine dehiscence. However, pain is not a constant feature of uterine rupture and may be absent in 10% of cases. In addition, severe pain may be present in the absence of uterine rupture. Finally, the pain of uterine rupture has been reported to 'break through' analgesia provided by modern, low-dose epidural techniques. In fact, many would consider epidural analgesia indicated in trial of scar since it may be readily converted to anaesthesia suitable for caesarean section if required (unless there is uterine rupture, in which case there may not be time to extend the epidural).

Management options

Women undergoing trial of scar (and often, their obstetricians) should have the potential advantages and disadvantages of regional analgesia explained to them. Pain that breaks through low-dose epidural analgesia or is present between contractions should raise the possibility of uterine dehiscence.

Key points

- Uterine rupture is the most important complication of trial of scar and occurs in ~3–4 cases per 1000.
- Epidural analgesia has previously been considered to be contraindicated but may have advantages.
- Pain in the presence of a working epidural may be a warning of impending uterine rupture.

Further reading

American College of Obstetricians & Gynecologists. ACOG Practice bulletin no. 115: Vaginal birth after previous cesarean delivery. *Obstet Gynecol* 2010; **116**: 450–63.

Cahill AG, Odibo AO, Allsworth JE, Macones GA. Frequent epidural dosing as a marker for impending uterine rupture in patients who attempt vaginal birth after cesarean delivery. *Am J Obstet Gynecol* 2010; **202**: 355.e1–5.

Guise JM, Denman MA, Emeis C, *et al.* Vaginal birth after caesarean: new insights on maternal and neonatal outcomes. *Obstet Gynecol* 2010; **115**: 1267–78.

Royal College of Obstetricians and Gynaecologists. Birth after previous caesarean birth. *Green-top 45.* London: RCOG 2007, http://www.rcog.org.uk/womens-health/clinical-guidance/birth-after-previous-caesarean-birth-green-top-45.

Chapter

64

Under-age pregnancy and advanced maternal age

Under-age pregnancy refers to pregnancy in girls under the age of consent (16 years in the UK). The term 'elderly' is applied to parturients over the age of 35. The UK has one of the highest teenage pregnancy rates in Europe, whereas the incidence of older women becoming pregnant is increasing in the developed world as a result of both maternal choice and infertility treatment.

Problems/special considerations

Under-age pregnancy

Those girls who are under-age when they present in pregnancy can be placed in the following groups:

- Those who have had normal antenatal care and have the full support of their family. This group usually have a parent available to give consent on behalf of the minor if that is felt appropriate, e.g. for epidural analgesia or for anaesthesia.
- Concealed pregnancy. This group may pose a problem with consent. Many will have had little or no antenatal care and may present to the hospital for the first time when they are in labour. Many present in advanced labour or to the Accident and Emergency Department with a life-threatening condition such as eclampsia, and there may not be time to find a parent or guardian before instituting treatment.

Overall, this is an 'at-risk' group who often need considerable support, including epidural analgesia.

Hypertension, anaemia, premature labour and low birth weight are all more common in under-age mothers.

Advanced maternal age

Miscarriage, fetal chromosomal abnormalities, multiple pregnancy, hypertension, ischaemic heart disease, diabetes, instrumental delivery, neonatal mortality and postpartum haemorrhage are more common in elderly mothers, who feature disproportionately in the Reports on Confidential Enquiries into Maternal Deaths.

Management options

In under-age mothers, it is important to remember at all times that the minor is the patient and must be involved in the decision making. In line with the Mental Capacity Act (in England and Wales), the child may make the decisions for her treatment if deemed competent. This may involve epidural analgesia and/or regional anaesthesia. Ideally, the support and consent of a parent or guardian should be sought although this may not be practical.

Elderly mothers require no special management other than an appreciation of the increased risks associated with advanced age. These women too should be considered an 'at-risk' group.

Key points

- Both under-age and elderly mothers are at-risk groups and have a higher incidence of complications.
- For minors, parental consent should be obtained when possible; if none is available, treatment should not be denied.
- Elderly mothers should be managed as routine, but the increased risk of complications should be remembered.

Further reading

Cleary-Goldman J, Malone FD, Vidaver J, et al. Impact of maternal age on obstetric outcome. *Obstet Gynecol* 2005; **105**: 983–90.

Joseph KS, Allen AC, Dodds L, et al. The perinatal effects of delayed childbearing. *Obstet Gynecol* 2005; **105**: 1410–18.

Placenta praevia

The placenta usually implants in the fundus of the uterus. An abnormally low placenta may be classified in many different ways:

- Low-lying (the placenta lies in the lower uterine segment); partial placenta praevia (partially overlies the cervical os); or total placenta praevia (fully overlies the os).
- Grade 1 (placenta is low-lying); grade 2 (reaches the os); grade 3 (asymmetrically covers the os); or grade 4 (symmetrically covers the os).
- Minor (leading edge of the placenta is in the lower uterine segment but not covering the os); or major (placenta lies over the os).

These classifications may be further subdivided into anterior or posterior. A low-lying placenta is noted in about 5% of early ultrasound scans, but most of these have moved into the fundus by the third trimester, and this finding is thus only regarded as significant after 27 weeks' gestation. The incidence at term is ~1:200–250. It occurs more frequently in mothers who have previously delivered by caesarean section (incidence is ~10% after four caesarean sections), and is also associated with increased parity, increasing maternal age and multiple gestation.

Vasa praevia refers to the presence of fetal vessels lying within the membranes over the os, unprotected by placental tissue or the umbilical cord, associated either with a velamentous cord insertion or a multi-lobed placenta. It occurs in 1:2000–6000 pregnancies.

In addition to the above, the placenta may be morbidly adherent; the terms placenta accreta, increta and percreta are used to describe placental penetration through the uterine decidua, into the myometrium, and through the myometrium, respectively. The incidence is ~1:2500 overall, increasing to ~5–9% in placenta praevia, 25–30% in placenta praevia with previous caesarean section, and 40–50% in placenta praevia with two previous caesarean sections.

Problems/special considerations

- *Diagnosis:* Antenatally, transabdominal ultrasound may suggest a low-lying placenta and its position may be more accurately identified by transvaginal ultrasound. High-resolution ultrasound, magnetic resonance imaging and colour flow Doppler imaging may define the degree of invasion of the placenta, although none is totally accurate.

  The mother who presents with late bleeding should undergo urgent ultrasonography to determine the position of the placenta. The differential diagnosis is of placental abruption, in which bleeding is normally accompanied by abdominal pain and tenderness. If there is uncertainty as to whether vaginal delivery is possible, then an examination in theatre may be performed with a view to proceeding to immediate caesarean section if necessary.

- *Presentation:* Placenta praevia usually presents as painless bleeding, with the first bleed commonly occurring at 27–32 weeks' gestation. Occasionally, bleeding may not be apparent until the mother goes into labour, which is more likely to be preterm. If there has been recurrent bleeding, the mother is usually kept in hospital, with cross-matched blood continuously available.

  Vasa praevia may present as abrupt onset of bleeding with rupture of the membranes and, since blood loss is entirely fetal, is associated with a high perinatal mortality.
- *Mode of delivery:* Although lesser degrees of placenta praevia, where the placenta does not encroach on the os, may be managed conservatively, caesarean section is the normal method of delivery. When the mother is actively bleeding, emergency caesarean section and delivery of the placenta may be essential to preserve the life of the mother and the baby. Placenta praevia may interfere with the development of the usually thin lower uterine segment and thus increase blood loss. Occasionally it may be necessary for the obstetrician to divide an anterior placenta praevia in order to gain access to the fetus, and this is usually accompanied by very heavy blood loss. If the placenta is morbidly adherent, placental separation may be difficult or even impossible to achieve, and torrential haemorrhage may occur, which can only be controlled by removing the uterus.

Management options

Immediate resuscitation

Management of the bleeding mother should follow basic principles of resuscitation. Two large-bore peripheral cannulae should be inserted and blood taken for haemoglobin estimation and emergency cross-match. The possibility of disseminated intravascular coagulation should be borne in mind if blood loss is very heavy, and coagulation factors should be replaced (fresh frozen plasma, cryoprecipitate, platelets) according to local haematological guidelines for massive transfusion.

Caesarean section

The presence of one or more consultant anaesthetist(s) and obstetrician(s) is mandatory for caesarean section with placenta praevia; other specialists (e.g. vascular surgeon, urologist) may be required for extreme cases of placenta percreta. Preparations should be made for major blood loss; this might include cell salvage, especially in elective cases.

Placenta praevia has commonly been regarded as an indication for general anaesthesia, because of the risk of heavy, uncontrolled bleeding. Regional anaesthesia has traditionally been contraindicated because of the perceived risk of vasodilating the patient who is, or is about to become, hypovolaemic.

However, in recent years, the use of regional anaesthesia in these circumstances has become more acceptable, and many senior anaesthetists would consider a regional technique for caesarean delivery, depending on each individual situation. Points that would tend to favour this approach would be a posterior placenta that will not interfere with delivery (although bleeding from a posterior placental bed may be more difficult to control), no or little active bleeding, prior cardiovascular stability, and a low risk of placenta accreta (no previous sections). However, the mother and her partner should be informed that conversion to general anaesthesia may occur. The patient who is bleeding heavily, who has an anterior placenta, or with a history of previous caesarean sections, may be best managed with general anaesthesia.

Recently, interventional radiology has been used in the prophylactic management of placenta praevia and accreta. In the elective situation, balloon catheters may be inserted prophylactically in the internal iliac/uterine arteries (or even aorta) via the femoral arteries before caesarean section, with a view to inflating the balloons should uncontrolled haemorrhage occur. The place of this technique is uncertain, largely because randomised trials have not been (and are unlikely to be) done, and there are risks associated with catheter placement. An alternative is to place femoral artery sheaths through which balloon or embolisation catheters can be passed should they be required subsequently. In the emergency situation, embolisation procedures may be performed after angiography to identify the bleeding vessels and this may be life-saving, though also not without risks – not least those associated with transferring a potentially unstable patient to the radiology suite.

Occasionally, when there are signs of acute placental insufficiency, the risks to the fetus of waiting for cross-matched blood must be balanced against the risk to the mother of proceeding without it; these are decisions that must be taken coolly and rationally, with full consultation between the parties.

Key points

- The chances of placenta accreta increase with number of previous caesarean sections.
- The risk of massive haemorrhage should be assessed when choosing an anaesthetic technique.
- Senior staff should be involved in obstetric and anaesthetic management.

Further reading

Heidemann B. Interventional radiology in the treatment of morbidly adherent placenta: are we asking the right questions? *Int J Obstet Anesth* 2011; **20**: 279–81.

Kuczkowski KM. A review of current anesthetic concerns and concepts for cesarean hysterectomy. *Curr Opin Obstet Gynecol* 2011; **23**: 401–7

Lilker SJ, Meyer RA, Downey KN, Macarthur AJ. Anesthetic considerations for placenta accreta. *Int J Obstet Anesth* 2011; **20**: 288–92.

Royal College of Obstetricians and Gynaecologists. Placenta praevia, placenta praevia accreta and vasa praevia: diagnosis and management. *Green-top 27*. London: RCOG 2011, http://www.rcog.org.uk/womens-health/clinical-guidance/placenta-praevia-and-placenta-praevia-accreta-diagnosis-and-manageme.

Sadashivaiah L, Wilson R, Thein A, *et al*. Role of prophylactic uterine artery balloon catheters in the management of women with suspected placenta accreta. *Int J Obstet Anesth* 2011; **20**: 282–7.

Snegovskikh D, Clebone A, Norwitz E. Anesthetic management of patients with placenta accreta and resuscitation strategies for associated massive hemorrhage. *Curr Opin Anesthesiol* 2011; **24**: 274–81.

Placental abruption

Placental abruption is defined as premature placental separation and occurs in around 1% of pregnancies. Major degrees of abruption have an incidence of 0.2%, with a perinatal mortality of 50%.

Risk factors for abruption are a previous history of abruption, an overdistended uterus (twins, polyhydramnios), pre-eclampsia, multiparity, greater maternal age, smoking, trauma and use of cocaine.

Problems/special considerations

- *Presentation:* The usual clinical picture is of bleeding in the third trimester which, unlike the differential diagnosis of placenta praevia, is associated with abdominal pain due to uterine distension. The uterus commonly starts contracting and this will exacerbate the underlying pain. The diagnosis of abruption is clinical, supported by ultrasound. Minor degrees of abruption may be diagnosed retrospectively after an uneventful delivery. Abruption that is retroplacental, as opposed to at the edge of the placenta, may be concealed; these patients may present with a hard, tense abdomen, hypovolaemic shock and even disseminated intravascular coagulation.
- *Blood loss:* It is easy to underestimate blood loss in abruption, especially if the membranes have not ruptured, since much of the bleeding will be concealed. Cardiovascular changes occur late, probably because of the sympathetic activity engendered by abdominal pain and because patients are generally young and fit.
- *Coagulopathy:* Coagulopathy is an early development in placental abruption, since coagulation factors are rapidly consumed by the intrauterine clot. Where abruption is severe enough to cause fetal death, the risk is as high as 50%. The risk of amniotic fluid embolism is also thought to be increased, especially in severe cases.

Management options

Management is dependent upon whether the fetus is still alive at presentation and upon the wellbeing of the mother. If there is no evidence of placental insufficiency, then the mother may be allowed to labour, with careful fetal and maternal monitoring. Basic fluid resuscitation is essential, and platelet count, coagulation tests and fibrin degradation products should be measured on admission and at regular intervals. Regional analgesic techniques are not contraindicated, but normovolaemia and unimpaired coagulation are of paramount importance if they are to be used. Blood should be cross-matched and available.

Early artificial rupture of the membranes may reduce the risk of coagulopathy and amniotic fluid embolism.

When the fetus has already died, then vaginal delivery is the technique of choice. Particular attention should be paid to the risk of coagulopathy.

Caesarean section

Caesarean section is indicated if there is fetal or maternal compromise. As with placenta praevia, general anaesthesia is the method of choice in the mother with cardiovascular decompensation, and should also be used in the presence of clotting disorders. If an epidural catheter is already *in situ*, then this should be used to provide anaesthesia unless there are major contraindications. Unlike placenta praevia, where the mother may be put at risk if caesarean section is carried out before blood is available, there are benefits for both fetus and mother in operating without delay in the case of abruption; coagulopathy may be prevented and the risk of causing massive bleeding by having to cut through the placenta is not an issue.

After delivery

Postpartum haemorrhage is far more common following abruption. This may arise as a result of coagulopathy or because the uterus fills with blood and cannot contract (Couvelaire uterus).

Key points

- Blood loss may be underestimated in abruption.
- Coagulopathy is common.
- Caesarean section should not be delayed once the mother has been resuscitated.

Further reading

Ananth CV, Oyelese Y, Yeo L, Pradhan A, Vintzileos AM. Placental abruption in the United States, 1979 through 2001: temporal trends and potential determinants. *Am J Obstet Gynecol* 2005; **192**: 191–8.

Oyelese Y, Ananth CV. Placental abruption. *Obstet Gynecol* 2006; **108**: 1005–16.

Tikkanen M. Placental abruption: epidemiology, risk factors and consequences. *Acta Obstet Gynecol Scand* 2011; **90**: 140–9.

Prolapsed cord

Cord prolapse occurs when the umbilical cord prolapses through the birth canal ahead of the presenting part, often before the cervix is fully dilated. It is generally more common when the fetus does not fully occlude the pelvic inlet and may follow artificial rupture of the membranes with a high presenting part. The incidence is 0.4% when the vertex is presenting, but this incidence rises to 0.5% in frank breech, 4–6% in complete breech and 15–18% in footling presentations.

Problems/special considerations

Prolapsed cord is a true obstetric emergency, since the almost invariable result is compression of the cord by the presenting part of the fetus, which effectively cuts off its own blood supply. Delivery must be achieved very rapidly to prevent hypoxic–ischaemic damage to the fetus, ideally within a few minutes of prolapse.

By definition, there is usually little, if any, warning of a cord prolapse. It usually occurs during procedures such as assessment of progress or artificial rupture of membranes, when it is detected by the appearance of the cord through the introitus, but it may present spontaneously as acute, severe fetal distress or the mother noticing 'something coming down'.

Management options

The successful management of prolapsed cord requires that there is a well established mechanism for performing immediate caesarean section with a minimum of notice. Guidelines should be established for handling emergencies of this nature. Regular simulated drills will highlight weak points in the process and ensure that all staff are familiar with their roles. Well recognised areas of delay include transfer of the patient to the operating theatre, gathering the theatre team, and waiting for inappropriate investigations or cross-matched blood.

The other danger of the need for rapid delivery is that important preparations may be overlooked in the rush, for example anaesthetic assessment, antacid premedication and removal of dentures. Damage to the bladder may occur if it is not emptied preoperatively.

However rapidly delivery can be achieved, every effort should be made to relieve the occlusion of the umbilical cord by manually lifting the presenting part off the cord. This can be difficult, and may be helped by maintaining a steep head-down tilt until delivery is imminent. Rapid transfer of the patient in this position, especially with a midwife supporting the fetus with her hand inside the birth canal, can be very fraught indeed. Instillation of saline into the bladder via a catheter has been claimed to assist this manoeuvre.

General anaesthesia

Caesarean section in these circumstances is often best managed by induction of general anaesthesia. It is a fast and reliable technique, and the manoeuvres needed to relieve the pressure on the cord often preclude positioning the patient for a *de novo* regional block. If general anaesthesia is to be used, a preoperative airway assessment is mandatory. If a problem with intubation is anticipated, the anaesthetist may have to make the difficult decision – in conjunction with the obstetrician – of whether an attempt at regional anaesthesia is appropriate. It is impossible to give general guidance for individual cases of this nature, but the main precept is that the mother's life should take priority over the fetus's.

Steps should always be taken to protect against aspiration of gastric contents (see Chapter 54).

Regional anaesthesia

Prolapsed cord does not necessarily rule out a regional block for caesarean section, especially if the mother already has a functioning epidural *in situ*. It is obviously better to avoid the risks of general anaesthesia in the unprepared patient if possible, and many mothers express a strong wish to be awake to witness the birth of their baby, if its viability is in doubt. The obvious problem with using an epidural block is the time delay whilst it takes effect, but various recipes for rapid top-up have been described (see Chapter 33, Epidural anaesthesia for caesarean section). Even if this is not fully effective by the time the operation starts, the first 2–3 minutes of surgery before the peritoneum is manipulated can be managed with a relatively low block. It is important in these circumstances for the anaesthetist to reassure the mother constantly (and often the partner as well); good, sympathetic communication may mean the difference between failure and success.

Spinal anaesthesia is not recommended for the inexperienced but a 'rapid sequence' technique has been reported in such cases. If it is attempted, a strict time limit should be applied and the clock watched by an independent observer. If a 3-minute cut-off point is used, and the mother is preoxygenated during the spinal attempt, then no time is lost if conversion to general anaesthesia is necessary. As with epidural anaesthesia, the mother may need support during the first few minutes before the block is fully established.

Key points

- The successful management of prolapsed cord depends on good communication and well-rehearsed guidelines.
- General anaesthesia may be the best option, but the risks to the mother should be borne in mind.
- Regional anaesthesia is often possible, but should not be allowed to delay delivery.

Further reading

Kinsella SM, Girgirah K, Scrutton MJ. Rapid sequence spinal anaesthesia for category-1 urgency caesarean section: a case series. *Anaesthesia* 2010; **65**: 664–9.

Lin MG. Umbilical cord prolapse. *Obstet Gynecol Surv* 2006; **61**: 269–77.

Lin MG. Royal College of Obstetricians and Gynaecologists. Umbilical cord prolapse. *Green-top 50*. London: RCOG 2008, http://www.rcog.org.uk/womens-health/clinical-guidance/umbilical-cord-prolapse-green-top-50.

Chapter 68

Fetal distress

Fetal distress is a loosely defined term used to indicate that the baby is compromised and in need of delivery.

Problems/special considerations

The main problem is that the diagnosis of 'fetal distress' can be difficult and must take into account many clinical parameters, together with the woman's previous obstetric history and her age. Although CTG and the presence of meconium are most commonly used to indicate fetal distress, fetal heart rate changes and meconium do not always correlate with acidosis or hypoxia, and the sensitivity and specificity for predicting a poor neonatal outcome are relatively low. In particularly high-risk cases, these signs may be more significant; in such cases antenatal diagnosis of impending fetal distress may be possible, based on ultrasound scans, Doppler blood flow studies and CTG monitoring.

Fetal distress is often used as a label to hasten operative delivery. The difficulty associating intrapartum signs with outcome means that the allowable time before delivery is uncertain. At one end of the spectrum is the baby that needs to be delivered as soon as possible since there is immediate threat to the life of the fetus, e.g. placental abruption. At the other end of the spectrum the baby needs to be delivered soon but there is time to plan the delivery. Most units' guidelines call for a maximum of 15–30 minutes between the decision to deliver by caesarean section and delivery itself, for urgent (grade-1) caesarean section. However, these times are derived largely from animal experiments over 30 years ago and their relevance is arguable, especially since most cerebral palsy is now known to be related to factors arising before labour. In addition, most units find it difficult to meet these time limits.

Delivery of babies who are diagnosed as being 'distressed' before labour (see Chapter 12, Antenatal care) often need the support of the neonatal unit; thus the time and place of delivery must also take account of neonatal cot availability. For women in labour, transfer to another unit is usually not possible.

For the above reasons, the term 'fetal distress' has fallen out of favour; for example, in UK national guidance on CTG monitoring, it is not used at all, and potentially abnormal CTG patterns are described as being 'non-reassuring', 'suspicious' or 'pathological'. In practice, though, the term is still often used to indicate a potentially compromised fetus.

Management options

It is most important that there is good communication between all members of the team, the mother and her partner. In particular, obstetricians should describe the clinical situation to their anaesthetic colleagues in more detail than just saying there is 'fetal distress' – and anaesthetists must be aware of the various signs that might indicate fetal compromise, so that they can put such descriptions into context. The choice of anaesthetic technique will depend on maternal factors and the degree of urgency of the case, the onus resting with the obstetrician to indicate the latter.

Given the uncertainty of the degree of 'distress' as outlined above, many apparently 'distressed' babies are born with good Apgar scores.

The ability to improve the fetus's condition whilst preparing for delivery is often forgotten. Intrauterine resuscitation includes ensuring the mother is in the left lateral position, giving her oxygen (although there is little hard evidence that this is beneficial), giving intravenous fluids and treating any hypotension, stopping oxytocic drugs and giving tocolytic drugs such as salbutamol or terbutaline 100–250 μg intravenously or glyceryl trinitrate 50 μg intravenously or 200–400 μg sublingually.

Fetal distress is a descriptive label for a variety of diagnoses and clinical situations, but if the anaesthetist understands that all fetal distress is not a life-threatening emergency, the care of the mother will improve. There are few situations in which there is not time to institute or extend a regional block to provide regional anaesthesia. For extreme cases, general anaesthesia is often used; although not necessarily faster than a spinal anaesthetic, it is generally more reliable if more hazardous.

Key points

- 'Fetal distress' is an ill-defined term, often erroneously used.
- Signs of 'fetal distress' are poorly correlated with poor neonatal outcome.
- Degree of urgency of delivery is a useful guide for anaesthetists to plan the anaesthetic technique, although definitions are vague.
- Anaesthetists must communicate with their obstetric and midwifery colleagues.
- Intrauterine resuscitation should always be remembered.

Further reading

Committee on Obstetric Practice, American College of Obstetricians & Gynecologists. ACOG Committee Opinion. Number 326, December 2005. Inappropriate use of the terms fetal distress and birth asphyxia. *Obstet Gynecol* 2005; **106**: 1469–70.

National Institute of Health and Clinical Excellence. The use of electronic fetal monitoring: the use and interpretation of cardiotocography in intrapartum fetal surveillance. London: NICE 2001.

Thurlow SL, Kinsella SM. Intrauterine resuscitation: active management of fetal distress. *Int J Obstet Anesth* 2002; **11**: 105–16.

Yentis SM. Whose distress is it anyway? 'Fetal distress' and the 30-minute rule. *Anaesthesia* 2003; **58**: 732–3.

Shoulder dystocia

Shoulder dystocia is an obstetric emergency and is defined as impaction of the fetal shoulder against the mother's symphysis pubis after the head has been delivered. The incidence is 0.6–1%. In 50% of cases, it is unanticipated and although it was thought to be associated with fetal weight, it may occur in fetuses with a normal birth weight. Risk factors include a previous history of shoulder dystocia, macrosomia, gestational diabetes, post-dates pregnancy and cephalopelvic disproportion. It is also associated with assisted deliveries.

It is important for obstetric anaesthetists to understand shoulder dystocia and its management, since they may be required to provide immediate assistance and prompt intervention may be lifesaving.

Problems/special considerations

- Fetal brachial plexus injury, most commonly Erb's palsy, occurs in 4–16% of cases. Most recover, usually within 6–12 months, but up to 10% of affected babies suffer some permanent damage. Humeral and clavicular fractures have also been reported.
- Fetal hypoxia may occur and if prolonged can lead to severe fetal morbidity or even death.
- Maternal soft tissue damage with extensive third or fourth degree tears have been reported. Uterine atony leading to massive obstetric haemorrhage and even uterine rupture is a complication.

Management options

Induction of labour or caesarean section is not recommended just because a woman has a history of shoulder dystocia. However, measures should be taken to anticipate this obstetric emergency if the mother has any associated risk factors.

The classic sign of shoulder dystocia is described as the 'turtle sign', in which the head appears on the peroneum and then retracts. Another is facial swelling caused by venous obstruction.

The use of the mnemonic HELPERR is encouraged in shoulder dystocia guidelines (Table 69.1).

Rarely, extreme measures such as deliberately fracturing the clavicle, maternal symphysiotomy or the Zavenelli manoeuvre (attempting to place the fetus's head back in the vagina and delivering the baby by caesarean section; it is considered a high-risk procedure for both mother and fetus) have been attempted, though their place has been questioned. Symphysiotomy is classically done under local anaesthesia but the Zavenelli manoeuvre requires general anaesthesia, which must be administered in the most difficult and fraught circumstances and therefore should not be undertaken lightly.

Table 69.1 The HELPERR mnemonic for managing shoulder dystocia

H	Call for help	
E	Evaluate for episiotomy	Episiotomy is not considered essential but may be helpful
L	Legs (McRoberts manoeuvre)	The McRoberts manoeuvre is the single most effective part of the management of shoulder dystocia, straightening the lumbosacral angle and rotating the pelvis cephalad. It has also been shown to increase intrauterine pressure and the force of contractions. The manoeuvre comprises flexion and abduction of the maternal hips, thus placing her thighs on her abdomen.
P	Suprapubic pressure	Suprapubic pressure may aid the McRoberts manoeuvre by allowing the anterior shoulder to pass under the symphysis pubis. It should be applied downwards and laterally to push the fetus's shoulder forwards i.e. towards its chest.
E	Enter manoeuvres (internal rotation)	These attempt to rotate the anterior shoulder into an oblique plane and under the symphysis pubis. A number have been described.
R	Remove posterior arm	The operator attempts to sweep the posterior arm forwards, over the fetus's chest, to make space for the body and thus release the anterior shoulder.
R	Roll the patient	The woman is placed on all fours.

Key points

- Shoulder dystocia is an obstetric emergency associated with significant fetal and maternal complications.
- Anticipation and preparation are paramount in cases where risk factors exist.
- The anaesthetist may be called upon to administer general anaesthesia in a situation which is stressful for all concerned.

Further reading

Gherman RB, Chauhan S, Ouzounian JG, et al. Shoulder dystocia: the unpreventable obstetric emergency with empiric management guidelines. Am J Obstet Gynecol 2006; 195: 657–72.

Gordon H. Shoulder dystocia. J Obstet Gynaecol 2008; 28: 371–2.

Lim GN, Gale A, Debroy B. Early resort to general anaesthesia in severe shoulder dystocia. J Obstet Gynaecol 2008; 28: 436–7.

Royal College of Obstetricians and Gynaecologists. Shoulder dystocia. Green-top 42. London: RCOG 2005, http://www.rcog.org.uk/womens-health/clinical-guidance/shoulder-dystocia-green-top-42.

Chapter 70

Intrauterine death

Most pregnancy loss occurs during the first trimester, and it is estimated that after 20 weeks' gestation fewer than 1% of all pregnancies end with fetal death. Of these, approximately a third occur with no explicable fetal or maternal cause.

Problems/special considerations

- Intrauterine death may cause major obstetric as well as psychological sequelae. It is unusual in the UK for intrauterine death to remain undiagnosed for several days but if this situation arises it is potentially life threatening, since the mother is at risk of developing disseminated intravascular coagulation (DIC) and sepsis.
- Fetal death occurring during the second half of pregnancy may be suspected by the mother when she fails to feel fetal movements. The diagnosis is confirmed by an absent fetal heartbeat on ultrasonography. In the majority of cases, the pregnancy will have been progressing apparently normally until shortly before fetal death occurs, and the diagnosis is devastating for the mother and her partner. The psychological as well as the medical wellbeing of the parents must be considered.
- Labour will normally be induced at the earliest possible opportunity after diagnosis of intrauterine death, and adequate analgesia must be provided. Tissue thromboplastin, a trigger factor for DIC, is not released from the fetus until 3–5 weeks after intrauterine death, but may be released from the placenta if there has been any placental separation. If there is intrauterine infection, this may also act as a trigger for developing a coagulopathy.
- All the potential complications of labour and delivery may occur, including slow progress in labour, difficulty with delivery and postpartum haemorrhage. Whilst the use of oxytocics is not limited by concerns about fetal welfare, the risk of overstimulating uterine contractions and causing uterine rupture must be considered, especially in the multiparous woman or the woman with a uterine scar. It may, very occasionally, be necessary for the obstetrician to perform destructive procedures to the fetus to achieve vaginal delivery, or alternatively to perform hysterotomy. Intrapartum care of the mother is stressful and traumatic for midwifery and medical staff.

Management options

Analgesia for labour should be discussed with the mother and her midwife before active labour begins. Parenteral opioids (usually diamorphine) are often used, sometimes with sedatives such as benzodiazepines. If opioid analgesia is used, consideration should be given to the use of patient-controlled analgesia.

Epidural analgesia can provide more effective pain relief without clouding maternal consciousness. Although this may appear distressing for the mother at the time, parents often appreciate memories of seeing and holding their baby. Epidural analgesia is contra-indicated if there is a coagulopathy, although DIC is rarely seen and only after the fetus has been dead for at least 1–2 weeks. Units should have guidelines on the management of these women, including the need for coagulation studies.

The anaesthetist should be aware of the possible risks of uterine rupture and postpartum haemorrhage in multiparous women.

Following delivery, the parents are usually encouraged to see and hold their dead baby. Photographs of the baby should be taken and kept with the medical records even if the parents do not wish to see the baby. The obstetric and midwifery staff should ensure that help is available for registering the stillbirth, discussing post-mortem examination and making any funeral arrangements.

Intrauterine death of one twin is a recognised risk of monochorionic twin pregnancy. Recommended management is usually conservative, although there have been recent reports that early delivery (by hysterotomy) of the dead twin improves outcome for the remaining twin. The psychological sequelae for both the parents and the surviving twin may be particularly difficult to deal with and may persist into the surviving twin's adult life.

Key points

- Intrauterine death is devastating for the parents; it is often completely unexpected and occurs towards the end of an apparently normal pregnancy.
- Standard obstetric management is induction of labour, with the aim of achieving vaginal delivery whenever possible.
- The obstetric anaesthetist should be able to advise about suitable analgesia and be available to deal with any complications of vaginal delivery.
- The situation demands the highest standard of communication skills and sensitivity from all medical and midwifery staff.

Further reading

Royal College of Obstetricians and Gynaecologists. Late intrauterine fetal death and stillbirth. *Green-top 55*. London: RCOG 2010, http://www.rcog.org.uk/womens-health/clinical-guidance/late-intrauterine-fetal-death-and-stillbirth-green-top-55.

Uterine inversion

Uterine inversion is a rare but potentially fatal complication of pregnancy. It may be incomplete or complete, depending on whether the fundus is delivered through the cervix. Nearly all occur within 24 hours of birth, although subacute (up to 4 weeks) and chronic forms have also been described.

The incidence is said to be between 1 in 2000 and 1 in 50 000 deliveries; this variation is thought to relate to the management of the third stage of delivery. Uterine inversion is more likely to occur when vigorous fundal pressure or cord traction is exerted before adequate placental separation. Coughing and vomiting and fundal insertion of the placenta are all thought to contribute to the risk of uterine inversion.

Problems/special considerations

Uterine inversion is an obstetric emergency. The presentation of the uterus through the cervix, usually with the placenta still attached, causes pain and severe vagal shock, the most important manifestation of which is bradycardia. This is often followed by severe haemorrhage.

Management options

Initial treatment is aimed at basic resuscitation, including intravenous fluids (including blood), oxygen and atropine to treat the bradycardia when indicated.

Replacement of the uterus should take place as soon as possible, since oedema quickly develops in the extruded uterus, hampering efforts to return it to its correct position. Urgent manual replacement may be successful without general anaesthesia in the first few minutes after the patient has collapsed, but general anaesthesia is usually required and should not be delayed. In the absence of shock or haemorrhage, regional anaesthesia may be suitable. Manual replacement of the uterus may be facilitated by uterine relaxation (see Chapter 58, Oxytocic and tocolytic drugs). Traditionally, deep halothane anaesthesia was used but this was associated with marked hypotension and prolonged uterine atony; more recently glyceryl trinitrate or β-adrenergic agonists have been used.

If the above method is not successful, hydrostatic pressure may be considered. In this technique, warm isotonic fluid is allowed to run into the uterus. Up to 5 litres of fluid may be required; therefore, there is a risk of systemic absorption. An open abdominal method of treatment has also been described but this is rarely required.

After the uterus has been replaced, oxytocic drugs are required straight away. It is important to remember that the relaxant effects of tocolytic drugs may persist for some time.

Key points

- Uterine inversion may present with collapse, severe bradycardia and haemorrhage.
- Anaesthesia is usually required for replacement of the uterus.
- Uterine relaxation may be required to enable its replacement.
- Good communication between anaesthetists and obstetricians is essential, with minimal delay in initiating treatment.

Chapter

72

Major obstetric haemorrhage

Successive Reports on Confidential Enquiries into Maternal Deaths have highlighted major obstetric haemorrhage as a significant direct cause of maternal mortality, although in the 2006–2008 recent report, there was a slight decrease in the number of deaths attributable to bleeding. In many cases, care is substandard: women at particular risk of haemorrhage are not identified beforehand, or else management is inadequate when bleeding does occur. A similar situation exists in other countries, especially developing ones, where haemorrhage is one of the leading causes of death, often related to a lack of resources.

Obstetric haemorrhage may be antepartum or postpartum. The most common causes of antepartum bleeding are placenta praevia and placental abruption. Postpartum haemorrhage is most commonly associated with uterine atony, trauma to the genital tract, ruptured uterus and caesarean section.

Problems/special considerations

- The extent of bleeding may be underestimated because it is concealed, for example in the vagina or bedclothes, between the legs (at caesarean section) or within the abdomen, or mistaken for bloodstained amniotic fluid.
- Pregnant women are generally healthy and tolerate blood loss well. The patient may therefore remain cardiovascularly stable even when there has been a significant decrease in her circulating blood volume. Consequently, the presence of hypotension, tachycardia and vasoconstriction in an obstetric patient represents severe hypovolaemia.
- Apparently moderate bleeding in obstetric patients may rapidly progress to major haemorrhage.

- Coagulopathy may be an underlying cause of haemorrhage, but severe haemorrhage may also result in impaired coagulation. Previously, coagulopathy as a result of haemorrhage was thought to be largely dilutional and although this may occur, it is thought that coagulopathy develops also as a result of a rapid consumption of clotting factors, in particular fibrinogen, as occurs in trauma. In certain conditions (e.g. placental abruption), disseminated intravascular coagulation may also occur.

Management options

The anaesthetist's first priority is resuscitation of the patient, but the management of major haemorrhage must involve the whole delivery suite as a team. The diagnosis and treatment of the cause of bleeding should be carried out during the primary resuscitation. The blood lost must be replaced urgently, and time should not be wasted placing monitoring lines. It is increasingly considered that blood products should be given early, as in trauma, and although baseline blood tests may be sent to the laboratory, resuscitation should not be delayed and/or based on the results of samples that have been sent 30–60 minutes previously. Many protocols for major obstetric haemorrhage have changed to follow those used in the armed forces where red cells and clotting factors are given in a ratio of 1:1 or 2:1. Since there is evidence that fibrinogen levels fall rapidly early on in obstetric haemorrhage, it has been suggested that cryoprecipitate or fibrinogen concentrate be given early.

If a surgical procedure is required (e.g. examination under anaesthesia, removal of retained placenta, caesarean section, hysterectomy, etc.), the presence of severe hypovolaemia combined with a possible coagulopathy usually precludes regional anaesthesia.

When major haemorrhage continues, aortic compression, uterine or internal iliac artery occlusion/ligation or hysterectomy (which may be life saving) should be considered. Embolisation of the uterine arteries under radiological control has been used but this requires special expertise.

Intraoperative cell salvage is well described now in obstetrics and the risk of infusing amniotic fluid into the mother's circulation is no longer a major concern. However, the benefit of using the intraoperative cell saver has been questioned in the emergency situation for obstetric haemorrhage; surveys in the UK have shown that the return of salvaged blood is often minimal and that its use is limited by the lack of availability of equipment and staff trained in its use. In addition, by the time it is set up much of the potentially salvageable blood may already have been lost.

Although the use of recombinant activated factor VII (rFVIIa; usual dose 75–100 µg/kg) in intractable haemorrhage has been reported, it is no longer advocated routinely as there have been case reports of thromboembolic events and also of non-responders. If it is given, any existing coagulopathy should be corrected first. Tranexamic acid (usual dose 0.5–1 g) has been advocated and has the advantages of being relatively cheap and non-prothrombotic.

Major obstetric haemorrhage guidelines must be available on all delivery suites and should be rehearsed regularly by all the delivery suite staff. Guidelines are published and recommended in the Confidential Enquiries reports although they may be adapted for local use. The guidelines should be brief, easily understood, with standard abbreviations and restricted to one A4 sheet so that they can be readily referred to in an emergency (Table 72.1).

Table 72.1 Example of a major obstetric haemorrhage guideline

Aims	To resuscitate the patient To treat the cause
Inform/summon	Obstetrician (including senior staff) Anaesthetist (including senior staff) Midwives Anaesthetic assistants and porters Haematologist (including senior staff)
Initial resuscitation	Airway/oxygenation Circulation (including 2 x 14 G intravenous cannulae)
Initial blood sample	Full blood count Coagulation screen/TEG/fast fibrinogen Cross-matching for at least six units of blood
Initial monitoring	Pulse rate Blood pressure Pulse oximetry
Initial fluids	Colloid usually recommended until blood ready In dire emergency, uncross-matched blood Patient's own ABO and Rh group if possible Uncross-matched O Rh negative if immediate transfusion is required
Subsequent monitoring	Central venous pressure Direct arterial blood pressure Arterial blood gas analysis Urine output Temperature
Specific obstetric management	May require general anaesthesia
Subsequent blood samples	As above, for assessment and guidance of therapy
Subsequent fluids	Blood/blood products according to condition. Fluids must be administered through warming equipment. A pressure bag or a rapid infusor device is required
Subsequent management	Early transfer to an intensive care unit should be considered

It is good practice for a delivery suite to have all the equipment that may be needed for massive haemorrhage collected together for easy access, preferably on a mobile trolley that can be quickly wheeled to the patient's bedside. This trolley should be checked and stocked on a daily basis.

Key points

- Obstetric haemorrhage continues to be a major contributor to maternal mortality.
- Major haemorrhage guidelines should be in place in all delivery suites and should be regularly rehearsed.

Further reading

Allam J, Cox M, Yentis SM. Cell salvage in obstetrics. *Int J Obstet Anesth* 2008; **17**: 37–45.

Bell SF, Rayment R, Collins PW, Collis RE. The use of fibrinogen concentrate to correct hypofibrinogenaemia rapidly during obstetric haemorrhage. *Int J Obstet Anesth* 2010; **19**: 218–23.

Cotton BA, Au BK, Nunez TC, *et al.* Predefined massive transfusion protocols are associated with a reduction in organ failure and postinjury complications. *J Trauma* 2009; **66**: 41–8.

Mercier FJ, Bonnet MP. Use of clotting factors and other prohemostatic drugs for obstetric hemorrhage. *Curr Opin Anesthesiol* 2010; **23**: 310–16.

Su LL, Chong YS. Massive obstetric haemorrhage with disseminated intravascular coagulopathy. *Best Pract Res Clin Obstet Gynaecol* 2012; **26**: 77–90.

Wise A, Clark V. Challenges of major obstetric haemorrhage. *Best Pract Res Clin Obstet Gynaecol* 2010; **24**: 353–65.

Chapter

73

Postpartum haemorrhage

Placental separation involves the sudden exposure of a vascular bed receiving up to 20% of the maternal cardiac output. Prevention of potentially massive haemorrhage requires contraction of uterine and arteriolar muscle, activation of circulating and endothelial clotting factors and platelet aggregation and deposition.

Postpartum haemorrhage (PPH) occurs in 2% of deliveries and is defined as a blood loss of over 500 ml after delivery of the placenta. A PPH occurring within 24 hours of childbirth is termed a primary PPH. A secondary PPH occurs within the next 6 weeks and is due to retained products of conception and/or infection.

Postpartum haemorrhage can be one of the most frightening obstetric emergencies and may be associated with maternal mortality.

Problems/special considerations

- There are a number of different causes of PPH (Table 73.1). Although initial management is the same (i.e. resuscitation), subsequent management depends on the cause, which may be difficult to ascertain in the face of continuing haemorrhage.
- After a normal delivery, attention is often focused on the baby, and thus moderate PPH may be unnoticed initially. This is compounded by the ability of normal pregnant women to compensate until hypovolaemia is severe (see Chapter 72, Major obstetric haemorrhage).

Table 73.1 Causes of postpartum haemorrhage

Obstetric	Uterine atony	Previous history of PPH
		Large placental site, e.g. multiple pregnancy
		Long or precipitous labour
		Prolonged oxytocic infusion
		Grandmultiparity
		Chorioamnionitis
		Retained products (placenta or membranes)
		Inverted or ruptured uterus
		Drugs, e.g. volatile anaesthetic agents, tocolytic drugs
	Trauma to the cervix, birth canal or perineum	
Non-obstetric	Primary coagulopathy, e.g. von Willebrand's disease	
	Secondary coagulopathy, e.g. disseminated intravascular coagulopathy, HELLP syndrome, post-massive transfusion coagulopathy, drugs	

- There may be few medical and midwifery staff in close attendance if PPH occurs without warning, especially following a spontaneous vaginal delivery in a delivery room. The severity of blood loss may be underestimated in such circumstances, and there may be a delay in resuscitation unless staff are well versed in the emergency management of such cases.

Management options

The first priority of the anaesthetist arriving at a PPH is resuscitation, followed by urgent assessment of the cause of bleeding.

The extent of haemorrhage is often underestimated. Any woman who has an unexplained tachycardia or a hypotensive episode in the postpartum period should be treated as having had a major blood loss until proven otherwise.

The most common cause of PPH is uterine atony. It is routine practice to administer oxytocics at the delivery of the anterior shoulder of the baby (see Chapter 58, Oxytocic and tocolytic drugs). This hastens placental separation and encourages uterine contraction in the third stage of labour. If the uterus fails to contract and bleeding continues, further oxytocic drugs may be given (Table 73.2), aided by manual rubbing of the uterus to stimulate contraction. If the uterus continues to relax, the possibility of retained products of conception should be considered, which necessitates exploration of the uterus. A retained placenta may involve the whole or part of the placenta, and manual removal of the placenta is indicated.

Genital tract trauma should be sought and this may require anaesthesia. Ideally, primary resuscitation of the patient, together with confirmation of preparation of blood for transfusion, should be established before anaesthesia is administered. It is often necessary to proceed to anaesthesia before the blood is available.

If there is continued uterine bleeding, the abdomen needs to be opened. Hysterectomy may sometimes be avoided by packing the uterus or using an intrauterine balloon, compression (B. Lynch) sutures, and ligation or embolisation of the uterine or internal iliac arteries or use of intravascular balloon catheters (depending on the expertise and proximity of the radiology department). Recent evidence suggests the incidence of peripartum

Table 73.2 Prevention and drug treatment of uterine atony causing postpartum haemorrhage (PPH)

Routine prophylaxis	Syntometrine (5 U Syntocinon with 0.5 mg ergometrine) intramuscularly at delivery of the anterior shoulder
PPH occurs	Syntocinon 5–10 U given slowly, intravenously, or an infusion containing 40–50 U Syntocinon/500 ml saline at a rate depending upon the clinical response but usually over a 4-h period
PPH persists	Ergometrine 125–250 µg intravenously, repeated as necessary
PPH unresponsive to the above	Carboprost (PGF2α) 250 µg given by deep intramuscular injection, repeated at intervals of ≥ 15 minutes, up to a total dose of 2 mg (8 doses). Direct injection into the myometrium is not recommended
Various*	Misoprostol 200–800 µg depending on the route: oral, sublingual, vaginal, rectal and intrauterine administration has been described

* Use of misoprostol may vary according to local protocols but it has been used to prevent as well as treat PPH.
N.B. Consider retained placenta, genital tract trauma and other causes of haemorrhage.
See Chapter 72, Major obstetric haemorrhage, for general management of haemorrhage.

hysterectomy in the UK is 4–5 per 10 000 births (ranging from 1:30 000 for a first vaginal delivery, through 1:220 for a third caesarean section, to 1:32 for placenta praevia).

Key points

- Any postpartum haemorrhage must be seen as a potential major obstetric haemorrhage and should be treated early and aggressively.
- Senior help should be sought at an early stage.
- Full resuscitation should not be regarded as being complete until the cause of the bleeding has been identified and treated.

Further reading

Ahonen J, Stefanovic V, Lassila R. Management of post-partum haemorrhage. *Acta Anaesthesiol Scand* 2010; **54**: 1164–78.

Kayem G, Kurinczuk JJ, Alfirevic Z, *et al.* Specific second-line therapies for postpartum haemorrhage: a national cohort study. *BJOG* 2011; **118**: 856–64.

Knight M; UKOSS. Peripartum hysterectomy in the UK: management and outcomes of the associated haemorrhage. *BJOG* 2007; **114**: 1380–7.

Liabsuetrakul T, Choobun T, Peeyananjarassri K, *et al.* Treatment for primary postpartum haemorrhage. *Cochrane Database Syst Rev* 2007; (1): CD003249.

Royal College of Obstetricians and Gynaecologists. Prevention and management of postpartum haemorrhage. *Green-top 52*. London: RCOG 2009, http://www.rcog.org.uk/womens-health/clinical-guidance/prevention-and-management-postpartum-haemorrhage-green-top-52.

Royal College of Obstetricians and Gynaecologists. The role of emergency and elective interventional radiology in postpartum haemorrhage. *Good Practice No. 6*. London: RCOG 2007, http://www.rcog.org.uk/womens-health/clinical-guidance/role-emergency-and-elective-interventional-radiology-postpartum-haem.

Collapse on labour ward

Although uncommon, collapse of a mother in the delivery suite may represent serious underlying pathology and demands rapid treatment; the mother may also rapidly respond to relatively simple measures, thus avoiding disaster.

Problems/special considerations

The management of a collapsed mother on the labour ward presents a challenge to all staff concerned. Typically, labour ward staff are less familiar with emergency equipment and drugs than staff in the operating theatres, so continuous support and education of staff is required; regular 'drills' have been recommended, though this may be difficult in a busy and possibly understaffed unit. In addition, the labour ward is often situated in an isolated or remote area of the hospital, so access to other key clinical areas, e.g. radiology suite and ICU, is not easy. Finally, pregnant women are usually fit and healthy and often clinical deterioration may occur unnoticed.

Collapse on labour ward may have several causes, some of which require specific investigation and/or management (Table 74.1).

Management options

Initial resuscitation in the undelivered patient is influenced by the risk of aortocaval compression and aspiration and the fact that the fetus is at risk. Thus the airway should

Table 74.1 Causes of collapse on labour ward

Cardiovascular	Haemorrhage (antenatal, e.g. placenta praevia, abruption; postnatal, e.g. splenic artery rupture)
	Regional anaesthetic sympathetic block
	Cardiac disease (congenital, acquired)
	Embolism (amniotic fluid, air, thrombus)
	Arrhythmias/vasovagal syncope
Neurological	Convulsion (eclampsia, epilepsy, local anaesthetic toxicity)
	Intracranial lesion (stroke, tumour)
Pharmacological	Local anaesthetics (toxicity, sympathetic block, total spinal)
	Opioids (systemic or especially spinal)
	Other (magnesium, antihypertensives, other sedatives, cocaine abuse, etc.)
Other	Anaphylaxis (drugs, latex)
	Airway obstruction (anaphylaxis, oedema)
	Sepsis

be secured, the lungs ventilated and the circulation supported with fluids, vasoactive drugs or cardiac massage as appropriate, with measures taken to displace the uterus or deliver the fetus if antepartum.

Concurrent with treatment is the need to determine the cause, with further management directed as appropriate.

All staff should be familiar with basic resuscitative techniques, and protocols should exist for the more important causes, e.g. eclampsia and haemorrhage. Rapid delivery of relevant information about the collapsed mother to the medical staff resuscitating her is also crucial in directing management towards a particular possible cause. This will be easier in delivery suites where there is good multi-professional communication about routine as well as problem cases.

Key points

- Collapse on labour ward has many causes including obstetric, anaesthetic and medical factors.
- Immediate management is as for the non-pregnant patient but with avoidance of aortocaval compression.

Further reading

Royal College of Obstetricians and Gynaecologists. Maternal collapse in pregnancy and the puerperium. *Green-top 56.* London: RCOG 2011, http://www.rcog.org.uk/womens-health/clinical-guidance/maternal-collapse-pregnancy-and-puerperium-green-top-56.

Chapter

75

Maternal cardiopulmonary resuscitation

Although the basic principles of cardiopulmonary resuscitation (CPR) are the same as in the non-pregnant state, the underlying causes of collapse are generally different, and the presence of the fetus has major implications for management and outcome.

Problems/special considerations

- *General management:* Because most mothers are healthy, cardiac arrest is rare in this group (estimated at 1:30 000) and thus resuscitative skills are easily forgotten, especially by those not regularly exposed to patients requiring cardiorespiratory support. There may be delay in recognising and responding to cardiorespiratory arrest. Midwives and obstetricians (and also anaesthetists) may be unfamiliar with protocols for life support and the drugs and equipment required, which may easily become faulty or out of date if not checked regularly. The maternity suite is often an unfamiliar place to the regular cardiac arrest team.

- *Cause of collapse:* In contrast to the situation in the non-pregnant population, most mothers are young and fit and thus unlikely to have ischaemic heart disease. However, the incidence of this condition has increased in recent years along with the incidence of risk factors such as older age, obesity and hypertension. In addition, cocaine abuse (especially problematic in the USA) may cause myocardial ischaemia. Most cases of peripartum cardiorespiratory arrest or collapse, however, will involve non-ischaemic causes (see Chapter 74, Collapse on labour ward). Thus actual cardiac arrest requiring artificial ventilation and cardiac massage is much more likely to be caused by hypovolaemia, embolism (with thrombus, air or amniotic fluid) and other conditions such as sepsis, electrolyte disturbances, anaphylaxis, drug abuse, etc.

- *Presence of the fetus:* In late pregnancy, CPR is ineffective if the woman is supine, and many reports have shown that outcome is improved by taking steps to avoid aortocaval compression. As long as the fetus stays within the uterus, there will thus be a conflict between the requirement for a stable and relatively supine chest in order to perform chest compressions effectively and the need to relieve aortocaval compression in order to improve cardiac output.

- *Airway management:* Depending on the gestation and particular details of the case, airway management may be difficult, as for any pregnant woman. The presence of a gravid uterus may hinder effective artificial ventilation and increase the risk of regurgitation by exerting pressure on the stomach. It may also increase the risk of injury to the liver, spleen and ribs because of the increased intra-abdominal pressure and altered shape of the chest. In addition, the fetus will consume oxygen and thus deprive the mother at a time when maternal oxygenation may be critical.

Management options

Some cases of cardiac arrest may be prevented by general training and drawing up of protocols in airway management and cardiovascular monitoring, identification of high-risk cases, good communication and organisation of facilities, equipment, etc.

All staff who work in the maternity suite must receive training and regular updates in CPR, including use of the defibrillator and other equipment. Drills have been shown to improve retention of skills although they may be very disruptive to a busy unit.

Actual management of cardiac arrest is as for the non-pregnant patient, although the different causes of collapse should be considered. The hands should be placed higher up the sternum than in the non-pregnant state, but transthoracic impedance (and thus the energy required for DC cardioversion) is the same. Relief of aortocaval compression is paramount; methods include manual displacement of the gravid uterus, placing a wedge under the mother's hip, or an assistant kneeling on the floor and using his/her thighs as a 'human wedge' under the mother's back. Cardioversion is less effective in the lateral position, as contact with the paddles and chest is reduced, but recently with the introduction of automated defibrillators, this is less problematic. If CPR is unsuccessful after 5 minutes, the fetus should be delivered by perimortem caesarean section. There are many reported cases of return of spontaneous cardiac output and maternal survival once delivery has been achieved, in cases where CPR has failed initially. Neonatal outcome is usually poor although this depends on the gestation, the cause of collapse, the delay before delivery and the effectiveness of CPR.

The risk of regurgitation and aspiration of gastric contents should be remembered and cricoid pressure applied, if hands are spare, until the trachea has been intubated.

If resumption of cardiac output does occur, there is some evidence that active hypothermia may improve neurological outcome in the non-pregnant population; as cardiac arrest in pregnancy is rare, the data are limited for this patient group.

Key points

- Ischaemic heart disease is unlikely in most mothers, and other causes (e.g. hypovolaemia, embolism) are more common.
- Regular training of staff and maintenance of equipment are required.
- Maternal cardiopulmonary resuscitation is impossible in late pregnancy unless aortocaval compression is relieved.

Further reading

Jeejeebhoy FM, Zelop CM, Windrim R, et al. Management of cardiac arrest in pregnancy: a systematic review. *Resuscitation* 2011; **82**: 801–9.

Soar J, Perkins GD, Abbas G, et al. European Resuscitation Council Guidelines for Resuscitation 2010 Section 8. Cardiac arrest in special circumstances: electrolyte abnormalities, poisoning, drowning, accidental hypothermia, hyperthermia, asthma, anaphylaxis, cardiac surgery, trauma, pregnancy, electrocution. *Resuscitation* 2010; **81**: 1400–33.

Suresh MS, LaToya Mason C, Munnur U. Cardiopulmonary resuscitation and the parturient. *Best Pract Res Clin Obstet Gynaecol* 2010; **24**: 383–400.

Vanden Hoek TL, Morrison LJ, Shuster M. 2010 American Heart Association Guidelines for Cardiopulmonary Resuscitation and Emergency Cardiovascular Care. Part 12: cardiac arrest in special situations. *Circulation* 2010; **122** (Suppl 3): S829–61.

Amniotic fluid embolism

Amniotic fluid embolism (AFE) has traditionally been estimated to occur in 1:8000–1:80 000 deliveries, the wide range reflecting the difficulty in its accurate diagnosis. More recent evidence suggests an incidence in the UK of ~1–2:100 000 births. Despite its rarity, AFE has been implicated in 10–12% of direct maternal deaths in the UK, making it one of the major causes of mortality.

The traditional explanation of AFE is that amniotic fluid enters the maternal circulation following forceful contractions, causing embolic obstruction similar to thromboembolism. However, the mechanism now proposed is systemic release of inflammatory mediators causing cardiovascular collapse, although the trigger for mediator release is still disputed (amniotic fluid, meconium, fetal cells or other substances having all been suggested). The role of amniotic fluid itself is uncertain since infusion of amniotic fluid may be well tolerated experimentally. Similarly, the traditional opinion that AFE is associated with certain risk factors, e.g. increased maternal age, induction of labour and multiparity, has been disputed Although AFE is most common during labour, it may also occur during caesarean section or even after delivery.

Problems/special considerations

Features of AFE are non-specific, including sweating, shivering, convulsions, unexplained fetal compromise (in 20% of cases), dyspnoea, cyanosis, cardiovascular collapse and disseminated intravascular coagulation (DIC). Collapse is typically profound, rapid and resistant to treatment. Thus the initial problem of AFE is its immediate management.

In addition, there are many causes of sudden collapse (see Chapter 74, Collapse on labour ward) and it may be difficult to diagnose the underlying condition. Although the diagnosis of AFE is often based on the demonstration of fetal squames in the maternal circulation or lung, this has been shown to be neither a sensitive nor a specific test, since normal mothers may demonstrate circulating fetal squames whilst 'classic' cases of AFE may not.

A final problem – and one that hinders development of effective methods of prevention and treatment – is the debate over the nature of AFE itself, even whether it represents a separate entity at all (the term 'sudden obstetric collapse syndrome' has been suggested as being more appropriate). Since the mechanism is so poorly understood, the condition remains an enigma.

Management options

Management is supportive, with basic resuscitative manoeuvres, management of bleeding and correction of DIC. There have been limited case reports of novel techniques being used successfully in the treatment of AFE, e.g. intravenous steroids, prostacyclin, plasma exchange, cardiopulmonary bypass and extracorporeal membrane oxygenation. A mortality rate of 60–80% was traditionally reported, but more recent reports suggest a lower mortality (~20%), suggesting that recognition and management of the syndrome has improved.

Key points

- Amniotic fluid embolism is probably a misnomer, but represents a catastrophic event on the labour ward.
- Features include convulsions, respiratory and cardiovascular collapse, disseminated intravascular coagulation and fetal compromise.
- There is no specific treatment but with prompt recognition and supportive therapy the prognosis is improved.

Further reading

Conde-Agudelo A, Romero R. Amniotic fluid embolism: an evidence-based review. *Am J Obstet Gynecol* 2009; **201**: 445.e1–13.

Gist RS, Stafford IP, Leibowitz AB, Beilin Y. Amniotic fluid embolism. *Anesth Analg* 2009; **108**: 1599–602.

Knight M, Tuffnell D, Brocklehurst P, Spark P, Kurinczuk JJ; UK Obstetric Surveillance System. Incidence and risk factors for amniotic fluid embolism. *Obstet Gynecol* 2010; **115**: 910–17.

Chapter

77

Cholestasis of pregnancy (obstetric cholestasis)

Cholestasis of pregnancy (intrahepatic cholestasis of pregnancy) is thought to result from an exaggerated cholestatic effect of oestrogens. It occurs in approximately 0.2% of pregnancies (except in Scandinavia and South America, where incidences of up to 10% have been reported) and is associated with multiple pregnancy. Its presenting symptom is pruritus, caused by the deposition of bile acids in the skin. Symptoms usually occur during the third trimester and may be sufficiently distressing to necessitate induction of labour. The condition is specific to pregnancy, and patients are invariably asymptomatic within 1–2 weeks of delivery. The condition tends to recur in subsequent pregnancies.

Problems/special considerations

Although symptoms usually occur in the third trimester, the condition may present at any stage of pregnancy. There is a personal or family history of jaundice whilst using the oral contraceptive pill, or during a previous pregnancy, in about 50% of cases.

Jaundice occurs in up to 50% of cases if untreated or undelivered. Clinical examination is otherwise normal except for scratch marks because of the severe itching. Fat malabsorption occurs, and the mother may complain of steatorrhoea. Malabsorption may result in vitamin K deficiency. Liver function tests reveal predominately conjugated bilirubinaemia, with markedly increased alkaline phosphatase and mildly increased transaminases.

There is an increased risk of preterm labour and fetal distress, presumed to be secondary to reduced placental blood flow or a direct effect of bile salts.

Management options

Treatment with cholestyramine, antihistamines or topical preparations has variable success. Corticosteroids have also been used, but most women are now treated with ursodeoxycholic acid, which has been shown to improve symptoms and reduce serum bile acid levels. Both the mother and the neonate should receive vitamin K therapy.

The mother's coagulation should be checked during the antenatal period and before considering insertion of an epidural or spinal needle, although coagulopathy is rare. If coagulation studies are within normal limits, the mother should be encouraged to have epidural analgesia for labour, since there is an increased incidence of caesarean section in women with cholestasis of pregnancy.

Key points

- Cholestasis of pregnancy is a benign and self-limiting condition for the mother but is associated with an increased incidence of preterm labour, fetal distress and caesarean delivery.
- Coagulopathy may occur secondary to vitamin K malabsorption.
- The only definitive treatment is delivery.
- Epidural analgesia should be encouraged unless contraindicated by coagulopathy.

Further reading

Joshi D, James A, Quaglia A, Westbrook RH, Heneghan MA. Liver disease in pregnancy. *Lancet* 2010; 375: 594–605.

Royal College of Obstetricians and Gynaecologists. Obstetric cholestasis. *Green-top 43*. London: RCOG 2011, http://www.rcog.org.uk/womens-health/clinical-guidance/obstetric-cholestasis-green-top-43.

Chapter 78

Acute fatty liver of pregnancy

Acute fatty liver of pregnancy is an uncommon (estimated 1 in 22 000 births in the UK) but serious complication of predominately primiparous women, especially those with multiple pregnancy. The condition was first reported in the literature in 1934 and traditionally the mortality for both mother and fetus has been reported to be as high as 85%. Current figures estimate maternal mortality to be about 10–20%, the improvement being attributed to earlier diagnosis and earlier delivery.

In some cases the condition may be associated with long-chain-3-hydroxyacyl-CoA dehydrogenase (LCHAD) deficiency; this is an enzyme that catalyses a reaction in the oxidation of fatty acids and if deficient, allows a build-up of fatty acids. Both parents have 50% of normal LCHAD activity and the fetus has no LCHAD activity, with the fetal liver dysfunction apparently causing fatty liver disease in the mother. Other enzyme deficiencies have also been correlated with acute fatty liver, so deficiency of LCHAD does not account for all the cases.

Symptoms usually present in the third trimester and tend to be non-specific: malaise, nausea and vomiting (which may be severe), headache and diffuse right upper quadrant or epigastric pain. Liver function may deteriorate rapidly leading to acute liver failure. There is overlap between acute fatty liver and pre-eclampsia, and it has been suggested that acute fatty liver is a manifestation of pre-eclampsia as is the HELLP (haemolysis, elevated liver enzymes and low platelet count) syndrome. It is often difficult to differentiate between HELLP and acute fatty liver.

The only treatment for acute fatty liver of pregnancy is termination of the pregnancy. As with pre-eclampsia, there may be a time lag of several days between delivery and clinical improvement.

Recovery is usually complete, with no evidence of chronic liver disease. Recurrence in subsequent pregnancies is said to be uncommon, although there have not been a large number of documented pregnancies in survivors of acute fatty liver. In cases associated with LCHAD deficiency the risk of acute fatty liver is 25% in each pregnancy.

Problems/special considerations

The differential diagnoses at initial presentation include pre-eclampsia, acute viral hepatitis, drug-induced hepatitis, cholestasis of pregnancy and biliary tract disease. Pruritus is uncommon in acute fatty liver and is highly suggestive of cholestasis.

- *Clinical examination:* The mother is usually, but not invariably, jaundiced. Although she may complain of abdominal pain it is unusual to find marked liver tenderness on examination, and this finding is suggestive of viral hepatitis or HELLP syndrome. If presentation occurs late, all the stigmata of acute liver failure may be present including hepatic encephalopathy, disseminated intravascular coagulation (DIC) and renal failure. The prognosis is poor if the disease presents in this advanced state.

- *Laboratory findings:* Serum alanine and aspartate transaminases levels are increased, but not as high as in viral hepatitis. Bilirubin is increased markedly in acute fatty liver compared with HELLP, as are uric acid and ammonia levels. Platelet counts fall, and there may be giant platelet formation. Prothrombin time is prolonged, and the more the liver damage the more deranged the coagulation profile becomes. There are reduced levels of antithrombin III, and DIC with low fibrinogen levels and increased fibrin degradation products occurs in severe disease. Haemoconcentration may occur secondary to hypovolaemia. There is frequently an increased white cell count and increased uric acid concentration. Hypoglycaemia is common.

- *Other investigations:* Liver biopsy provides confirmation of the diagnosis, but it may be contraindicated on clinical grounds. The findings are of fibrin deposition, haemorrhage and microvesicular fatty infiltration. Both computerised tomography and ultrasonography have been used with some success to demonstrate fatty infiltration of the liver.

Management options

Acute fatty liver of pregnancy is uncommon but has a high mortality if the diagnosis is delayed. A high index of clinical suspicion is needed for the non-specifically unwell mother with pre-eclampsia, especially if there is any indication that she may be jaundiced.

Once the diagnosis is confirmed the mother should be stabilised as necessary and delivered. Operative delivery is not indicated unless the obstetrician considers that successful vaginal delivery is unlikely to be achieved. Regional analgesia and anaesthesia are contraindicated in the presence of any coagulopathy.

Medical support is likely to include administration of glucose, blood, clotting factors and platelets. Hypertension associated with pre-eclampsia should be controlled. If regional analgesia is contraindicated, analgesia for labour can be provided by using cautious doses of opioid drugs, preferably by a patient-controlled intravenous route. Adjuvant sedative drugs such as promazine and promethazine should not be given. Because of impaired metabolism, atracurium is the preferred neuromuscular blocking drug for general anaesthesia. Elimination of opioid drugs is likely to be prolonged.

If operative delivery is needed, persistent bleeding from surgical sites should be anticipated and prophylactic wound drains are advisable. Close observation is essential following delivery, and intensive care management including multi-organ support may be required. Mildly affected mothers should have a low protein diet and scrupulous fluid and electrolyte management until clinical and laboratory findings return to normal.

Key points

- Acute fatty liver of pregnancy potentially has a very high mortality unless diagnosed and treated promptly.
- Some cases are caused by long-chain-3-hydroxyacyl-CoA dehydrogenase (LCHAD) deficiency and have an increased risk of recurrence.
- Delivery of the fetus is the only definitive treatment.

- Acute liver failure and multi-organ derangement can occur rapidly. Regional analgesia and anaesthesia are usually contraindicated because of abnormal clotting studies.
- Pre-eclampsia frequently co-exists with acute fatty liver, and it is possible that acute fatty liver is a variant of pre-eclampsia.

Further reading

Joshi D, James A, Quaglia A, Westbrook RH, Heneghan MA. Liver disease in pregnancy. *Lancet* 2010; **375**: 594–605.

Knight M, Nelson-Piercy C, Kurinczuk JJ, Spark P, Brocklehurst P; UK Obstetric Surveillance System. A prospective national study of acute fatty liver of pregnancy in the UK. *Gut* 2008; **57**: 951–6.

Rajasri AG, Srestha R, Mitchell J. Acute fatty liver of pregnancy (AFLP) – an overview. *J Obstet Gynaecol* 2007; **27**: 237–40.

Chapter

79

HELLP syndrome

HELLP (haemolysis, elevated liver enzymes and low platelet count) syndrome is one of the presentations of pre-eclampsia and may occur before or soon after delivery. Severe HELLP syndrome is associated with disseminated intravascular coagulation (DIC) and placental abruption and may progress to multi-organ failure. It is associated with a high fetal and maternal morbidity and mortality.

Problems/special considerations

- The mother with HELLP syndrome may not necessarily have presented with symptoms or signs of pre-eclampsia. The main presenting feature may be abdominal pain, perhaps with nausea and vomiting, so a high index of suspicion is needed. The first presentation may be a seizure.
- Mild changes in liver function tests have been reported in up to 50% of women with pre-eclampsia, but more serious dysfunction may occur, including periportal haemorrhage and hepatic infarction. There have also been several reported cases of liver rupture associated with severe HELLP syndrome. Acute fatty liver of pregnancy is also considered by many authorities to be part of the spectrum of pre-eclampsia/eclampsia.
- Other complications of HELLP syndrome include renal failure, DIC, pulmonary oedema, pleural effusions, acute respiratory distress syndrome, retinal detachment and

cerebral oedema. About 16% of women who are undelivered and who develop HELLP syndrome present with placental abruption.

Management options

The treatment of HELLP syndrome is supportive; delivery of the placenta is the definitive treatment.

Women should be delivered as soon as the maternal condition has been optimised, usually by caesarean section. Recommendations vary regarding pre- or perioperative platelet transfusion, with some centres suggesting platelet transfusion if the platelet count is below 50×10^9/l and others not giving platelets until the count falls below 20×10^9/l.

The benefits of invasive pressure monitoring must be balanced against the potential hazards. Careful fluid balance is important, and may be guided with central venous pressure monitoring and urine output. However, many anaesthetists believe that the hazards of central venous lines and their use on the labour ward for fluid balance outweigh the benefits, and there is little evidence in the literature supporting an improved outcome.

Regional anaesthesia is relatively contraindicated in the presence of thrombocytopenia, but ultimately the anaesthetist must choose the anaesthetic technique that he or she judges to be the safest in the circumstance. The choice of regional anaesthesia in a woman with a platelet count of less than 75×10^9/l should only be made by an experienced consultant obstetric anaesthetist.

If general anaesthesia is used, attempts must be made to attenuate the hypertensive response to intubation, usually by use of an intravenous opioid as part of the induction sequence (see Chapter 80, hypertension, pre-eclampsia and eclampsia). Tracheal intubation should be carried out as atraumatically as possible.

There is no specific treatment for HELLP syndrome other than symptomatic treatment of the associated complications, although there is some evidence to support steroid therapy, e.g. two doses of dexamethasone 10 mg 12 hours apart followed by 5 mg at 24 and 36 hours. Plasma exchange has been reported to be useful anecdotally although the evidence for it is weak. Women with HELLP syndrome should be managed in a high-dependency or intensive therapy environment. Postnatal management is entirely supportive.

Key points

- HELLP syndrome is part of the spectrum of pre-eclampsia/eclampsia and may present without prodromal symptoms and signs of pre-eclampsia.
- It may present before or after delivery and is associated with significant maternal and fetal morbidity and mortality.
- Epigastric pain, nausea and vomiting are common presenting features, and a high index of suspicion is essential in every pregnant woman presenting with abdominal pain.
- Treatment consists of delivery and supportive management of the associated complications.

Further reading

Haram K, Svendsen E, Abildgaard U. The HELLP syndrome: clinical issues and management. A review. *BMC Pregnancy Childbirth* 2009; **9**: 8.

Sibai BM. Diagnosis, controversies, and management of the syndrome of hemolysis, elevated liver enzymes, and low platelet count. *Obstet Gynecol* 2004; **103**: 981–91.

Hypertension, pre-eclampsia and eclampsia

Hypertension in pregnancy is diagnosed either by raised absolute values of systolic or diastolic pressure (>140 mmHg or >90 mmHg respectively) or by increases in systolic or diastolic pressures above those at booking (>30 mmHg or >15 mmHg respectively). Pressures should be raised on two separate occasions using appropriate methods of measurement (see below).

Hypertensive disorders of pregnancy are divided into chronic hypertension, gestational hypertension and pre-eclampsia.

Chronic hypertension and gestational hypertension

Chronic hypertension occurs in 3–5% of pregnancies though the incidence is increasing in the UK as maternal age increases. It is diagnosed by pre-existing hypertension or hypertension that occurs before 20 weeks' gestation, although the diagnosis may be masked by the normal slight fall in blood pressure that occurs in early pregnancy, and pre-eclampsia may rarely present earlier than 20 weeks. The risk of pre-eclampsia is approximately doubled, and there is also a greater risk of abruption and fetal growth restriction, but if the blood pressure is controlled women with chronic hypertension would be expected to have good outcomes.

Gestational hypertension describes hypertension after 20 weeks' gestation without any features of pre-eclampsia, and occurs in 6–7% of pregnancies. The risk of pre-eclampsia is increased slightly, this risk increasing the earlier the hypertension develops. Blood pressure usually returns to normal within 1–2 months of delivery.

Pre-eclampsia

Pre-eclampsia is usually defined as hypertension and proteinuria that develops after 20 weeks' gestation in a previously normotensive and non-proteinuric woman (oedema is now omitted from the definition although it is often present), with the involvement of one or more organ systems. Because of practical difficulties in quantifying 24-hour proteinuria, measurement of a random urine protein:creatinine ratio (PCR) is often done instead, a PCR > 30 mg/mmol correlating with a 24-hour protein excretion > 300 mg. It is possible to develop non-proteinuric pre-eclampsia and also to have eclamptic seizures with minimal or even no hypertension. Pre-eclampsia occurs in 5–6% of pregnancies overall (up to 25% in patients with pre-existing hypertension).

Pre-eclampsia/eclampsia is a major direct cause of maternal death worldwide. The pathophysiology of pre-eclampsia is still only partially understood, but it is known that failure of placentation occurs early in pregnancy and this leads to vascular endothelial cell damage and dysfunction. The endothelial cell damage is thought to lead to release of vasoactive substances, which promote generalised vasoconstriction and reduced organ perfusion. This is exacerbated by an increased sensitivity to circulating catecholamines. Pre-eclamptic women demonstrate an imbalance of the normal thromboxane/prostacyclin ratio and increased free radical activity.

Pre-eclampsia encompasses HELLP (haemolysis, elevated liver enzymes and low platelet count) syndrome, eclampsia and possibly acute fatty liver of pregnancy. Although the disease is progressive, a mother may be asymptomatic until she presents with an eclamptic fit, and although pre-eclampsia is a disease of pregnancy, terminated only by delivery, pre-eclampsia, HELLP syndrome and eclampsia may all present for the first time after delivery.

There have been many attempts to prevent development of pre-eclampsia, e.g. with dietary vitamins, antioxidants and minerals, with no clear benefit found. The large international CLASP (Collaborative Low-dose Aspirin Study in Pregnancy) trial failed to show universal benefit from low-dose aspirin, suggesting instead that aspirin may be beneficial in selected high-risk women.

Problems/special considerations

- *Measurement:* Blood pressure measurements should be made with the mother sitting (or on her side in late pregnancy) to avoid aortocaval compression. Most automated blood pressure measuring devices have not been validated in pregnancy and many tend to under-read blood pressure, especially in pre-eclampsia, giving a false sense of security (though they can be used to monitor trends, so long as manual measurements are taken at intervals). If manual methods of measurement are used, it is now recommended that Korotkoff phase V sounds should be used to measure diastolic pressure, not phase IV, since the former are more reproducible and better correlated with true diastolic pressure in pregnancy.

- *Clinical features:* Pre-eclampsia is frequently asymptomatic despite significant disease. Symptoms are often non-specific and include headache, visual disturbance and epigastric pain. The most commonly occurring signs are hypertension, oedema and hyperreflexia, although the latter is subjective and unreliable as a prognostic indicator (though sustained clonus is pathological). Women may also present with the clinical features of pulmonary oedema, cerebral haemorrhage, impaired liver function, placental abruption or coagulopathy. Oedema may also affect the airway. Investigations may reveal abnormal renal and hepatic function, coagulation disorders and pleural and pericardial effusions. Occasionally the clinical presentation may be dramatic – ruptured liver has been reported.

  A particular complication that may be seen is the posterior reversible encephalopathy syndrome (PRES), that although is not specific to pregnancy or to pre-eclampsia, is increasingly described in association with the latter. It is characterised by headache, convulsions, confusion and visual loss, with T2-weighted MRI imaging typically revealing bilateral hyper-intensities, predominantly in the parieto-occipital region. Recovery usually takes several days, though neurological deficits may persist.

- *Fetal effects:* Chronic impairment of uteroplacental blood flow causes intrauterine growth retardation and this may be one of the first signs of pre-eclampsia. There is an increased risk of prematurity.

- *Haemodynamic changes:* The normal expansion of blood volume that takes place in early pregnancy fails to occur in pre-eclamptic women and there is therefore a relatively hypovolaemic state. This is exacerbated by leaky capillaries, which allow inappropriate fluid shifts between compartments. Colloid osmotic pressure is low in pre-eclamptic women, and any increased hydrostatic pressure due to iatrogenic fluid overload, impaired left ventricular function or postpartum fluid shifts may therefore readily precipitate pulmonary oedema.

  Results of the numerous studies (both invasive and non-invasive) of the haemodynamic changes occurring in pre-eclampsia are confusing. There is generalised vasoconstriction and therefore systemic vascular resistance is usually increased. Cardiac index and cardiac output may be high, low or normal but this is frequently a reflection of drug therapy. In severe pre-eclampsia, especially if there is pulmonary oedema, right atrial pressure may not accurately reflect pulmonary artery pressure, and central venous pressure monitoring may therefore be an unreliable guide to treatment.

- *Convulsions:* In the UK, approximately 1–2% of pre-eclamptic women develop eclampsia (~2–3 per 10 000 births), though the incidence is higher in the developing countries. Forty per cent of eclamptic fits occur after delivery, most commonly within the first 3 days and rarely more than one week postpartum. In approximately a third of cases, there are minimal prodromal signs or symptoms, and only ~40% have proteinuria or hypertension in the preceding week. Recurrent seizures are associated with increased maternal morbidity and mortality. Twenty per cent of eclamptic patients experience pre-eclampsia in the next pregnancy, and 2% have eclampsia.

Management options

The management of chronic and gestational hypertension consists of antihypertensive drugs and close monitoring for development of pre-eclampsia or intrauterine growth retardation.

The Report on Confidential Enquiries into Maternal Deaths in the United Kingdom strongly recommends that every obstetric unit should have written guidelines for the management of pre-eclampsia and eclampsia. There have also been recommendations that every obstetric unit should have an 'eclampsia pack' containing everything necessary to treat eclamptic women with magnesium.

Women with mild to moderate disease and without major fetal compromise are usually offered a trial of vaginal delivery, whilst those with severe pre-eclampsia (especially < 37 weeks' gestation) are likely to be delivered by caesarean section (although some evidence exists to support expectant care). The anaesthetist should assess the mother, paying particular attention to any symptoms of pre-eclampsia, drug treatment, the airway, the level of hypertension, the results of haematological and biochemical investigations, and the proposed mode of delivery.

Hypertension

Treatment of hypertension does not modify the course of the underlying disease process but may reduce the morbidity and mortality attributable to uncontrolled hypertension. Whether treatment of mild hypertension during pregnancy is worthwhile is unclear, but because of the risk of haemorrhagic stroke most guidelines suggest treating a systolic blood pressure of 160 mmHg or more.

The first-line treatment of hypertension includes methyldopa, which has a long safety record for the fetus, labetalol, nifedipine and other β-adrenoreceptor blockers such as metoprolol and propranolol. Patients already receiving angiotensin converting enzyme inhibitors or anti-angiotensin receptor agents should have them withdrawn because of their fetotoxic effects.

Hydralazine is the most commonly used agent for management of acute hypertension. Administration of small repeated intravenous boluses (e.g. 5 mg) is preferable to continuous infusion. Hydralazine acts primarily as a vasodilator and should therefore be used with caution and preferably in conjunction with gentle volume replacement, since acute vasodilatation may cause an uncontrolled fall in blood pressure and thus provoke fetal distress. (Reduction in maternal blood pressure is associated with a significantly greater percentage reduction in uteroplacental perfusion.)

Labetalol (10 mg boluses) may be used parenterally in the acute situation, and oral nifedipine (5–10 mg) has also been used, acting within 15–30 minutes. Although there have been concerns over sublingual nifedipine and the risk of uncontrolled hypotension, particularly in combination with magnesium sulphate, this is not thought to be a common problem, especially with slow-release preparations.

Nitroprusside and glyceryl trinitrate may be used for acute control of hypertension but are not commonly used in the UK.

Angiotensin converting enzyme inhibitors are contraindicated in pre-eclampsia as their use is associated with unacceptably high fetal morbidity and mortality.

Convulsions

Magnesium sulphate has been shown to reduce the incidence of eclampsia in pre-eclampsia by approximately half, although whether it should be offered routinely to pre-eclamptics is controversial since only 1–2% of the latter go on to develop pre-eclampsia in the UK, and a significant proportion of eclamptics cannot be identified beforehand (see Chapter 81, Magnesium sulphate).

In women who have had a convulsion, magnesium sulphate reduces the incidence of recurrent convulsions by about half compared with phenytoin and diazepam, and 'magnesium packs' should be available on every labour ward.

The optimum treatment of convulsions themselves is less clear; both magnesium sulphate and diazepam have been used, though some authorities claim that eclamptic fits are self-limiting and that no treatment other than initiation of the magnesium sulphate regimen is needed.

Analgesia for labour

Regional analgesia is the method of choice, since it prevents hypertensive episodes associated with contraction pain and may be beneficial to the compromised fetus by improving uteroplacental perfusion. Although epidural analgesia may lower blood pressure it should not be considered a treatment for hypertension. A combination of low-dose local anaesthetic and opioid may be given by continuous epidural infusion or intermittent boluses, and this can be supplemented as necessary should instrumental or operative delivery be required. The platelet count should be measured before insertion of the epidural (if trends suggest that platelet numbers are decreasing significantly, a platelet count should be repeated immediately before epidural insertion; otherwise, a platelet count within the last ~4 hours is usually considered adequate). Current opinion suggest that a platelet count of at least $75 \times 10^9/l$ is advisable before instituting central neural blockade, although any stated lower safe limit is entirely arbitrary, and the relative risks and benefits of regional analgesia and anaesthesia must be considered for each patient. Several studies have confirmed that if the platelet count is at least $100 \times 10^9/l$ there is no need to perform further coagulation studies. In some centres, thromboelastography or similar techniques are used to assist decision making concerning epidural insertion. Bleeding time is rarely used since a normal range for bleeding time has not been established in pregnancy and there is considerable inter- and intra-observer variability in its measurement.

If epidural analgesia is contraindicated, it is important to control the blood pressure by using appropriate agents (hydralazine, nifedipine, labetalol) and to provide alternative analgesia. Patient-controlled intravenous opioids offer the mother the psychological benefit of being in control of her analgesia and are more predictable than intramuscular opioids.

Anaesthesia for caesarean section

Regional anaesthesia

Regional is preferable to general anaesthesia, both for the mother and for the fetus. Although the use of spinal anaesthesia in pre-eclampsia was traditionally avoided because of the fear of causing severe hypotension, there is now evidence that so long as there is no hypovolaemia, cardiovascular stability is maintained better in pre-eclamptic patients than in non pre-eclamptic ones. Furthermore, there is evidence that uterine artery velocity and neonatal condition are unaffected by spinal anaesthesia if systolic arterial pressure remains at least 80% of baseline.

Combined spinal–epidural anaesthesia confers the benefits of dense anaesthesia (especially of the sacral nerve roots) with the flexibility of epidural anaesthesia and postoperative analgesia.

The untreated pre-eclamptic mother may exhibit greater sensitivity to vasoconstrictors than the normotensive mother. Adrenaline-containing epidural solutions are sometimes avoided in severe cases although their use appears to be safe.

General anaesthesia

General anaesthesia may be necessary if there is great urgency to deliver the mother or if regional anaesthesia is contraindicated by coagulopathy or major haemorrhage. Extreme prematurity does not contraindicate regional anaesthesia and nor does eclampsia.

The additional risks of general anaesthesia for caesarean section are compounded in the pre-eclamptic woman by the potential for a significantly compromised airway and the hypertensive response to intubation and extubation. There may also be potential drug interactions, especially between magnesium sulphate and neuromuscular blocking agents.

Laryngeal oedema is uncommon but may be sufficient to obscure all normal anatomy at laryngoscopy. Each obstetric theatre should include small-sized tracheal tubes on the intubation trolley for this eventuality.

Uncontrolled hypertension in response to tracheal intubation may provoke cardiac arrhythmias, myocardial ischaemia or cerebrovascular catastrophe. Numerous agents have been used to attenuate this response, but the most commonly used agents in the UK are fentanyl 1–4 µg/kg or alfentanil 7–10 µg/kg and labetalol 10–20 mg. Other opioids, β-blockers and lidocaine may be used; magnesium sulphate 30 mg/kg also appears to be effective.

Monitoring and fluid therapy

All women with moderate or severe pre-eclampsia should have continuous electronic fetal monitoring. Direct arterial pressure monitoring is more accurate than non-invasive methods, because of the inaccuracy of most non-invasive monitors. The relative benefits of intra-arterial monitoring must be balanced against the familiarity of midwifery staff with its use. Central venous pressure catheters may provide guidance for fluid administration during regional anaesthesia, although their use is uncommon in the UK. Access via the antecubital fossa rather than via neck veins is sometimes recommended, especially in the undelivered mother. Pulmonary artery catheterisation is rarely used.

All pre-eclamptic women should have a urinary catheter inserted and an accurate hourly fluid balance recorded. Fluid management is controversial. The risks of volume overload and iatrogenic pulmonary oedema must be balanced against the risk of hypotension if vasodilators are given without concomitant volume replacement. In general, the emphasis has shifted away from liberal use of fluids in order to encourage urine output, towards careful restriction, since long-term problems from renal failure are rare, whereas deaths from pulmonary oedema are well reported.

Postoperative management

The risks of deterioration in blood pressure control, of HELLP syndrome and of eclampsia do not end immediately with delivery of the placenta. Women with moderate and severe pre-eclampsia should be monitored in a high-dependency environment for at least 24–48 hours after delivery. Invasive monitoring and antihypertensive treatment should be continued during this time.

Key points

- Hypertensive disorders of pregnancy are divided into chronic hypertension, gestational hypertension and pre-eclampsia.
- Pre-eclampsia and eclampsia are a major cause of maternal death.
- Although the classic presentation of the disease is hypertension, proteinuria and oedema occurring after 20 weeks of pregnancy, pre-eclampsia is a multisystem disease and may present atypically.
- HELLP syndrome is part of the spectrum of pre-eclampsia and may not be preceded by significant pre-eclampsia.
- Pre-eclampsia can only be effectively treated by delivery of the placenta, although symptomatic treatment attenuates maternal morbidity.
- Effective control of hypertension in pre-eclampsia reduces cardiovascular and cerebrovascular morbidity and mortality.
- Eclampsia may occur without premonitory symptoms or signs, and 40% of eclamptic fits occur after delivery.

Further reading

Dennis AT. Management of pre-eclampsia: issues for anaesthetists. *Anaesthesia* 2012; **67**: DOI: 10.1111/j.1365-2044.2012.07195.x.

Duley L, Gülmezoglu AM, Henderson-Smart DJ, Chou D. Magnesium sulphate and other anticonvulsants for women with pre-eclampsia. *Cochrane Database Syst Rev* 2010; (11): CD000025.

Gogarten W. Preeclampsia and anaesthesia. *Curr Opin Anesthesiol* 2009; **22**: 347–51.

Knight M; UK Obstetric Surveillance System (UKOSS). Eclampsia in the United Kingdom 2005. *BJOG* 2007; **114**: 1072–8.

National Institute for Health and Clinical Excellence. The management of hypertensive disorders during pregnancy. *Clinical Guideline 107*. London: NICE 2010, http://guidance.nice.org.uk/CG107.

Steegers EAP, von Dadelszen P, Duvekot JJ, Pijnenborg R. Pre-eclampsia. *Lancet* 2010; **376**: 631–44.

Chapter

Magnesium sulphate

81

Magnesium was first reported to be effective in preventing further fits in eclamptic women in 1925. The Collaborative Eclampsia Trial, reporting in 1995, confirmed that magnesium sulphate is significantly more effective than either diazepam or phenytoin in preventing recurrence of fits in eclamptic women.

The MAGPIE Trial, reporting in 2002, showed that magnesium sulphate was also effective in reducing (by about half) the incidence of eclampsia when given to pre-eclamptic women. However, since the incidence of eclampsia in the UK is low ($\sim$1–2% of pre-eclamptic cases), the number needed to treat in order to prevent a single woman having a convulsion is $\sim$110 in the UK. This has led to controversy about whether magnesium should be routinely given to all pre-eclamptics in the UK, especially since there was no overall effect on maternal and neonatal morbidity and mortality in the trial. In populations in which the incidence is higher, e.g. the African subcontinent, or in those with severe pre-eclampsia, the number needed to treat is lower, so administration to such cases is less controversial. However, even in these cases it is impossible to predict which women will go on to develop eclampsia.

These two studies have changed clinical practice around the world but especially in the UK, where magnesium used to be infrequently used for pre-eclampsia/eclampsia.

Magnesium sulphate is widely used in the USA as a tocolytic agent in preterm labour but randomised trials have failed to confirm its efficacy for this purpose.

Magnesium has a number of other uses outside obstetrics but these are not discussed further here.

Site of action

Magnesium is essential for potassium and calcium metabolism. It acts as a calcium antagonist, probably reducing systemic and cerebral vasospasm via action at calcium channels and intracellular sites. It is a cofactor in the sodium–potassium–ATPase system and is also an

Table 81.1 Signs and symptoms of magnesium toxicity at various blood levels

Symptoms	Magnesium level mg/dl	mmol/l
Normal adult levels	1.7–2.4	0.7–1.1
Therapeutic range	4–8	2–4
Loss of patellar reflexes, warmth, flushing, somnolence	9.5–12	4.2–5
Respiratory depression	12–16	5–6.5
Muscle paralysis	15–17	6.2–7
Cardiac conduction defects	> 18	> 7.5
Cardiac arrest	30–35	12.5–14.5

N-methyl-D-aspartate (NMDA) receptor antagonist; it is thought that its anticonvulsant action is mediated through these systems.

Production of endothelial prostacyclin is increased by magnesium and this may help to restore the thromboxane–prostacyclin imbalance that occurs in pre-eclampsia.

Magnesium sulphate relieves the cerebral vasospasm associated with pre-eclampsia and eclampsia; transcranial Doppler studies have demonstrated an increase in cerebral blood flow.

Side effects

Magnesium sulphate has widespread effects, not all of which are beneficial. Its use has been associated with increased obstetric haemorrhage (presumably due to generalised vasodilatation and uterine atony), increased length of labour and increased rate of caesarean section. Prophylactic use of magnesium sulphate before induction of general anaesthesia for caesarean section (e.g. in severe pre-eclampsia) can prolong the effects of neuromuscular blocking agents; use of a peripheral nerve stimulator is mandatory.

Toxicity is possible during infusion although this is unlikely in usual dosage unless there is concomitant renal impairment. Symptoms/signs of toxicity occur as blood levels increase (see Table 81.1). Magnesium toxicity is reversed by intravenous calcium gluconate (10 ml of 10% solution, given by slow intravenous injection), and calcium should always be available when magnesium therapy is given.

Dose

The Collaborative Eclampsia Trial and MAGPIE Trial used an intravenous loading dose of 4–5 g magnesium sulphate (given over 5–15 minutes) followed by either 5 g intramuscularly into each buttock and a further 5 g intramuscularly every 4 hours for 24 hours, or an intravenous infusion of 1–2 g/h after the intravenous loading dose.

There is controversy about whether an intravenous maintenance infusion of 1 g/h produces adequate plasma levels, with some studies suggesting that 3 g/h is required to guarantee therapeutic levels (4–8 mg/dl). The Collaborative Eclampsia group has stated that use of higher doses would increase the risk of toxicity without conferring proven benefit and in the MAGPIE Trial, side effects occurred in a quarter of cases.

Monitoring

If the regimen used in the two above trials is used, clinical monitoring is considered to be adequate. Quarter-hourly measurement of respiratory rate, assessment of patellar tendon reflexes and hourly monitoring of urine output should be performed. Monitoring of plasma levels is advisable if larger doses of magnesium sulphate are used, if there is impaired renal function, if symptoms/signs of toxicity occur or a convulsion occurs despite therapy.

Key points

- Magnesium sulphate is the only drug proven to be effective in preventing recurrence of fits in eclampsia.
- Magnesium sulphate reduces the incidence of eclamptic fits before they occur but its use for this purpose is controversial because there is no reliable method of predicting eclampsia.
- Both intramuscular and intravenous regimens are effective, and clinical monitoring is adequate.
- Calcium gluconate should be available at the bedside of every woman receiving magnesium sulphate.

Further reading

Duley L, Gülmezoglu AM, Henderson-Smart DJ, Chou D. Magnesium sulphate and other anticonvulsants for women with pre-eclampsia. *Cochrane Database Syst Rev* 2010; (11): CD000025.

Duley L, Henderson-Smart DJ, Chou D. Magnesium sulphate versus phenytoin for eclampsia. *Cochrane Database Syst Rev* 2010; (10): CD000128.

Duley L, Henderson-Smart DJ, Walker GJ, Chou D. Magnesium sulphate versus diazepam for eclampsia. *Cochrane Database Syst Rev* 2010; (12): CD000127.

Duley L, Matar HE, Almerie MQ, Hall DR. Alternative magnesium sulphate regimens for women with pre-eclampsia and eclampsia. *Cochrane Database Syst Rev* 2010; (8): CD007388.

Hyperemesis gravidarum

Nausea and vomiting during early pregnancy occurs in about 70–90% of women although in most cases it is not severe and has diminished by the mid-second trimester. Rarely, severe vomiting continues throughout pregnancy and may require hospitalisation in about 3–10 per 1000 women. It is more common in first pregnancies and with younger maternal age, obesity, multiple pregnancy, previous history of hyperemesis, metabolic disorders and eating disorders. The aetiology is unknown but hormonal (particularly oestrogen and human chorionic gonadotrophin), metabolic and psychological factors have been implicated.

Anaesthetists may be asked to advise on antiemetic therapy or to assist in establishing peripheral or central venous access for fluid replacement and/or nutrition. They may also be involved in providing analgesia or anaesthesia for delivery or, rarely, for termination of pregnancy if hyperemesis is very severe.

Problems/special considerations

Clinical symptoms are non-specific and it is important to consider other causes of nausea and vomiting. There may be evidence of malnutrition and/or dehydration, with associated biochemical and metabolic derangement including renal and particularly hepatic impairment and mineral/vitamin deficiency, e.g. Wernicke's encephalopathy. The muscle bulk is virtually always reduced in severe cases and there may be fetal growth retardation. Because of the importance of psychological factors, these patients may need psychological/psychiatric support, which may be difficult in the maternity suite; in early pregnancy they are often managed on general gynaecological wards.

Management options

Diagnosis

The diagnosis of hyperemesis gravidarum should be one of exclusion since there are other conditions that should be considered in severe vomiting in pregnancy (Table 82.1).

Treatment

Initially, non-pharmacological methods of management are usually proffered, such as frequent small snacks (e.g. dry crackers), ginger root tea, hypnosis and use of

Table 82.1 Causes of vomiting in pregnancy

Infective	Gastroenteritis
	Urinary tract infection
	Hepatitis
Surgical	Intra-abdominal pathology
	Primary gastrointestinal
	Severe reflux oesophagitis
Neurological	Increased intracranial pressure
	Migraine
Metabolic	Diabetes
	Hypercalcaemia
	Uraemia
	Acute fatty liver of pregnancy
Drug-related	Antibiotics
	Analgesics
	Alcohol
Psychogenic	

acupressure bands or acupuncture to stimulate an area on the ventral surface of the wrist between the long flexor tendons. Electrolyte replacement drinks and oral nutritional supplements, if tolerated, are advocated. The evidence for the more esoteric treatments is somewhat mixed although is probably strongest for acupressure or acupuncture for its general (as opposed to obstetric) antiemetic effect. Psychological support is generally advocated.

Standard antiemetics such as metoclopramide, prochlorperazine and cyclizine are usually tried first; promazine has traditionally been used. Domperidone and ondansetron are also used. It should be remembered that the effects of these drugs on the fetus are unclear and that few are licensed for use in pregnancy.

There is some evidence to support the use of steroids as treatment (e.g. intravenous hydrocortisone 100 mg, twice daily, then prednisolone 45–50 mg/day, reduced to the lowest possible dose). The use of diazepam has been studied in randomised trials and its success is thought to be a result of its sedative properties. However, sedative drugs are not routinely recommended because of their addictive properties and also because of possible adverse effects on the fetus.

In cases where dehydration is apparent, hospitalisation and intravenous rehydration (and occasionally resuscitation) is required; use of glucose-containing solutions may provide a small amount of calorific intake but excessive administration may result in hyponatraemia. Vitamin and mineral supplementation is advisable, especially with thiamine. Enteral nasogastric nutrition has been used. In very severe cases, parenteral nutrition may be required; in fact use of parenteral nutrition has been advocated as a treatment in its own right and there are several reports of its apparent success, occasionally on repeated occasions throughout the same pregnancy.

Oesophagitis may be severe and is treated by using standard methods.

Key points

- Nausea and vomiting occurs in about 75% of pregnancies.
- Hospitalisation is required in about 3–10 per 1000 women.
- Urea and electrolyte disturbances and hepatic impairment may occur.
- There are few randomised controlled trials of therapy but many different non-pharmacological and pharmacological therapies have been used.

Further reading

Jarvis S, Nelson-Piercy C. Management of nausea and vomiting in pregnancy. *BMJ* 2011; **342**: d3606.

Jueckstock JK, Kaestner R, Mylonas I. Managing hyperemesis gravidarum: a multimodal challenge. *BMC Med* 2010; **8**: 46.

Matthews A, Dowswell T, Haas DM, Doyle M, O'Mathúna DP. Interventions for nausea and vomiting in early pregnancy. *Cochrane Database Syst Rev* 2010; (9): CD007575.

Chapter

83

Maternal mortality

There has been continuous audit of maternal deaths in England and Wales since 1952 (and the whole of the UK since 1984), the results of which have been published every three years as the Report on Confidential Enquiries into Maternal Deaths (CEMD). The organisation of the Enquiry has changed in recent years, being administered by the Confidential Enquiry into Maternal and Child Health (CEMACH) and then the Centre for Maternal and Child Enquiries (CMACE). The most recent triennial report, published by CMACE in 2011 and covering the years 2006–08, found the following:

- The UK maternal mortality rate (equals no. of indirect + direct deaths per 100 000 maternities; see below) was 11.4, down from 14.0 previously.
- The Maternal Mortality Rate (MMR, the international definition: equals no. of indirect + direct deaths (from birth certificates only) per 100 000 live births) was 6.7, down from 7.0 (comparable with other Northern European countries; in the USA, MMR was 17 in 2008; in sub-Saharan Africa it is around 1000).
- Cardiac disease was the leading cause of maternal death, followed by neurological disease, sepsis, hypertensive disorders and thromboembolism (Fig. 83.1).

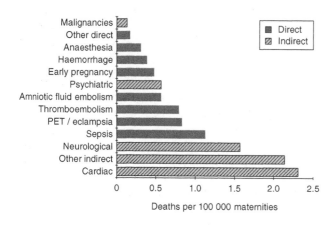

Fig. 83.1 Major causes of death in the CEMD report 2006–08.

During a review of the entire confidential enquiries programme, cases have continued to be reported via a portal administered by the Healthcare Quality Improvement Partnership (HQIP), which now oversees the programme. In 2012 a new consortium, MBRRACE-UK (Mothers and Babies – Reducing Risk through Audits and Confidential Enquiries across the UK) was appointed by HQIP to run the maternal and perinatal death enquiries.

Other countries have established reviews of maternal deaths but none are as well established or complete as the CEMD.

Definitions and data collection

A maternal death is any death occurring during or within 42 days of the pregnancy ending. The enquiry into any maternal death is initiated by local reporters in each unit and organised by regional offices. Each death is assessed by obstetric anaesthetic, midwifery and pathology assessors as appropriate.

Maternal deaths are classified as:

- Direct (resulting from obstetric complications of pregnancy) – 107 cases in 2006–08.
- Indirect (deaths resulting from previous existing disease or disease that developed during pregnancy and that was not due to direct obstetric causes but was aggravated by the physiological effects of pregnancy) – 154 cases in 2006–08.
- Late (occurring after 42 days and within one year of the pregnancy ending) – 33 cases in 2006–08.
- Coincidental (from unrelated causes, such as road traffic accident) – 50 cases in 2006–08.

Since 1994–96 the number of indirect deaths has outnumbered that of direct deaths. Deaths may be associated with substandard care, a term used not only to denote failure of clinical care, but also to indicate failure of the woman to take responsibility for her own health (such as refusal of blood transfusion or refusal to be admitted) and inadequate resources for staffing, intensive care and back-up services. The triennial reports make recommendations for improved care; these tend to include the same themes, e.g.:

Table 83.1 Anaesthetic deaths since 1985 in the CEMD reports

Triennium	Direct anaesthetic deaths	Proportion of direct deaths	Rate per 100 000 maternities
1985–87	6	4.3%	0.26
1988–90	4	2.8%	0.17
1991–93	8	6.3%	0.35
1994–96	1	0.7%	0.05
1997–99	3	2.8%	0.14
2000–02	6	5.7%	0.30
2003–05	6	4.5%	0.28
2006–08	7	6.5%	0.31

- The importance of early recognition of critically unwell parturients.
- The importance of early involvement of senior clinicians and referral to other relevant specialists.
- The need for local provision of intensive care (not necessarily on the intensive care unit).
- The need for protocols for common, potentially serious conditions, e.g. pre-eclampsia, major haemorrhage.
- The need for regular drills and training in life-threatening emergencies.
- The need for better record keeping and communication generally.

Anaesthetic deaths

Although anaesthesia is no longer one of the three leading causes of maternal death, as it was in the 1980s, there are still lessons to be learnt from the deaths associated with anaesthesia and the cases in which anaesthesia was felt to have contributed to the death. In the 2006–08 report, there were seven direct anaesthetic deaths (Table 83.1): two failures of ventilation; four postoperative complications (one involving inappropriate administration of Syntocinon, one incompatible blood transfusion, one aspiration of gastric contents, and one presumed opioid overdose); and one case of leukoencephalitis following spinal anaesthesia. Difficulties in airway management including tracheal intubation are regularly highlighted, even though the number of failed intubations is now low.

Key points

- Obstetric anaesthesia is high-risk anaesthesia.
- The severity of co-existing medical disease is easily underestimated.
- Adequate monitoring equipment and trained anaesthetic assistance are required for obstetric anaesthesia.
- Intensive care facilities may be required.
- The anaesthetic record is a legal document and is essential for adequate evaluation of morbidity and mortality.

Further reading

Centre for Maternal and Child Enquiries (CMACE). Saving mothers' lives: reviewing maternal deaths to make motherhood safer: 2006–2008. The eighth report of the Confidential Enquiries into Maternal Deaths in the United Kingdom. *BJOG* 2011; **118** (Suppl 1): 1–203.

Kinsella SM. Anaesthetic deaths in the CMACE (Centre for Maternal and Child Enquiries) Saving Mothers' Lives report 2006–08. *Anaesthesia* 2011; **66**: 243–6.

Yentis SM. From CEMD to CEMACH to CMACE to…? Where now for the confidential enquiries into maternal deaths? *Anaesthesia* 2011; **66**: 859–60.

Allergic reactions

Patients may be mildly allergic to many substances and this may become better or worse during pregnancy. Severe reactions, however, are rare on labour ward. Although divided into anaphylactic (release of histamine and other inflammatory mediators from mast cells via cross-linkage of IgE molecules on the cell surface by the antigen, after prior exposure), anaphylactoid (direct release of mediators from mast cells via interaction of molecules (e.g. drugs) with the cell surface) and others (e.g. direct complement activation), the distinction is largely academic since the clinical presentation is identical.

Most severe reactions on labour ward are caused by drugs, especially antibiotics, intravenous anaesthetic drugs (particularly suxamethonium) and oxytocin. Traditionally, up to 10% of individuals with true penicillin allergy have been thought to be allergic to cephalosporins; more recent estimations put this figure at 1% for cross-reactivity with first-generation cephalosporins, and a negligible risk with third- and fourth-generation cephalosporins. Allergy to amide local anaesthetic drugs is rare but has been reported, as has allergy to preservatives used in local anaesthetic and other drug preparations. Non-steroidal anti-inflammatory drugs and paracetamol often cause rashes but these are usually mild following brief oral/rectal courses, although severe reactions have been reported following intravenous administration. Reactions may also follow administration of gelatine intravenous fluids and blood. Latex allergy is more common in subjects with multiple exposures to latex such as medical or nursing staff, cleaners, those with neurological disease requiring repeated bladder catheterisation, e.g. spina bifida, and those with allergy to certain foodstuffs including avocados, bananas, kiwi fruit and chestnuts. Finally, other conditions not primarily allergic may also present in a similar way, e.g. amniotic fluid embolism.

Patients may have a history of previous allergic reactions to drugs or other substances, although many patients who give only a vague history are not truly allergic.

Problems/special considerations

Features range from mild skin rashes to severe urticaria, hypotension, bronchospasm, abdominal pain, diarrhoea, a 'feeling of impending doom' and cardiovascular collapse. Initial hypotension is largely related to profound vasodilatation, which is followed by leakage of intravascular fluid into the interstitium. Cardiac depression (thought to be caused by circulating inflammatory mediators) may also contribute to hypotension. The cardiovascular effects are exacerbated by aortocaval compression.

Features usually occur within a few seconds or minutes of exposure to the allergen. During caesarean section in latex allergic subjects, anaphylaxis typically occurs 10–15 minutes after induction of anaesthesia and once surgery has started, since the most provocative stimulus is exposure via mucous membranes.

Since clinical features may develop at a time of great physiological change, e.g. during caesarean section or during/after delivery, it may be difficult to assess the situation and determine what has happened. Administration of many different drugs together or within a short time is common and this may hinder the diagnosis (and is suspected of increasing the risk of a reaction).

Management options

Immediate management of severe reactions consists of intravenous adrenaline 100 μg boluses and fluids, with management of the airway and administration of oxygen. Aortocaval compression must be avoided at all times. Adrenaline may cause uteroplacental vasoconstriction and uterine hypotony, which may contribute to fetal hypoxia and postpartum haemorrhage respectively. Intravenous chlorpheniramine 10 mg and hydrocortisone 200 mg may be given to reduce the effects of subsequent inflammatory mediator release. For less severe reactions (e.g. urticaria only), chlorpheniramine alone may suffice.

In an acute reaction, blood should be taken for tryptase levels as soon as possible and at 1–2 and 24 hours. The enzyme is normally present in mast cells and in miniscule amounts in the plasma; an increase in plasma concentration therefore represents mast cell degranulation (but does not distinguish between anaphylactic and anaphylactoid reactions). Immunoglobulin and complement levels may be suggestive, but not diagnostic, of an allergic response. If a severe reaction is suspected, the patient should be referred for testing at least 4–6 weeks later; normally this will involve skin tests (prick testing ± intradermal testing). Further tests may be performed on plasma (e.g. radioallergoabsorbent test (RAST) looking for concentrations of specific antibody, e.g. to latex) or occasionally basophils or other cellular components, if skin testing is not diagnostic. The patient should be advised to obtain a 'MedicAlert' bracelet and given written details of all the drugs tested and the results, in case she should require a subsequent anaesthetic. A copy of the letter should also be sent to her general practitioner.

It is important that mothers with a previous history of severe allergic reactions are identified antenatally. Wherever possible, the previous anaesthetic record should be obtained and a plan for her care documented. Management of the known allergic case includes a general state of readiness and awareness as well as the obvious avoidance of any known allergens. Latex allergic patients may be identified from the history in most cases by asking about food allergies and skin reactions after exposure, e.g. rubber gloves, condoms, etc. If patients have had a previous severe reaction where the allergen is unknown, pretreatment with H_1- and H_2-antagonists ± steroids should be considered, although whether this should be routinely done if the allergen is known and can be avoided, is controversial. Routine screening of all women by using skin or blood testing is generally not indicated, since precautions should be taken on the basis of a strong history even if testing produces negative results.

Key points

- In severe allergic reactions, immediate management is with oxygen, adrenaline and intravenous fluids.
- Hydrocortisone and chlorpheniramine are second-line drugs.
- Blood should be taken for mast cell tryptase levels as early as possible and at 1–2 and 24 hours.
- Subsequent testing should include skin testing.

Further reading

Association of Anaesthetists of Great Britain & Ireland. Management of a Patient with Suspected Anaphylaxis During Anaesthesia. London: AAGBI 2009, http://www.aagbi.org/sites/default/files/ana_web_laminate_final.pdf.

Dewachter P, Mouton-Faivre C, Emala CW. Anaphylaxis and anesthesia: controversies and new insights. *Anesthesiology* 2009; **111**: 1141–50.

Harper NJ, Dixon T, Dugué P, *et al.* Suspected anaphylactic reactions associated with anaesthesia. *Anaesthesia* 2009; **64**: 199–211.

Soar J, Perkins GD, Abbas G, *et al.* European Resuscitation Council Guidelines for Resus- citation 2010 Section 8. Cardiac arrest in special circumstances: electrolyte abnor- malities, poisoning, drowning, accidental hypo- thermia, hyperthermia, asthma, anaphylaxis, cardiac surgery, trauma, pregnancy, electrocution. *Resuscitation* 2010; **81**: 1400–33.

Chapter

85

Cardiovascular disease

In the 2006–08 Confidential Enquiries into Maternal Deaths, cardiac disease was the leading overall cause of maternal death in the UK. The spectrum of pre-existing cardiac disease affecting pregnant women has changed in the UK as rheumatic heart disease has become less common (though it is still a major problem in other parts of the world) and congenital heart disease more common, partly related to the improved survival of girls with congenital heart disease who undergo surgery during infancy and childhood.

The most common acquired heart disease in the UK is ischaemic heart disease. Possible epidemiological factors include an increased prevalence of risk factors, e.g. smoking amongst younger women, increased age and obesity.

Problems/special considerations

Although different sorts of cardiac disease require different management, there are general principles that are applicable to this heterogeneous group. Many of these have been highlighted in recent Reports on Confidential Enquiries into Maternal Deaths, which have found the following:

- There is a general failure fully to understand the impact of the normal physiological changes of pregnancy on pre-existing cardiovascular pathology (see Chapter 11, Physiology of pregnancy).

Table 85.1 Risk of death or severe morbidity resulting from certain cardiac lesions in pregnancy

Low risk (mortality 0.1–1%)	Most repaired lesions Uncomplicated left-to-right shunts Mitral valve prolapse; bicuspid aortic valve; aortic regurgitation; mitral regurgitation; pulmonary stenosis; pulmonary regurgitation
Intermediate risk (mortality 1–5%)	Metal valves Single ventricles Systemic right ventricle; switch procedure Unrepaired cyanotic lesions Mitral stenosis; aortic stenosis; severe pulmonary stenosis
High risk (mortality 5–30%)	NYHA III or IV Severe systemic ventricular dysfunction Severe aortic stenosis Marfan's syndrome with aortic valve lesion or aortic dilatation Pulmonary hypertension (N.B. mortality 30–50%)

- Management of women with cardiac disease is often undertaken by inappropriately experienced medical staff. Consultants from all relevant specialties should be involved in management from early pregnancy onward, and should be prepared to seek advice from (and if necessary to refer patients onwards to) specialist cardiological units.
- There may be failure to carry out essential investigations such as chest radiography, where the radiation risks to the fetus are minimal but the information gained from the investigation may be life-saving.
- There may be failure to communicate with other specialties involved in a woman's care and failure to organise clear written plans for management of labour and delivery.
- The severity of the mother's condition may be underestimated, either because of the above or because symptoms are mild or absent, or because they are mistaken for those of pregnancy.

Management options

The pregnant woman with cardiac disease, whether congenital or acquired, should be seen as early as possible in her pregnancy. Ideally, she should be seen for preconceptual counselling when her risks (Table 85.1) and those of her baby can be fully discussed.

A full history and examination should be performed during the first trimester of pregnancy, and baseline cardiological investigations should be arranged. These may include electrocardiography, chest x-ray, echocardiography and possibly cardiac catheterisation. Severity of cardiac disease is frequently assessed by using the New York Heart Association (NYHA) classification, which although originally described for heart failure is a useful overall measure of severity:

- *NYHA I:* No limitation of physical activity and no objective evidence of cardiovascular disease.
- *NYHA II:* Slight limitation of normal physical activity and objective evidence of minimal disease.

- *NYHA III:* Marked limitation of physical activity and objective evidence of moderately severe disease.
- *NYHA IV:* Severe limitation of activity including symptoms at rest and objective evidence of severe disease.

Women with cardiovascular disease graded NYHA I and II usually tolerate the physiological changes of pregnancy well, though it should be remembered that certain conditions (e.g. mitral and aortic stenosis, pulmonary hypertension and complex lesions) may be dangerous even in the absence of symptoms.

Studies suggest that cardiac complications (pulmonary oedema, arrhythmia, stroke or cardiac death) are more likely in women who have the following predictors: a history of previous cardiac events or arrhythmia; NYHA class IV or cyanosis; left heart obstruction; and left ventricular systolic dysfunction – with complications occurring in around a quarter of women with one predictor and three quarters of women with more than one predictor.

Consideration should be given to the appropriate place for both subsequent antenatal management and delivery. Referral to a local teaching hospital with facilities for cardiac surgery may be indicated, and in some cases it may be in the woman's best interests to be referred to a supraregional unit.

Routine antenatal care is not adequate for women with cardiac disease. Antenatal appointments need to be more frequent; there must be clear communication with the general practitioner and the community midwife and also with the woman herself, who should receive instructions about symptoms that demand immediate medical attention. Serial investigations and careful documentation of symptoms should alert medical staff to any deterioration in cardiac health, and it may be useful to admit women with cardiac disease for 24–48 hours towards the end of the second trimester of pregnancy in order to repeat investigations and arrange multidisciplinary review. Women require careful monitoring for development of pre-eclampsia, since it may be poorly tolerated in the presence of cardiac disease.

Elective admission to hospital in the third or even second trimester may be useful to ensure the mother can rest, with due attention to antithrombotic prophylaxis and regular assessments. Continuous oxygen therapy may also be given if required.

As a general rule, operative delivery should only be carried out if indicated for obstetric reasons or deteriorating maternal condition, and not just because the mother has cardiac disease. Regional analgesia and anaesthesia can be safely provided for the majority of women with cardiac disease, even in those with fixed cardiac output (although this is more controversial), although this may be precluded by anticoagulation in certain cases. Analgesia and anaesthesia should only be carried out in units familiar with the management of such high-risk patients. The risk of endocarditis should be remembered; although recent UK guidance suggests prophylactic antibiotics may not be indicated, many clinicians with experience of managing such patients still elect to give them because the consequences of endocarditis can be so devastating.

The puerperium is a time of high risk for many women with cardiac disease, and vigilance should be maintained. The mother with cardiac disease should be nursed on the delivery suite or high-dependency unit until all medical staff involved in her care agree that she can be safely returned to the general postnatal ward. Haemodynamic parameters have usually returned to normal within 3–5 days but may take longer in severe cases, and rarely may never return to pre-pregnancy values.

Key points

- Women with cardiovascular disease should be identified and assessed early in pregnancy, and referred to specialist units when necessary.
- Good communication between specialties is mandatory.
- Clear management plans should be written.
- Vigilance should be maintained into the puerperium.

Further reading

Curry R, Swan L, Steer PJ. Cardiac disease in pregnancy. *Curr Opin Obstet Gynecol* 2009; **21**: 508–13.

ESC Guidelines on the management of cardiovascular diseases during pregnancy: the Task Force on the Management of Cardiovascular Diseases during Pregnancy of the European Society of Cardiology (ESC). *Eur Heart J* 2011; **32**: 3147–97.

Malhotra S, Yentis SM. Reports on Confidential Enquiries into Maternal Deaths: management strategies based on trends in maternal cardiac deaths over 30 years. *Int J Obstet Anesth* 2006; **15**: 223–6.

Royal College of Obstetricians and Gynaecologists. Cardiac disease and pregnancy. *Good Practice No. 13*. London: RCOG 2011, http://www.rcog.org.uk/cardiac-disease-and-pregnancy-good-practice-no-13.

Chapter

86 Arrhythmias

During pregnancy there is an increased incidence of both benign arrhythmias and arrhythmias associated with cardiac disease. If the abnormal rhythm causes haemodynamic instability, there is potential for fetal compromise and treatment should be instituted.

Problems/special considerations

- Sinus tachycardia is normal during pregnancy. Superimposed supraventricular ectopic beats occur commonly, particularly in association with caffeine and alcohol consumption, and may cause palpitations and anxiety. Underlying organic disease is extremely unlikely in these women, and they should be reassured and given advice about avoiding likely precipitators of the arrhythmia.
- Paroxysmal supraventricular tachycardia is more common in pregnancy and rarely indicates underlying organic disease. Palpitations, dizziness and syncope may occur, and although attacks may terminate spontaneously with rest, persistent tachycardia should

be treated acutely with either suitable antiarrhythmic agents (adenosine or verapamil) or with DC cardioversion. In persistent cases, His bundle studies and subsequent ablation of abnormal conduction pathways may be indicated, although it is usual to wait until after delivery for such management.

- Atrial fibrillation is usually associated with mitral valve disease and less commonly with cardiomyopathy. The major risks from atrial fibrillation in pregnancy are thromboembolic disease and pulmonary oedema. Prophylactic anticoagulants should be used, and it may be necessary to consider full anticoagulation in some situations, such as during and immediately following DC cardioversion. Pregnancy does not alter medical management of atrial fibrillation. It is particularly important to confirm that therapeutic plasma levels of antiarrhythmic agents are achieved throughout the pregnancy.
- Ventricular ectopic beats are relatively common during pregnancy and may be either asymptomatic or noticed by the patient as palpitations. No treatment is necessary other than reassurance that there is no sinister underlying cause.
- Ventricular tachycardia or fibrillation may occur in association with severe organic cardiac disease, such as myocardial infarction. In such situations, pregnancy is of secondary concern, since the arrhythmia is usually life threatening, and the primary goal of treatment is termination of the arrhythmia by whatever means is effective.
- Conduction disorders require referral for cardiological opinion, since some cardiologists recommend aggressive management (permanent pacing) of even first degree heart block during pregnancy, although this is disputed.

Management options

In general, pregnant women with cardiac arrhythmias should be assessed and treated in the same way as those who are not pregnant. Underlying causes such as heart disease and medical conditions such as thryotoxicosis should not be forgotten, and women should be investigated appropriately. Women with known predisposing cardiac conditions, e.g. Wolff–Parkinson–White syndrome, should be referred early for cardiological advice, and plans made both for management during delivery and should an acute arrythmia occur. During an acute episode, it is especially important to avoid aortocaval compression since this will exacerbate any circulatory embarrassment.

All commonly used antiarrhythmics cross the placenta (and indeed may be administered to the mother to treat a fetal arrhythmia). There are published case reports of the use of most antiarrhythmic drugs during pregnancy but few well designed controlled studies. Previous anxieties that β-blocking drugs caused intrauterine growth retardation appear to have been largely discounted, and problems were mainly associated with atenolol. However, maternal β-blockade may cause fetal bradycardia and make interpretation of the fetal heart rate trace difficult. Consensus opinion recommends using the smallest dose of the most well established drug that will achieve a therapeutic effect.

If DC cardioversion is performed during pregnancy, it is important to safeguard the airway and to remember the risks of aortocaval compression. In practice, this means using rapid sequence induction of general anaesthesia and tracheal intubation, together with uterine displacement for women in the second half of pregnancy. Prophylactic anticoagulation should be considered during and after DC cardioversion because of the increased risk of thromboembolic disease during pregnancy.

Agents that are associated with increased heart rate (e.g. oxytocin, ephedrine, terbutaline/salbutamol) should be avoided or used very cautiously if needed, in women at risk of tachyarrhythmias.

Key points

- No antiarrhythmic drug is considered completely safe for use in pregnancy, but any cardiac arrhythmia compromising haemodynamic stability requires urgent treatment.
- Use of older and well-established antiarrhythmics is generally recommended for first-line management, but newer drugs should not be withheld if other means are unsuccessful.
- Relief of aortocaval compression is essential.

Further reading

Ferrero S, Colombo BM, Ragni N. Maternal arrhythmias during pregnancy. *Arch Gynecol Obstet* 2004; **269**: 244–53.

Lewis N, Dob DP, Yentis SM. UK Registry of High-risk Obstetric Anaesthesia: arrhythmias, cardiomyopathy, aortic stenosis, transposition of the great arteries and Marfan's syndrome. *Int J Obstet Anesth* 2003; **12**: 28–34.

Nelson-Piercy C, Adamson DL. Managing palpitations and arrhythmia during pregnancy. *Postgrad Med J* 2008; **84**: 66–72.

Chapter

87

Pulmonary oedema

The pregnant mother may be at increased risk of developing pulmonary oedema because her cardiac output and blood volume are increased considerably compared with pre-pregnancy values. This increase is greater in the mother with multiple pregnancy. Colloid osmotic pressure is also reduced in pregnancy.

Problems/special considerations

- Acute pulmonary oedema in the pregnant woman may mimic an acute asthmatic attack. Attempts to treat the latter will tend to exacerbate the former.
- There are multiple aetiologies of pulmonary oedema in pregnancy, but a careful history will usually provide a diagnosis of the underlying cause. Pulmonary oedema may occur:

(i) As a complication of co-existing cardiac disease.
(ii) Secondary to complications of pregnancy, e.g. pre-eclampsia, major obstetric haemorrhage, intrauterine fetal death, amniotic fluid embolism, peripartum cardiomyopathy.
(iii) Secondary to aspiration of gastric contents.
(iv) Secondary to major sepsis.
(v) Following therapeutic or recreational drug administration, e.g. β-adrenergic agonists, glucocorticoids, oxytocics, cocaine.
(vi) Following excessive administration of intravenous fluid.
- Hypoxaemia caused by oedema is exacerbated by the increased oxygen demand of pregnancy and the reduced functional residual capacity and oxygen reserve.

Management options

Women who are known to be at increased risk of developing cardiac failure should receive antenatal and intrapartum care in an obstetric unit with high-dependency and intensive care facilities on site. Pulse oximetry is particularly useful since a fall in saturation may be an early sign of pulmonary oedema.

Women receiving β-adrenergic agonists must have fluid balance and electrolytes monitored rigorously, and supplementary oxygen therapy should be considered. Invasive monitoring of central venous pressure should be considered if regional analgesia or anaesthesia is used in a woman who has been receiving β-agonists.

Appropriate investigations should be performed, including chest radiography, since this carries negligible risk to the fetus.

In the absence of any obvious cause for cardiac failure, it is important to consider the use of illicit drugs.

Invasive cardiovascular monitoring will guide diagnosis and treatment, and the mother should be transferred to a high-dependency or intensive care unit at the earliest possible opportunity.

Oxygen therapy is invariably beneficial. Delivery of the fetus reduces oxygen demand and relieves the physical effect of the gravid uterus on the diaphragm and lungs. Dexamethasone, given to improve neonatal respiratory function, may worsen fluid retention.

Key points

- Pulmonary oedema is uncommon in pregnancy but may be fatal.
- Chest radiography should not be withheld.
- Delivery of the fetus may be indicated.
- The mother should be managed in a high-dependency or intensive care unit.

Further reading

Dennis AT, Solnordal CB. Acute pulmonary oedema in pregnant women. *Anaesthesia* 2012; **67**: 646–59.

Sciscione AC, Ivester T, Largoza M, *et al.* Acute pulmonary edema in pregnancy. *Obstet Gynecol* 2003; **101**: 511–15.

Cardiomyopathy

Pregnant women may have a pre-existing cardiomyopathy or may develop cardiomyopathy of pregnancy (peripartum cardiomyopathy – PPCM).

- The causes of pre-existing cardiomyopathy are diverse and include infection, systemic disease such as sarcoidosis, infiltrative disease such as amyloid, toxins such as alcohol and cocaine, ischaemic heart disease and congenital cardiomyopathies. Of this group, the most commonly encountered in the antenatal clinic are the congenital hypertrophic obstructive cardiomyopathies (HOCMs).
- The aetiology of PPCM is unknown, but viral or autoimmune myocarditis, or an exaggerated response to the haemodynamic stresses of pregnancy, have been suggested. The classic criteria for diagnosis of PPCM are:
  (i)   Development of cardiac failure in the last month of pregnancy or within 5 months of delivery
  (ii) Absence of other aetiology for cardiac failure
  (iii) Absence of cardiac disease prior to the last month of pregnancy
  (iv) Echocardiography criteria have subsequently been added: ejection fraction $< 45\%$ and/or fractional shortening $< 30\%$, and end-diastolic dimension > 2.7 cm/m^2 body surface area.

  It has been suggested that the definition should be extended to include cardiac failure developing within the third trimester of pregnancy for which no other cause can be found. The incidence of PPCM is estimated to be 1 in 3000 pregnancies.

  Functionally, patients with HOCM have an obstructive cardiomyopathy, whilst those with PPCM have a dilated cardiomyopathy.

Problems/special considerations

- Patients with obstructive cardiomyopathy have a hypertrophied left ventricle and interventricular septum. Mitral regurgitation is often present. Any factors that increase myocardial contractility (β-agonists, circulating catecholamines) or decrease preload or afterload (vasodilatation, hypovolaemia) will cause an increase in left ventricular outflow obstruction. Tachycardias reduce the time for diastolic filling, and atrial arrhythmias are particularly poorly tolerated.
- The obstructive component of HOCM varies considerably. Women with minimal obstruction usually tolerate pregnancy well, although the more severe the degree of left ventricular hypertrophy the greater the risk of myocardial ischaemia, particularly in response to the stress of pregnancy and delivery.

- Patients with dilated cardiomyopathy have reduced myocardial contractility. The left ventricle is hypokinetic, ejection fraction is less than 0.4 and there is usually mitral and/or tricuspid regurgitation. Pressures in the right side of the heart are raised, and cardiac or pulmonary artery catheterisation usually confirms pulmonary hypertension. Any factors that depress myocardial contractility or increase afterload will further compromise cardiovascular stability.

  Women with PPCM usually present with the classic signs of left ventricular or congestive cardiac failure. There is a high associated risk of embolic phenomena.

Management options

Obstructive cardiomyopathy

Women with HOCM have usually been diagnosed before pregnancy, and baseline cardiological investigations should be available. If β-blocking drugs are being used these should be continued during pregnancy.

Serial cardiological investigations (electrocardiography (ECG), echocardiography) should be performed during pregnancy. Tachycardias should be treated with suitable β-blockers, and esmolol has been recommended for use in the acute situation. Cardioversion may be required to terminate supraventricular tachycardia; amiodarone is recommended for ventricular tachycardias. Nitrates should not be used to treat angina because the consequent vasodilatation and afterload reduction further aggravates left ventricular outflow obstruction.

There is no indication to deliver women by caesarean section unless there are obstetric reasons to do so or unless the maternal condition deteriorates. Continuous ECG and arterial blood pressure monitoring should be used throughout labour and delivery and continued into the early postnatal period.

Traditionally, regional analgesia has been considered contraindicated because of the risk of acute reduction in afterload. However, provision of high quality analgesia is beneficial, particularly for preventing pain-induced tachycardia. Intrathecal opioid analgesia is not accompanied by sympathetic blockade but is of limited efficacy in advanced labour. Epidural or combined spinal–epidural analgesia, using low-dose ($<0.1\%$ bupivacaine) epidural local anaesthetic with fentanyl, offers good analgesia with minimum haemodynamic disturbance.

Maintenance of adequate hydration – intravenously if necessary – is important. Phenylephrine is preferable to ephedrine for treatment of hypotension because the α effects of phenylephrine have less effect on myocardial contractility and heart rate than the mixed α and β effects of ephedrine.

Dilated cardiomyopathy/PPCM

The majority of cases of PPCM present in the peripartum or immediate postpartum period. Treatment includes use of positive inotropes such as digoxin (and parenteral inotropes such as dopamine and dobutamine in the acute situation), oxygen and diuretics, vasodilators to reduce afterload (but not angiotensin converting enzyme inhibitors before delivery), bed rest and anticoagulants (because of the risk of thromboembolic disease). Heart or heart–lung transplantation may be needed in severe cases that fail to respond to maximal medical therapy.

If PPCM presents antenatally, delivery is indicated as soon as the woman's condition has been optimised. Caesarean section may be necessary unless conditions are favourable for induction of labour.

Regional analgesia and anaesthesia are thought to be beneficial for the patient with dilated cardiomyopathy, since the cardiodepressant effects of most general anaesthetic drugs are avoided, and afterload is beneficially reduced. Hypotension should be treated with drugs with predominantly β activity, which stimulate myocardial contractility (ephedrine) rather than pure α-agonists (phenylephrine) which increase systemic vascular resistance.

PPCM has a high recurrence rate, and some authorities consider further pregnancies to be contraindicated following PPCM. Others suggest that another pregnancy can be considered if there is no residual cardiomegaly by 6 months postpartum. Case series suggest that if left ventricular function is still impaired one year after delivery there is a ~20% risk of death in the next pregnancy.

Key points

- Hypertrophic obstructive cardiomyopathy is usually inherited, and presents with variable left ventricular outflow obstruction.
- Treatment is directed at reduction of myocardial contractility and increasing preload and afterload.
- Tachyarrhythmias and myocardial ischaemia are particular hazards.
- Peripartum cardiomyopathy usually presents in the peripartum or early postpartum period.
- Treatment is symptomatic and is directed at maintaining myocardial contractility and reducing afterload.

Further reading

Blauwet LA, Cooper LT. Diagnosis and management of peripartum cardiomyopathy. *Heart* 2011; **97**: 1970–81.

Curry R, Swan L, Steer PJ. Cardiac disease in pregnancy. *Curr Opin Obstet Gynecol* 2009; **21**: 508–13.

Pyatt JR, Dubey G. Peripartum cardiomyopathy: current understanding, comprehensive management review and new developments. *Postgrad Med J* 2011; **87**: 34–9.

Stergiopoulos K, Shiang E, Bench T. Pregnancy in patients with pre-existing cardiomyopathies. *J Am Coll Cardiol* 2011; **58**: 337–50.

Chapter 89

Coarctation of the aorta

Coarctation of the aorta occurs in approximately 5% of patients with congenital heart disease and may occur as an isolated lesion or in association with other cardiovascular defects. Preductal coarctation is associated with patent ductus arteriosus, ventricular septal defect, bicuspid aortic valve and (in about 10% of cases) transposition of the great vessels. The majority of cases of preductal coarctation present with congestive cardiac failure in the neonatal period and are diagnosed and corrected surgically in infancy.

Postductal coarctation of the aorta may not be diagnosed until adolescence or adult life. There are associated berry aneurysms of the circle of Willis in approximately 10% of cases, and bicuspid aortic valve in 50% of patients.

Problems/special considerations

- Undiagnosed coarctation may present for the first time in pregnancy. There is invariably hypertension and this may be accompanied by congestive cardiac failure, caused by inability to compensate for the increased blood volume and cardiac output of pregnancy. The generalised peripheral vasodilatation and consequent reduction in systemic vascular resistance that occur in pregnancy may also precipitate cardiac failure.
- Pregnancy in women with an uncorrected aortic coarctation is associated with a maternal mortality of 3–9%, and a fetal mortality of up to 20%. Pregnancy or labour may be complicated by aortic dissection or rupture. Corrected coarctation is considered a low-risk lesion in pregnancy, unless there are associated abnormalities such as those described above, or aortic dilatation.
- There is a risk of aortic rupture or dissection if blood pressure increases acutely, e.g. because of severe pain or following use of certain drugs, e.g. ergometrine, vasopressors. Increased shearing forces associated with swings in blood pressure may also be dangerous.
- Hypertension is limited to the arms, and blood pressure may be reduced in the legs; palpation of the peripheral pulses frequently reveals absent foot pulses and radiofemoral delay. An aortic systolic murmur is heard on auscultation of the chest, and there may also be audible bruits over the intercostal and internal mammary vessels, which carry collateral flow to the lower limbs. A chest x-ray may show rib notching caused by the collateral vessels, and left ventricular hypertrophy.

Management options

Women with corrected coarctation should be assessed early in pregnancy, and any associated abnormalities noted.

There is no proven benefit of operative delivery for women with uncorrected coarctation, although anxiety about undiagnosed aneurysms of the circle of Willis may lead to recommendations for epidural analgesia and elective instrumental delivery. There is also no evidence that allowing the woman to labour increases her risks of aortic dissection or rupture. Minimising haemodynamic disturbance is the main aim of management of delivery. Cardiac output is relatively fixed; tachycardia secondary to uncontrolled pain may precipitate cardiac failure, but bradycardia and acute reduction in systemic vascular resistance are also hazardous. Hypovolaemia leads to compromised left ventricular filling.

Invasive systemic arterial pressure monitoring allows close attention to changes in blood pressure and facilitates analgesic and anaesthetic management. Central venous pressure monitoring may also be useful. Epidural or combined epidural–spinal techniques can provide safe and effective pain relief in labour. Although the main risk is from hypertension, it is also important to avoid hypotension.

For caesarean section, both regional and general anaesthesia may be suitable, although many practitioners would avoid single-shot spinal anaesthesia because of the risk of uncontrolled hypotension. Combined spinal–epidural, continuous spinal or epidural techniques allow gradual extension of the anaesthetic level cephalad and minimise the risks of rapid onset of profound hypotension. If general anaesthesia is used, steps should be taken to prevent the hypertensive response to tracheal intubation.

Postoperative management in a high-dependency environment is essential; invasive monitoring should be continued postoperatively and adequate analgesia should be ensured by using either the epidural route or patient-controlled intravenous analgesia.

Key points

- Women with corrected coarctation do not usually pose any particular problem in pregnancy, although there may be other associated cardiovascular abnormalities.
- Uncorrected coarctation may be associated with aortic dissection or rupture.
- Both general and regional anaesthesia are acceptable options but both may be hazardous.
- Invasive arterial ± central venous pressure monitoring is recommended.

Further reading

ESC Guidelines on the management of cardiovascular diseases during pregnancy: the Task Force on the Management of Cardiovascular Diseases during Pregnancy of the European Society of Cardiology (ESC). *Eur Heart J* 2011; **32**: 3147–97.

Chapter

90

Prosthetic heart valves

Most women with a prosthetic heart valve presenting to a UK antenatal clinic will have had the valve inserted because of congenital heart disease, although immigrants from the Indian subcontinent and some parts of eastern Europe still have a high incidence of acquired valve disease.

Women with corrected congenital heart disease and a prosthetic heart valve have increased morbidity in pregnancy, especially if they are anticoagulated.

Problems/special considerations

The relative risk of pregnancy in women with prosthetic heart valves is dependent not only on the underlying cardiac abnormality and residual impairment of cardiac function but also on the type of valve replacement used. Prosthetic heart valves may be mechanical, porcine or human allograft (homograft). Women with valves inserted before the end of the 1970s are almost certain to have mechanical valves. Homograft valves have only been widely available since the end of the 1980s.

- *Mechanical valves:* The most important risks for women with mechanical valves are the risks associated with anticoagulation during pregnancy and the risk of endocarditis. Both warfarin and heparin therapy are associated with significant maternal morbidity and fetal morbidity and mortality; warfarin is better for maternal health but worse for the fetus, while heparin is better for the fetus and worse for the mother.

  Warfarin is teratogenic, causing mental retardation, short stature and multiple facial abnormalities. Its use in the second trimester of pregnancy is associated with fetal blindness, microcephaly and mental retardation. There is also an increased risk of fetal internal haemorrhage. Spontaneous abortion, maternal haemorrhage and stillbirth are also increased in women receiving warfarin.

  Although less common, administration of heparin during pregnancy is also associated with increased rates of spontaneous abortion, fetal and maternal haemorrhage and stillbirth. Prolonged use of heparin may also cause maternal osteoporosis and heparin-induced thrombocytopenia, though these are less common with low molecular weight heparins. However, the main risk with heparin is thromboembolism involving the heart valves, increasing maternal morbidity and mortality. Traditionally, British practice has been to convert women to heparin for the first trimester of pregnancy and then maintain them on warfarin before reverting to heparin for the last few weeks of pregnancy and for delivery, while practice in the USA has been to heparinise women throughout pregnancy. In particular high-risk cases, low-dose aspirin may be added to heparin therapy in an attempt to improve maternal outcome.

- *Porcine valves:* The major risks of porcine valves are thromboembolic events and valve failure. The rate of valve degeneration at 10 years is estimated at 50–60%. There is some evidence that pregnancy accelerates the degeneration of porcine valves, and it is therefore imperative to follow these women closely during pregnancy and immediately to investigate any possibility of deteriorating cardiac function.

  Although the advantage of porcine compared with mechanical valves is that anticoagulation is not needed routinely, women with atrial fibrillation or a history of a thromboembolic event are likely to require full anticoagulation, with its attendant risks.

- *Homograft valves:* These valves are used primarily for aortic replacement, and the available evidence suggests that they are associated with a significantly lower pregnancy morbidity than either porcine or mechanical valves. There is no need for anticoagulant therapy and there do not appear to be the same risks of degenerative change as with porcine valves.

  Women with aortic valve replacement tolerate the physiological changes of pregnancy relatively well, but those with mitral valve replacement have a relatively fixed cardiac output and are at risk of developing cardiac failure during pregnancy. They also have an increased risk of atrial fibrillation; if this occurs it should be treated promptly, by cardioversion if necessary.

Management options

Pre-pregnancy counselling should be offered to women with prosthetic valves, firstly to advise those with congenital heart disease of the increased risks of congenital heart disease in their offspring, and secondly to advise those who are dependent on anticoagulants of the risks of such therapy in pregnancy. Valve function and cardiac status should also be assessed before pregnancy if possible.

All women with prosthetic heart valves should be regarded as having high-risk pregnancies and should be delivered in large maternity units, preferably in or near to centres with facilities for cardiac surgery. Cardiac function should be assessed early in the first trimester of pregnancy and at regular intervals throughout the pregnancy. It is particularly important for women with prosthetic valves to receive regular dental care during pregnancy, and any dental treatment should be preceded by prophylactic antibiotics. Similarly, any intercurrent infection during pregnancy should be aggressively treated.

The presence of a prosthetic heart valve is not in itself an indication for operative delivery. There are obvious advantages in planned induction of labour in the anticoagulated woman, since she can be converted to prophylactic rather than therapeutic doses of heparin over the period of induction and delivery. This enables regional analgesic and anaesthetic techniques to be used (following laboratory assessment of coagulation status) if appropriate. If regional analgesia is contraindicated, patient-controlled intravenous opioid analgesia is the most appropriate alternative for labour and also for provision of postoperative analgesia if general anaesthesia has been used for caesarean section.

Most units continue to give prophylactic antibiotics to cover delivery in women with prosthetic heart valves, despite recent guidelines suggesting this is unnecessary.

In general, management and monitoring will depend on the severity of residual cardiac disease and the underlying lesion, and the requirements of each woman must be determined on an individual basis.

Key points

- Women with prosthetic heart valves are not a homogeneous group. They differ in their underlying cardiac disease, degree of impairment of cardiac function and type of prosthetic valve.
- Pre-pregnancy counselling is recommended whenever possible.
- Antenatal care and delivery should be undertaken in a hospital with facilities for high-dependency care.
- Regular assessment of cardiac function during pregnancy is important.

Further reading

Bates SM, Greer IA, Middeldorp S, *et al.* VTE, thrombophilia, antithrombotic therapy, and pregnancy: antithrombotic therapy and prevention of thrombosis, 9th edn: American College of Chest Physicians Evidence-Based Clinical Practice Guidelines. *Chest* 2012; **141** (2 Suppl): e691S–736S.

European Society of Cardiology. Recommendations for the management of patients after heart valve surgery. *Eur Heart J* 2005; **26**: 2463–71.

ESC Guidelines on the management of cardiovascular diseases during pregnancy: the Task Force on the Management of Cardiovascular Diseases during Pregnancy of the European Society of Cardiology (ESC). *Eur Heart J* 2011; **32**: 3147–97.

Stout KK, Otto CM. Pregnancy in women with valvular heart disease. *Heart* 2007; **93**: 552–8.

Chapter

91

Congenital heart disease

About 70–80% of children with congenital heart disease (CHD) now reach adult life (16 years and over) and thus reproductive age. Unfortunately, there is still a significant mortality rate amongst young adults with corrected CHD. In the pregnant population, cyanotic CHD is associated with a higher maternal and fetal morbidity and mortality than non-cyanotic disease, but both groups of women should be regarded as high-risk patients.

Problems/special considerations

- Patients primarily with disorders of cardiac output may experience cardiac failure as pregnancy progresses, because of the increased demands placed on the cardiovascular system and the increased oxygen demand. Patients with cyanotic (or potentially cyanotic) disorders may experience worsening cyanosis as the decreasing systemic

Table 91.1 Risk of neonatal cardiac lesions when at least one parent has congenital heart disease

Tetralogy of Fallot	2–3%
Persistent ductus arteriosus; aortic coarctation	4%
Atrial septal defect	5–11%
Pulmonary stenosis	6–7%
Ventricular or atrioventricular septal defect	10–16%
Aortic stenosis	15–18%
Marfan's/Di George's syndrome	50%

vascular resistance encourages shunting of blood across the heart; this is compounded by increased oxygen demand. Both types of patients are prone to arrhythmias and venous thromboembolism, and tolerate hypovolaemia poorly.

- A maternal haematocrit of greater than 60%, arterial oxygen saturation of less than 80%, right ventricular hypertrophy and episodes of syncope are all considered poor prognostic factors. Women with cyanotic disease have higher rates of spontaneous abortion and these are said to correlate with haematocrit.
- Conditions associated with particularly high risk in pregnancy are:
  (i) Pulmonary hypertension (residual or primary)
  (ii) Systemic right ventricle
  (iii) Moderate and severe aortic stenosis
  (iv) Marfan's syndrome with aortic dilatation
  (v) Complex surgery such as Fontan or Mustard procedures.
  Women with corrected septal defects are usually asymptomatic but some may have conduction disorders and there may still be residual pulmonary hypertension. A large Canadian study found that the presence of more than one of the following predictors was associated with an estimated risk of pulmonary oedema, arrhythmia, stroke, cardiac arrest or cardiac death of 75%: New York Heart Association classification > II or cyanosis; previous cardiac event or arrhythmia; left heart obstruction; and left ventricular systolic dysfunction.
- Regardless of the maternal cardiac condition, the fetus of the mother with CHD has an increased risk of CHD (Table 91.1).
- Bolus doses of Syntocinon cause a transient but sometimes profound fall in arterial blood pressure; the drug should be given by intravenous infusion if at all. Ergometrine causes a sharp rise in arterial, central venous and intracranial pressures and should generally be avoided in women with CHD, although it may be preferable to Syntocinon in certain fixed output states without pulmonary hypertension. If caesarean section is performed, the need for oxytocics may be avoided by performing a brace suture through the uterus to provide mechanical, rather than pharmacological, uterine compression.
- Women may be receiving therapeutic doses of anticoagulants and this may preclude regional analgesia and anaesthesia, though the latter is still possible if timed appropriately.

Management options

Women with CHD must be identified early in pregnancy (preferably seen for preconception counselling) and managed jointly by the obstetrician, cardiologist and obstetric anaesthetist. Appropriate investigations and plans should be instituted (see Chapter 85, Cardiovascular disease) and placed clearly in the patient's notes. Some units have a register in which high-risk patients approaching term delivery can be entered.

Caesarean section is not indicated for women with CHD unless there are obstetric indications or worsening maternal condition. Planned induction of labour may appear to have obvious benefits, but carries the risk of an increased likelihood of obstetric intervention.

Invasive arterial and/or central venous pressure monitoring is generally recommended except for mild conditions; the use of pulmonary artery catheters is controversial and is usually impractical outside the intensive care unit.

Cautious use of low-dose epidural bupivacaine (0.1% or less) in combination with an opioid (usually 2.0–2.5 μg/ml fentanyl) provides optimal analgesia for women with CHD. Intrathecal opioids and continuous spinal analgesia have also been used. The use of high concentrations of bupivacaine (0.25–0.5%) in labour is contraindicated because of the risk of rapid and uncontrolled decrease in cardiac output.

Elective instrumental delivery avoids the fall in cardiac output that accompanies pushing, and should be recommended for most cases, although a maximum of 15–30 minutes' pushing can be allowed for mild cases.

Anaesthesia for caesarean delivery in women with CHD carries high risks. The options are for slow induction of regional anaesthesia (e.g. epidural, continuous spinal or combined spinal–epidural with a very small spinal component) or a 'cardiac' general anaesthetic (which usually necessitates some hours of postoperative ventilatory support). There are no absolute rules; the relative risks and benefits in each individual case must be considered. A consultant anaesthetist with expertise in the management of high-risk pregnancy should be involved in the decision making.

Management of intrapartum anticoagulation should be discussed with both the haematologist and cardiologist. Recent guidelines have not recommended routine prophylactic antibiotic cover for labour but many centres continue to give this, usually amoxycillin and gentamicin. All drug therapy should be discussed with a cardiologist with expertise in the management of CHD.

Key points

- Cyanotic congenital heart disease is associated with high maternal and fetal morbidity and mortality.
- Multidisciplinary antenatal and intrapartum care is essential.
- Regional analgesia for labour is usually beneficial; choice of anaesthetic technique for caesarean section is controversial.

Further reading

Curry R, Swan L, Steer PJ. Cardiac disease in pregnancy. *Curr Opin Obstet Gynecol* 2009; **21**: 508–13.

ESC Guidelines on the management of cardiovascular diseases during pregnancy: the Task Force on the Management of Cardiovascular Diseases during Pregnancy of the European Society of Cardiology (ESC). *Eur Heart J* 2011; **32**: 3147–97.

Head CEG, Thorne SA. Congenital heart disease in pregnancy. *Postgrad Med J* 2005; **81**: 292–8.

Sermer M, Colman J, Siu S. Pregnancy complicated by heart disease: a review of Canadian experience. *J Obstet Gynaecol* 2003; **23**: 540–4.

Stout K. Pregnancy in women with congenital heart disease: the importance of evaluation and counseling. *Heart* 2005; **91**: 713–14.

Chapter

92 Pulmonary hypertension and Eisenmenger's syndrome

Primary pulmonary hypertension is associated with an extremely high maternal mortality (40–60%) and is one of the few remaining maternal conditions in which pregnancy is considered absolutely contraindicated.

Secondary pulmonary hypertension may occur as a result of chronic pulmonary disease, e.g. connective tissue disease, or congenital heart disease such as severe aortic/mitral stenosis, or more usually, chronic left-to-right shunt. These conditions are also associated with high maternal mortality, particularly left-to-right shunt leading to Eisenmenger's syndrome (reversal of the shunt when pulmonary pressures exceed systemic pressures).

Although women are advised against pregnancy, many do not heed this advice.

Problems/special considerations

- Pulmonary artery pressures may be close to systemic arterial pressures and are associated with a high pulmonary vascular resistance. There is right ventricular hypertrophy and a relatively fixed low cardiac output. Increases in pulmonary vascular resistance, decreases in systemic vascular resistance or falls in cardiac output can all have catastrophic and potentially fatal consequences. In Eisenmenger's syndrome, peripheral vasodilatation increases shunt across the heart and thus worsens hypoxaemia.
- The increased cardiac output that occurs during pregnancy is poorly tolerated, since it causes further increase in pulmonary artery and right ventricular pressures, and volume overload. Right ventricular dilatation and tricuspid regurgitation may occur, and left ventricular function and cardiac output may become increasingly impaired. The major haemodynamic changes occurring during parturition and the puerperium can prove fatal. Major haemorrhage causing hypovolaemia, or autotransfusion with the third stage of labour causing volume overload, are both poorly tolerated.

Management options

Close antenatal monitoring is essential, and women with pulmonary hypertension are frequently admitted for inpatient care in the third trimester of pregnancy or even earlier – most women resting more in hospital than is possible at home. Prophylactic anticoagulation is controversial, but prophylactic heparin is often given in addition to simple anti-thromboembolism measures such as graduated compression stockings. Care must be taken to avoid prolonged immobility in hospital. The risks of aortocaval compression if women adopt supine or semi-supine positions are not confined to labour, and the lateral position should be adopted for any antenatal examinations of mother or fetus.

Pulmonary hypertension itself is not considered an indication for caesarean section, though it may be required should maternal condition deteriorate or if there is fetal compromise. The advantages of choosing to deliver by caesarean section include avoiding a prolonged second stage and the adverse effects of bearing down, and also avoiding uncontrolled vaginal haemorrhage. Continuous oxygen therapy may be beneficial for both mother and fetus. The mother may describe 'funny spells' and these should be taken seriously as potential indicators of episodes of severe pulmonary hypertension. Induction of labour is an option if the cervix is favourable, but is associated with a higher rate of operative delivery than spontaneous labour.

For delivery, maternal monitoring should include electrocardiography and invasive right atrial and arterial blood pressure measurement. Use of a pulmonary artery catheter is more controversial and has been associated with an increased risk of thrombosis; other methods of cardiac output monitoring have been used intraoperatively. Scrupulous care must be taken to avoid accidental injection of air because of the risk of systemic embolism in women with shunts.

Oxygen is a readily available and easily administered pulmonary vasodilator and should be given continuously throughout labour and delivery. Hypoxia, hypercarbia and acidosis all tend to increase pulmonary artery pressure and pulmonary vascular resistance. Prolonged labour, use of systemic opioids and inadequate hydration are all, therefore, risk factors for these women.

Regional analgesia has been used successfully; epidural infusions or intermittent boluses of low concentrations of local anaesthetic and opioid (0.0625–0.1% bupivacaine with fentanyl 2.0–2.5 µg/ml; alternatively opioid alone) provide good analgesia without compromising haemodynamic stability. Combined spinal–epidural analgesia is a suitable alternative but offers little advantage over low-dose epidural analgesia, except possibly more profound analgesia if opioids alone are used. Use of air to identify the epidural space should be avoided because of the risk of air embolism.

Although general anaesthesia has traditionally been recommended for women with pulmonary hypertension, regional anaesthesia has been successfully used for both Eisenmenger's syndrome and primary pulmonary hypertension. It is imperative to use a slow titration technique and invasive central monitoring if regional anaesthesia is chosen.

General anaesthesia offers potentially greater haemodynamic stability, and the opportunity to minimise oxygen consumption by eliminating the work of breathing and maximise arterial oxygen saturation. It is also easier to administer inhaled pulmonary vasodilators such as 100% oxygen, nebulised prostacyclin or nitric oxide; use of the latter two has been described, although their place in improving oxygenation is still uncertain. However, the cardiodepressant effects of general anaesthesia with associated reduction in cardiac output are still hazards for these women, as is the potentially increased risk of thromboembolism. A high-dose opioid 'cardiac' general anaesthetic provides maximal haemodynamic stability. There is no particular advantage in elective ventilation postoperatively, but high-dependency or intensive care nursing is mandatory.

Postoperative and post-delivery analgesia can be provided by patient-controlled intravenous opioids or by epidural or intrathecal opioids. Invasive monitoring must be continued for several days; women with pulmonary hypertension are frequently successfully delivered, only to die during the first 2 weeks after delivery. Mortality is associated with thromboembolism or refractory right heart failure.

Key points

- Pregnancy is extremely hazardous for women with pulmonary hypertension.
- Maternal mortality may be as high as 60%.
- The physiological changes of normal pregnancy are poorly tolerated by women with pulmonary hypertension.
- Hypovolaemia and any increase in pulmonary vascular resistance must be avoided.
- Cautious use of regional analgesia for vaginal delivery with full invasive cardiovascular monitoring is recommended.
- Both general and epidural anaesthesia have been used for operative delivery; both have significant risks.

Further reading

Bildirici I, Shumway JB. Intravenous and inhaled epoprostenol for primary pulmonary hypertension during pregnancy and delivery. *Obstet Gynecol* 2004; **103**: 1102–5.

Bonnin M, Mercier FJ, Sitbon O, *et al.* Severe pulmonary hypertension during pregnancy: mode of delivery and anesthetic management of 15 consecutive cases. *Anesthesiology* 2005; **102**: 1133–7.

Curry R, Swan L, Steer PJ. Cardiac disease in pregnancy. *Curr Opin Obstet Gynecol* 2009; **21**: 508–13.

Lane CR, Trow TK. Pregnancy and pulmonary hypertension. *Clin Chest Med* 2011; **32**: 165–74.

Madden BP. Pulmonary hypertension and pregnancy. *Int J Obstet Anesth* 2009; **18**: 156–64.

Chapter 93

Ischaemic heart disease

Myocardial infarction (MI) during pregnancy is uncommon, with a reported incidence of 1 in 10 000–35 000 pregnancies. There have been an increasing number of case reports of MI during pregnancy and delivery, and it is possible that the incidence is now higher. Ischaemic heart disease in the antenatal population is frequently related to smoking and obesity, but may also be associated with the use of illegal drugs, particularly crack cocaine. Postpartum MI has been reported as a complication of pre-eclampsia. Women who have had previous MI, with or without previous coronary artery bypass grafting, may also present to the obstetrician and obstetric anaesthetist.

Problems/special considerations

- A high index of suspicion is necessary. Myocardial ischaemia may not be considered in the differential diagnoses of a pregnant woman presenting with chest pain, and the presentation may be atypical. The woman who has been using cocaine is frequently an unreliable historian, and may conceal or deny her drug abuse. Clinical examination and investigations may be difficult to interpret; a systolic murmur is common during pregnancy, and it should be remembered that left axis deviation with non-specific ST and T wave changes is commonly seen in the healthy pregnant patient. Cardiac troponin I is a useful investigation since it is unaffected by pregnancy, labour and delivery.
- Maternal mortality of acute MI during pregnancy has been reported to be as high as 30–50%, with the highest mortality associated with MI during the third trimester of pregnancy and also if a woman delivers within two weeks of an MI. Recent studies suggest a lower mortality rate of under 10%.
- Myocardial ischaemia and infarction caused by cocaine are associated with a high incidence of cardiac arrhythmias.
- Antenatal considerations include: the use of anticoagulants; planning of place, time and mode of delivery; use of intrapartum invasive monitoring; and choice of analgesia and anaesthesia for delivery.

Management options

These women should be managed by a multidisciplinary team. Reported treatments include the use of intra-aortic balloon counterpulsation and percutaneous transluminal coronary angioplasty.

Mode of delivery

There is no consensus of opinion in the literature about the preferred mode of delivery of a woman who has had antenatal MI, nor about the method of anaesthesia. Vaginal delivery eliminates the stress of surgery and the need to provide anaesthesia. The risk of peripartum thromboembolism is also reduced, as is the potential for obstetric haemorrhage. However, induction of labour carries an increased risk of further obstetric intervention, whereas allowing spontaneous onset of labour is unpredictable. Caesarean delivery can be optimally timed to permit senior staff from all concerned specialties to be involved. There is adequate time to institute full invasive monitoring and to organise cardiovascular support, but surgical intervention increases the risks of complications.

Monitoring

Most authorities suggest using intra-arterial pressure monitoring, pulse oximetry and continuous electrocardiographic monitoring. The use of pulmonary artery pressure monitoring is more controversial and is associated with significant risks that may outweigh potential benefits.

Analgesia and anaesthesia

For analgesia in labour, epidural analgesia minimises haemodynamic instability caused by the pain and stress of labour. Use of low-dose local anaesthetic and opioid infusions or boluses avoids the risk of hypotension. Combined spinal–epidural analgesia would also be a suitable alternative.

Both 'cardiac' (high-dose opioid) general anaesthesia and epidural anaesthesia have been used successfully for caesarean section. The major concerns with general anaesthesia are the uncontrolled hypertensive response to tracheal intubation, the risks of potentially life-threatening arrhythmias (particularly in cocaine users) and the need for postoperative ventilatory support because of the high doses of opioids used.

The major concern with regional anaesthesia is haemodynamic instability caused by rapid onset of sympathetic blockade. For this reason, single-shot spinal anaesthesia is not recommended; if a regional technique is chosen a slow incremental epidural technique should be used (continuous spinal and combined spinal–epidural anaesthesia have also been used successfully).

Oxytocic drugs

Ergometrine causes acute hypertension and is contraindicated in women with ischaemic heart disease. Large intravenous boluses (> 5 U) of Syntocinon cause transient hypotension and may compromise coronary filling; it is therefore preferable to use an intravenous infusion of Syntocinon during management of the third stage of labour.

Puerperium

The fluid shifts that occur during the early postpartum period contribute to potential haemodynamic instability at this time. High-dependency nursing and medical care is mandatory; intensive cardiovascular monitoring should be maintained for at least 24–48 hours after delivery. Epidural opioids are recommended for provision of postoperative analgesia. The use of prophylactic anticoagulants should be considered for 3–6 months post-delivery.

Key points
- Myocardial infarction during pregnancy has a high maternal mortality.
- The association between myocardial infarction and cocaine consumption should be considered.
- Management of labour and delivery is based on maintaining haemodynamic stability and minimising myocardial oxygen consumption.

Further reading
Kealey A. Coronary artery disease and myocardial infarction in pregnancy: a review of epidemiology, diagnosis, and medical and surgical management. *Can J Cardiol* 2010; **26**: 185–9.

Ladner HE, Danielsen B, Gilbert WM. Acute myocardial infarction in pregnancy and the puerperium: a population-based study. *Obstet Gynecol* 2005; **105**: 480–4.

Roth A, Elkayam U. Acute myocardial infarction associated with pregnancy. *J Am Coll Cardiol* 2008; **52**: 171–80.

Chapter

94

Endocrine disease

The most common endocrine disorder affecting pregnancy is diabetes mellitus, which is considered separately. Although there are several other conditions that may have obstetric implications, most have little specific obstetric anaesthetic relevance over and above considerations applicable to the non-pregnant state.

Special considerations/management options
- *Thyroid disease:* Anaesthetic implications are as for non-pregnant patients. Goitre may increase in size in pregnancy. Acute hyperthyroidism ('thyroid storm') may cause premature labour and fetal loss (and rarely, fetal hyperthyroidism). Rarely, the fetus may be affected by anti-thyroid treatment; goitre has been reported. Neonatal encephalopathy is more common if the mother has thyroid disease.
- *Adrenal disease:* Hypoadrenalism is a rare cause of collapse on the labour ward. Patients receiving steroid therapy may require extra dosage peripartum (see Chapter 141, Steroid therapy).

  Phaeochromocytoma is a rare but well recognised cause of hypertension in pregnancy. Medical management is classically with α-blockade first and then β-blockade; it is important to ensure adequate fluid replacement. Magnesium therapy has also been used to control pre- and intraoperative hypertension. Regional anaesthesia has been safely used for labour and vaginal delivery. Combined caesarean section and excision of the tumour has been reported using both regional and general anaesthesia, with appropriate monitoring. More recently there have been reports of an elective two-step procedure being used whereby patients are treated medically first, followed by caesarean section and then the tumour is excised. Phaeochromocytoma may be a part of the multiple endocrine neoplasia syndrome.

- *Neurological endocrine disease:* Most of the anaesthetic implications relate to the effects of any intracranial space-occupying lesion. Specific hormonal conditions are managed as for non-pregnant patients. Sheehan's syndrome is pituitary infarction caused by severe hypotension ('pituitary apoplexy'), originally described in association with placental abruption. Pregnant women are thought to be particularly susceptible to this phenomenon because the pituitary gland enlarges during pregnancy and its blood supply is consequently more critical.
- *Other conditions:* These are managed as for non-pregnant patients.

Key points

- Diabetes mellitus is the most common and important endocrine disease in pregnancy.
- General management of endocrine disease is as for non-pregnant patients.

Further reading

Amin A, Robinson S, Teoh TG. Endocrine problems in pregnancy. *Postgrad Med J* 2011; **87**: 116–24.

Kennedy RL, Malabu UH, Jarrod G, *et al*. Thyroid function and pregnancy: before, during and beyond. *J Obstet Gynaecol* 2010; **30**: 774–83.

Chapter

95

Diabetes mellitus

In the general population, diabetes mellitus is present in about 2% of individuals, in about half of them undiagnosed. In pregnancy, insulin requirements increase as peripheral sensitivity to insulin decreases (thought to be caused by the opposing action of placental hormones); thus known diabetics may become unstable, and otherwise normal subjects may reveal themselves as having gestational diabetes if they cannot meet the increased demands (the latter occurs in up to 2–5% of pregnancies). Most gestational diabetics recover after pregnancy although most relapse in subsequent pregnancies at an earlier gestational age, and there is a 50% risk of developing type-2 diabetes in later life. Gestational diabetes is associated with older age, ethnicity, obesity, a family history of diabetes and poor previous obstetric history.

Screening of pregnant women for gestational diabetes is controversial and even amongst those that advocate it, there is disagreement about the cut-off points and definitions used. Most programmes involve initial random blood glucose testing with referral for a mini-glucose tolerance test (GTT) typically at 26 weeks' gestation if abnormal. The mini GTT involves a challenge of 50 g oral glucose followed by a blood glucose estimation one hour later; a concentration of ≥ 7.8 mmol/l constitutes abnormality. The full GTT includes a 75 g glucose challenge and has more specific divisions into normal/gestational diabetes/diabetes subgroups depending on fasting and GTT results.

Problems/special considerations

- *Effect of diabetes on the mother:* Diabetes has many effects on most organ systems, the most immediately important being renal impairment, cardiovascular disease and central and peripheral neurological disease. Women with long-standing type-1 diabetes, depending on their overall glycaemic control, may already manifest these complications, whereas those women with gestational or type-2 diabetes are usually younger than 40–45 years and systemic effects tend to be less common.
- *Control of blood sugar:* This is important during pregnancy since poor control is associated with increased incidence of fetal abnormalities (see below). In pregnancy, insulin requirements increase by up to 50% at term.

    During labour, it is important to avoid hyper- or hypoglycaemia, the former because it results in maternal and fetal acidosis and the latter because of the risk of impaired neurological function. Insulin requirements may decrease in the first stage but increase in the second stage of labour, although this may depend on other factors such as length of labour, pre-labour state, etc.
- *Effect of diabetes on pregnancy:* Diabetics have an increased incidence of miscarriage, pregnancy-induced hypertension, polyhydramnios, caesarean section and preterm labour (the last may not hold for gestational diabetes). There is also an increased incidence of neonatal hypoglycaemia and hyperbilirubinaemia. In type-1 diabetes, there is a 5–10-fold incidence of congenital malformation if glycaemic control during pregnancy is poor, with a 5-fold increase in stillbirth rate and 4–5-fold increase in perinatal death rate. Good glycaemic control reduces the incidence of congenital malformation to 2%, about twice the normal. Macrosomia occurs about 4–6 times as commonly in diabetics as non-diabetics, depending on the definition used; it is thought to be caused by reactive fetal insulin secretion in response to maternal hyperglycaemia and/or transfer of maternal insulin to the fetus. It may result in obstructed labour.

Management options

Before conception, known diabetics should be counselled and their care optimised (ideally, glycosylated haemoglobin concentration $< 7\%$).

Table 95.1 Sample sliding scale for insulin during labour in diabetics

Blood glucose concentration (mmol/l)	< 3.9	4.0–5.9	6.0–8.9	9.0–11.9	12.0–14.9	15.0–17.9	> 18
Insulin infusion rate (U soluble insulin/h)	0.5	1	2	3	4	5	6

During pregnancy, careful dietary advice ± pharmacological intervention aim to maintain normal blood glucose concentrations. Ideal glucose levels are 3.5–5.9 mmol/l and below 7.8 mmol/l postprandial. Close follow-up of pregnant diabetics is required, with monitoring of glycaemic control as well as screening for infections, since diabetic ketoacidosis may be precipitated by infection as in the non-pregnant state. Monitoring of fetal wellbeing and growth is also important. Increasing insulin requirements in pregnancy may reflect reduced placental function and may be an indication for induction of labour. Women with absent warning signs of hypoglycaemia should be advised against driving (pregnancy may alter awareness of hypoglycaemia, which occurs particularly in the first trimester). With regards to the fetus, women with diabetes should be offered antenatal examination of the fetal heart at 18–20 weeks' gestation.

During labour, most authorities advocate continuous glucose/insulin infusions; a suitable regimen comprises a 5% glucose infusion plus 20 mmol/l potassium chloride with a continuous insulin infusion using a sliding scale, according to regular (30–60 minute) blood glucose concentration monitoring (Table 95.1). The aim is to maintain blood glucose concentrations at 4–6 mmol/l; if this cannot be achieved the entire insulin infusion scale is increased by 1 U/h. If blood glucose concentration repeatedly falls below 4 mmol/l the 5% dextrose may be changed for 10% glucose. Urine should be tested, e.g. 4-hourly, for glucose and ketones. Avoidance of glucose during labour has been popular previously, but leads to maternal and fetal acidosis. Most authorities advise continuous fetal monitoring through-out labour, and a paediatrician should attend all deliveries, with neonatal unit admission prepared. For elective caesarean section, the same intravenous regimen is started in the morning, the patient having been nil by mouth since midnight and having omitted her usual morning insulin.

Insulin requirements fall rapidly once delivery has occurred, and the insulin infusion rate should be halved once the baby has been born. Most gestational diabetics do not need insulin postpartum; insulin-dependent diabetics may be given a subcutaneous dose of soluble insulin (e.g. 5 U) when ready to eat and drink, and the infusion stopped 60 minutes later.

Management as far as regional or general anaesthesia is concerned is along standard lines, although the former is especially desirable. In labour, regional analgesia is thought to be beneficial by reducing catecholamine levels and thus avoiding anti-insulin effects and the propensity for acidosis. Care should be taken to assess the mother for the complications of diabetes, as above. In addition, of especial relevance to general anaesthesia, autonomic neuropathy may be associated with reduced gastric emptying, and a syndrome of stiff joints has been described in which difficult tracheal intubation has featured. The syndrome is suggested by the 'prayer sign' in which the patient is unable to lay the palmar surfaces of her index fingers fully flat against one another when pressing her palms together as if praying; when viewed from the side there is a space between the proximal phalangeal joints. The syndrome has also been implicated in causing reduced compliance of the epidural space, with the risk of spinal cord ischaemia when large volumes are injected epidurally.

Fluid therapy should be separate from intravenous dextrose/insulin; thus two intravenous cannulae are usually required if anaesthetic intervention is needed. Hartmann's solution may result in a small increase in blood glucose concentration caused by gluconeogenesis from lactate metabolism, although this is rarely a problem in practice. Patients should receive adequate diabetic follow-up postpartum. Patients who have presented with gestational diabetes in particular should be followed up with a 6-week fasting plasma glucose check, and this should be checked annually thereafter.

Key points

- Diabetes mellitus is associated with increased incidence of fetal malformations, macrosomia and death, especially if diabetic control is poor.
- Pregnant diabetics should be closely followed throughout pregnancy and peripartum.
- Regional analgesia and anaesthesia are especially desirable.
- Insulin and glucose infusions are used in labour.
- Insulin requirements fall rapidly after delivery.

Further reading

Confidential Enquiry into Maternal and Child Health/Obstetric Anaesthetists' Association. *The CEMACH/OAA Diabetes Project: A national audit of anaesthetic records and care for women with type 1 or type 2 diabetes undergoing caesarean section.* London: CEMACH/OAA 2010, http://www.oaa-anaes.ac.uk/assets/_managed/editor/File/Reports/CMACE_OAA_diabetes_report_2010.pdf.

Kamalakannan D, Baskar V, Barton DM, Abdu TAM. Diabetic ketoacidosis in pregnancy. *Postgrad Med J* 2003; **79**: 454–7.

National Institute for Health and Clinical Excellence. Diabetes in pregnancy: management of diabetes and its complications from pre-conception to the postnatal period. *Clinical Guideline 63.* London: NICE 2008, http://guidance.nice.org.uk/CG63.

Chapter 96

Anaemia and polycythaemia

Pregnancy is associated with an increase in red cell mass and a greater increase in plasma volume. Circulating plasma volume can increase by 30–50% in single pregnancies but may double in multiple pregnancies. Red cell mass increases by 20–30%. There is therefore a physiological dilutional 'anaemia'. This increase in red cell mass and the needs of the developing fetus increase requirement for iron and folate, which often need to be supplemented. Normal iron absorption is around 1–2 mg a day; however, requirements in pregnancy may be as high as 6.6 mg a day. Many women start pregnancy with depleted iron stores and a low haemoglobin concentration, and the likelihood of this increases with subsequent pregnancies. In some cases of extreme iron deficiency, parenteral iron may be required.

Polycythaemia in pregnancy is rare and is usually secondary to other disease processes such as cyanotic heart disease. The underlying problem is usually more significant than the haemoglobin concentration itself. Primary polycythaemia (rubra vera) is a neoplastic disease usually seen in older patients than in the childbearing population.

Problems/special considerations

Anaemia

Normal vaginal delivery of a single fetus is associated with a blood loss of around 500 ml, but this may double with twin deliveries. Caesarean section is associated with a blood loss of 500–1000 ml. Following delivery, there is a fall in plasma volume caused by diuresis; this partially compensates for the drop in haemoglobin concentration resulting from blood loss.

Mothers who are already anaemic have less reserve than normal and may thus be more susceptible to the effects of haemorrhage. Since they rely on an even greater increase in cardiac output than normal to maintain oxygen delivery, cardiac depression (e.g. caused by general anaesthesia) may have profound effects on maternal and fetal oxygenation. Maternal myocardial ischaemia is also more common. Haemorrhage in Jehovah's Witnesses is a particular problem and an important cause of maternal death.

Pernicious anaemia is extremely rare in pregnancy but the presence of a macrocytic anaemia may prompt investigation. Folate and B_{12} deficiency may cause congenital malformations in the neonate, abruption and haemorrhage. Maternal complications include neurological complications such as subacute combined degeneration of the cord. Aplastic anaemia has been reported in pregnancy and in some cases has resolved following delivery.

Polycythaemia

There have been few published cases of polycythaemia complicating pregnancy. There may be associated thrombocytopenia or thrombocythaemia. Thrombocytopenia may be dilutional and may not reflect function. Thrombotic events (arterial and venous) do occur and prophylactic aspirin and heparin have been given to prevent them.

In cyanotic heart disease, a haemoglobin concentration greater than 16 g/dl is associated with poor fetal outcome; this probably represents both a marker of severity of the underlying disease and impairment of uteroplacental oxygenation resulting from increased blood viscosity.

Coagulation times may be artefactually prolonged in severe polycythaemia.

Management options

As long as the above potential problems are considered, anaesthetic management in general is routine. In anaemia, the threshold for transfusion should be lower than normal. Newer formulations of parenteral iron (iron-sucrose) have been used postpartum to restore haemoglobin concentration more rapidly than oral iron, and are associated with few adverse reactions unlike iron-dextran and sodium ferric gluconate preparations. Erythropoietin has been used in Jehovah's Witnesses – management of whom must include senior staff.

In polycythaemia, regional analgesia and anaesthesia may be precluded by recent administration of heparin, although the benefits usually outweigh the risk of epidural haematoma.

Key points

- A drop in haemoglobin concentration during pregnancy is normal.
- Postpartum diuresis partially compensates for peripartum blood loss.
- Polycythaemia in pregnancy is usually secondary to underlying disease.

Further reading

Goonewardene M, Shehata M, Hamad A. Anaemia in pregnancy. *Best Pract Res Clin Obstet Gynaecol* 2012; **26**: 3–24.

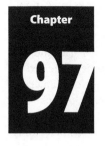

Chapter

97 Deep-vein thrombosis and pulmonary embolism

For many years, thromboembolism has been the most common direct cause of death in pregnancy in the UK; in the 2006–08 Confidential Enquiries into Maternal Deaths report, there was a significant reduction in the number of women dying from thromboembolism and this is thought to be related to the issuing of guidelines in 2004 on thromboembolism prophylaxis during and after pregnancy (a similar but smaller reduction occurred after guidance on post-caesarean section thromboembolism, issued in 1995). Apart from pregnancy itself, risk factors include bed rest, dehydration, coincident thrombophilia, preeclampsia, greater maternal age, patient/family history, smoking, obesity and caesarean section (the last by up to eight times).

Untreated calf vein thrombosis causes a mortality of 15%. Iliofemoral thrombosis (which is more common in pregnancy) may be associated with an even greater mortality. Untreated pulmonary embolus (PE) in pregnancy may recur and is associated with a mortality of 25%.

Problems/special considerations

- Physiological changes in pregnancy favour coagulation. Pregnant women are therefore far more likely to develop thromboembolism than non-pregnant women. In addition, obesity and the gravid uterus may cause venous stasis whilst supine and encourage thrombus formation.
- Diagnosis of deep-vein thrombosis (DVT) in pregnancy may be difficult; however, a high index of suspicion is required since mortality audits have identified patients with classic symptoms and signs who were not treated effectively. Not only is the diagnosis often not considered in pregnancy, but women may be denied appropriate investigation because of their pregnant state.

Management options

Treatment of thromboembolism in pregnancy

Suspected DVT in pregnancy should be investigated with duplex ultrasonography and venography if necessary. A raised concentration of d-dimers or other fibrin degradation products may not be helpful since both may be raised in normal pregnancy; however, low levels make the diagnosis unlikely. Suspected PE in pregnancy should be investigated with chest radiography, arterial blood gas analysis and electrocardiography, followed by a ventilation/perfusion scan or computed tomography pulmonary angiogram depending on local protocols/availability. Magnetic resonance imaging and specialised echocardiography have also been used to diagnose PE. Bilateral duplex lower limb ultrasonography should be performed if necessary.

Treatment of thromboembolism is with heparin; intravenous unfractionated heparin has now largely been replaced by subcutaneous low molecular weight heparin and this should not be delayed whilst awaiting investigation. Heparin therapy is preferred to warfarin because of the latter's fetal effects. Full anticoagulation precludes regional analgesia and anaesthesia (see Chapter 99, Coagulopathy) and can be a problem when pregnancy is complicated by ante- or postpartum bleeding.

Massive PE may require dispersion under radiological control or open embolectomy. Administration of potent intravenous fibrinolytic drugs may result in massive obstetric haemorrhage.

The use of vena caval filters in pregnancy has not been properly evaluated. Although there have been reports of the successful use of vena caval filters in pregnancy, many authors feel that their use is not justified because of the high risk of angulation and movement as a result of the pressure of the gravid uterus. However, they could be of use in women in whom anticoagulation is contraindicated.

Thromboprophylaxis in pregnancy

Increasing numbers of women are being given prophylaxis against arterial or venous thrombosis in pregnancy. Some women have a hereditary or acquired thrombophilia or a past medical history of thrombosis. In addition, some obstetricians treat women with a history of stillbirth, intrauterine death and miscarriage with prophylactic doses of antithrombotics such as aspirin, heparin or both. Other women require continuation of pre-pregnancy therapeutic doses of antithrombotics, such as those with prosthetic heart valves. Warfarin is teratogenic when used in the first trimester; it is now rarely used in pregnancy. Women with metal heart valves are at particular risk of valve thrombosis and are therefore an exception. Evaluation of women who may require anticoagulation should ideally be done before pregnancy.

Thromboprophylaxis following caesarean section

Venous thromboembolism occurs in around 1% of women following vaginal delivery and 2–3% following caesarean section. A significant proportion of fatal PE occurs 2–6 weeks postpartum.The Royal College of Obstetricians and Gynaecologists has issued guidance on the prophylaxis of venous thromboembolism following caesarean section, listing risk factors for which prophylactic low molecular weight heparin should be given. Many units prefer to treat all women as high-risk and give prophylaxis routinely unless there is a contraindication, in order to reduce the chance of omitting prophylaxis accidentally.

Increased doses of heparin are required in pregnancy. Neither warfarin nor heparin is excreted in breast milk.

Key points

- Venous thromboembolism is the most common cause of death in pregnancy.
- If untreated, thromboembolism carries a high mortality.
- Low molecular weight heparin is the treatment of choice for venous thromboembolism.
- Prophylaxis against thromboembolism should be considered in all women undergoing caesarean section.

Further reading

Bates SM, Greer IA, Middeldorp S, et al. VTE, thrombophilia, antithrombotic therapy, and pregnancy: antithrombotic therapy and prevention of thrombosis, 9th edn: American College of Chest Physicians Evidence-based Clinical Practice Guidelines. Chest 2012; 141 (2 Suppl): e691S–736S.

Durán-Mendicuti A, Sodickson A. Imaging evaluation of the pregnant patient with suspected pulmonary embolism. Int J Obstet Anesth 2011; 20: 51–9.

Royal College of Obstetricians and Gynaecologists. The acute management of thrombosis and embolism during pregnancy and the puerperium. Green-top 37b. London: RCOG 2007, http://www.rcog.org.uk/womens-health/clinical-guidance/thromboembolic-disease-pregnancy-and-puerperium-acute-management-gre.

Royal College of Obstetricians and Gynaecologists. Reducing the risk of thrombosis and embolism during pregnancy and the puerperium. Green-top 37a. London: RCOG 2009, http://www.rcog.org.uk/womens-health/clinical-guidance/reducing-risk-of-thrombosis-greentop37a.

Chapter

98

Thrombophilia

Thrombophilia has been defined as a familial or acquired abnormality of haemostasis likely to predispose to thrombosis. Up to 30–50% of patients with a history of venous thromboembolism may have a congenital thrombophilia and others may have a detectable phospholipid autoantibody. This is a developing area, which may yet demonstrate further congenital or acquired factors explaining a propensity to thrombosis.

Problems/special considerations

- Pregnancy is associated with a physiological hypercoagulable state. When a pre-existing thrombophilia is present, thrombosis may occur within the uterus causing failure of implantation; within the placenta causing fetal loss, abruption, pre-eclampsia, intrauterine growth retardation and fetal distress in labour; or in the systemic circulation. Patients with thrombophilia may thus present with subfertility, with a personal or family history of venous and arterial thromboses or with thromboses in pregnancy or in the puerperium.
- Diagnosis is difficult in pregnancy because of the changes in clotting factor profile associated with pregnancy.
- The usual treatment of thrombophilia complicating pregnancy is prophylactic subcutaneous low molecular weight heparin combined with low-dose aspirin. This has implications for the timing of regional analgesia and anaesthesia (see Chapter 99, Coagulopathy).

Thrombophilias can be classified into congenital and acquired.

Congenital thrombophilias

These deficiencies are not heterogeneous; factors may be reduced quantitatively or qualitatively, underlying the importance of haematological input in their management. Subtle, subclinical deficiencies of these factors are very much more common than the figures quoted below (around 1 in 200):

- *Activated protein C resistance (APCR):* The circulating anticoagulant protein C, when activated by thrombin, inactivates factors V and VIII. APCR occurs normally in pregnancy associated with an increase in factor VIII. This makes diagnosis in pregnancy difficult. In congenital APCR, factor V is more resistant to cleavage by protein C. Factor V Leiden occurs in about 5–7% of the European population and is associated with a rate of thrombosis in pregnancy in about 1 in 400–500. Factor V Leiden is much more sinister when in the homozygous form or when combined with another thrombophilia.

In the absence of other risk factors such patients should not need thromboprophylaxis in pregnancy.

- *Antithrombin III (ATIII) deficiency:* This is a rare defect occurring in 1 in 5000 women but may account for up to 12% of thromboembolic events in pregnancy. In untreated affected women, 55–68% of pregnancies are complicated by venous thromboembolism. Anticoagulant prophylaxis may be required throughout pregnancy and for at least 3 months postpartum. Discontinuation of heparin at the time of delivery and administration of ATIII concentrate has been advocated by some authors, but this is controversial.

- *Protein C or protein S deficiency:* This occurs in 1 in 15 000 pregnancies and is associated with a rate of venous thrombosis of up to 25% (protein S is a cofactor for protein C). Treatment with heparin throughout pregnancy and the puerperium is controversial. The risk of thrombosis is greatest postpartum in both protein C and S deficiencies and several authors suggest thromboprophylaxis for this period only.

- *Other causes:* These include hyperhomocystinaemia and mutations of the prothrombin gene.

Acquired thrombophilia

The antiphospholipid syndrome is the most common cause of acquired thrombophilia. Autoantibodies against cell membrane phospholipids, including lupus anticoagulant and anticardiolipin antibodies, may lead to intravascular thrombosis which may lead to fetal loss. There is some evidence that other as yet unidentified autoantibodies may also cause thrombosis and miscarriage.

The lupus anticoagulant is so called because it causes a prolongation of the activated partial thromboplastin time even when diluted (because the autoantibody binds to phospholipid in the assay). However, it is associated with a thrombotic tendency. It may occur on its own (hence antiphospholipid syndrome) but may also occur as part of various autoimmune diseases, e.g. systemic lupus erythematosus. Anticardiolipin antibodies are detected by using an immunoassay.

Of women with recurrent miscarriage (three or more), 15% have persistently positive results for phospholipid antibodies. If untreated, 90% will have spontaneous abortions or stillbirths in subsequent pregnancies. Lupus anticoagulant is detected in ~30% of cases and anticardiolipin antibodies in ~70%. Clinical features of the antiphospholipid syndrome are recurrent fetal loss, thrombosis (arterial and venous), thrombocytopenia, haemolytic anaemia, hypertension, pulmonary hypertension and livedo reticularis. Antiphospholipid syndrome is associated with a 5% incidence of thromboembolism or cerebrovascular accident in pregnancy. Rarely, a severe generalised thrombotic state may lead to multi-organ failure.

Management options

Women with a strong personal or family history of thrombosis and a poor obstetric history should be screened for known causes of thrombophilia.

Patients are at high risk of obstetric intervention in labour and may benefit from epidural analgesia and regional anaesthesia for delivery and caesarean section. The decision to site an epidural should be based on the dose and interval after heparin administration and the potential benefit to the patient. Ideally, women who are likely to be receiving heparin at the time of delivery should discuss a management plan with an anaesthetist in an assessment clinic. In the majority of cases the benefits of regional analgesia and anaesthesia far outweigh the risk of epidural haematoma.

Key points
- Thrombophilias are a significant cause of fetal loss in pregnancy.
- The adverse effects on maternal and fetal health are treatable.
- The risks and benefits of regional analgesia and anaesthesia should be considered antenatally if possible.

Further reading

Bates SM, Greer IA, Middeldorp S, et al. VTE, thrombophilia, antithrombotic therapy, and pregnancy: antithrombotic therapy and prevention of thrombosis, 9th edn: American College of Chest Physicians Evidence-based Clinical Practice Guidelines. *Chest* 2012; **141** (2 Suppl): e691S–736S.

Danza A, Ruiz-Irastorza G, Khamashta M. Antiphospohlipid syndrome in obstetrics. *Best Pract Res Clin Obstet Gynaecol* 2012; **26**: 65–76.

Gray G, Nelson-Piercy C. Thromboembolic disorders in obstetrics. *Best Pract Res Clin Obstet Gynaecol* 2012; **26**: 53–64.

Ruiz-Irastorza G, Crowther M, Branch W, Khamashta MA. Antiphospholipid syndrome. *Lancet* 2010; **376**: 1498–509.

Chapter

99

Coagulopathy

Normal coagulation is important to the obstetric anaesthetist for two reasons: firstly because of the potential risk of spinal haematoma following regional analgesia and anaesthesia, and secondly because of the risk of postpartum haemorrhage.

Problems/special considerations

In general terms, increased bleeding may arise from defects in the function of:
- Blood vessels, e.g. caused by severe infections, metabolic disease (such as hepatic failure, renal failure) or congenital structural abnormalities.
- Platelets, caused by reduced numbers (e.g. thrombocytopenia, disseminated intravascular coagulation (DIC)) or impaired function (e.g. antiplatelet drugs).

- The coagulation system, caused by congenital disorders (e.g. haemophilia, von Willebrand's disease), acquired coagulation factor dysfunction (e.g. anticoagulant therapy, hepatic failure, vitamin K deficiency, DIC) or increased fibrinolysis.

Von Willebrand's disease is associated with blood vessel and platelet defects as well as coagulation factor dysfunction. Massive blood transfusion may result in dilution of both platelets and coagulation factors. In major obstetric haemorrhage, this dilution may also be associated with a consumptive process leading to early, rapid depletion of fibrinogen.

Management options

Specific disorders should be managed according to the underlying pathology and in conjunction with haematologists. Coagulation studies should always be performed before considering regional analgesia and anaesthesia, although the ideal test or combination of tests and the 'safe' limits for those tests, are unknown (see Chapter 80, Hypertension, pre-eclampsia and eclampsia; Chapter 102, Thrombocytopenia). It has been suggested that regional blockade can be performed providing the activated partial thromboplastin time ratio or International Normalised Ratio is less than 1.5, although this is controversial. Symptoms of excessive bruising or bleeding should be sought since they may signify increased risk of bleeding in borderline cases. Newer coagulation tests such as thromboelastography/thromboelastometry (TEG/ROTEM) and the platelet function analyser have received much attention lately. Although TEG/ROTEM have been useful in assessing preoperative coagulation in cardiac and liver surgery, they have yet to be validated in pregnancy. The platelet function analyser has been suggested as a replacement for bleeding time but its ability to predict postoperative bleeding has yet to be determined.

Increasing numbers of women are presenting in pregnancy taking anticoagulant therapy. Whereas full anticoagulation is a contraindication to regional analgesia and anaesthesia, it should be possible to time regional analgesia and anaesthesia for prophylactic regimens. Low-dose aspirin is generally felt to pose minimal risk, although the numbers of mothers who have been studied (receiving both aspirin and regional blockade) are small compared with the rarity of the outcome (spinal haematoma). Other antiplatelet drugs are less commonly used in pregnancy and experience with them is limited.

Prophylactic heparin (especially low molecular weight heparin) has been associated with spinal haematoma in non-pregnant patients who receive regional analgesia and anaesthesia, although many of these cases have been associated with relatively large doses in high-risk patients. The risk of therapeutic levels of heparin activity following a supposedly prophylactic dose in pregnancy is unknown. In addition, heparin pharmacokinetics are altered in pregnancy and larger doses are required than in non-pregnant patients, so data from series in which standard (non-pregnant) doses of heparin were used may be misleading. Most obstetric anaesthetists would follow the guidelines recommended for non-pregnant patients, in which regional analgesia and anaesthesia or removal of an epidural catheter should be avoided for 6 hours after a prophylactic dose of unfractionated heparin (12 hours after low molecular weight heparin), and heparin should only be given 2–4 hours after a regional block or catheter removal. In particular cases where the risks of general anaesthesia are increased (e.g. obesity, cardiac disease), an epidural may still represent a safer option than general anaesthesia, even within these time limits.

Key points

- Specific coagulation disorders should be managed with involvement of haematologists.
- Low-dose aspirin therapy is considered to represent minimal risk.
- The risks and benefits of regional analgesia and anaesthesia should be considered for women who are receiving prophylactic heparin therapy. In general, guidelines prohibiting regional blockade or catheter removal within certain periods of heparin administration should be followed.

Further reading

Choi S, Brull R. Neuraxial techniques in obstetric and non-obstetric patients with common bleeding diatheses. *Anesth Analg* 2009; **109**: 648–60.

Pacheco LD, Costantine MM, Saade GR, *et al.* von Willebrand disease and pregnancy: a practical approach for the diagnosis and treatment. *Am J Obstet Gynecol* 2010; **203**: 194–200.

Thornton P, Douglas J. Coagulation in pregnancy. *Best Pract Res Clin Obstet Gynaecol* 2010; **24**: 339–52.

Chapter

100

Von Willebrand's disease and haemophilia

Von Willebrand's disease (vWD) is a heterogeneous group of mainly autosomal dominant disorders in which there is reduced or abnormal circulating von Willebrand factor (vWF); it is the most common inherited bleeding disorder. Von Willebrand factor has two functions: firstly, it combines with factor VIII in vivo to produce a pro-coagulant complex (VIIIc) that protects factor VIII from premature destruction. Hence, factor VIII activity may be reduced in vWD. Secondly, vWF assists platelet adhesion to exposed subendothelium of damaged capillaries and is excreted by endothelium and activated platelets. Deficiency of vWF therefore affects platelet adherence and the clotting cascade itself. It ranges from a mild disease of little significance, seen in up to 1% of the population, to a very severe form in which vWF is absent.

Haemophilia A and B (factor VIII and IX deficiency respectively) are X-linked disorders and classically do not affect the female population. As many as 1 in 10 female carriers, however, may have a clinically significant clotting deficiency.

Problems/special considerations

Von Willebrand's disease

This is classified into three main variants:

- *Type I (80–90% of cases):* vWF is normal but present in diminished quantities. In pregnancy, vWF increases and may even return to normal; following delivery, VIIIc levels can fall dramatically (though this change may be delayed until late in the puerperium), and there is an increased incidence of postpartum haemorrhage. Levels of VIIIc can be increased by the administration of desmopressin (DDAVP) intravenously.

- *Type II (9–15% of cases):* There is an abnormal vWF; hence additional release of abnormal vWF following administration of DDAVP is unlikely to improve the coagulopathy. Clotting does not improve in pregnancy. In the IIb subtype, abnormal vWF clumps inactivated platelets and causes thrombocytopenia. In this variant, DDAVP exacerbates the coagulopathy because increased amounts of abnormal vWF worsens the thrombocytopenia. A new variant of vWD type IIN (Normandy) has been described in which there is an isolated decrease in factor VIII concentration because of decreased affinity of the abnormal vWF for factor VIII, which results in increased factor VIII consumption. Thus it can be confused with haemophilia A.

- *Type III (autosomal recessive; < 1% of cases):* vWF is undetectable and factor VIIIc concentration is very low. The bleeding abnormality is severe and does not respond to DDAVP.

No consensus exists regarding the safe levels of FVIII:C and vWF for using neuraxial techniques, and the literature consists only of case reports and series.

Haemophilia

A concentration of factor VIII or IX of 30% of normal is considered acceptable for vaginal delivery. For planned operative delivery, factor concentrations are usually increased to normal. Half of all fetuses will be affected and therefore fetal blood sampling and forceps or ventouse deliveries should be avoided unless chorionic villous sampling or amniocentesis has shown the fetus to be unaffected. After delivery, factor VIII level can fall abruptly resulting in secondary haemorrhage.

Management options

Close liaison with haematologists is necessary throughout pregnancy. A management plan, including treatment for significant haemorrhage, is helpful. An epidural is rarely contra-indicated in type I vWD, but specialist interpretation of laboratory tests (particularly VIIIc concentration) is required. Owing to the sometimes precipitous drop in vWF and VIIIc following delivery, removal of the epidural catheter postpartum may be more of a problem; it is advisable either to remove epidural catheters immediately or to wait until the bleeding diathesis can be assessed.

The usual dose of DDAVP is 20 μg (0.3 μg/kg) in 50 ml of saline given over 30 minutes. DDAVP also stimulates fibrinolysis so tranexamic acid is often given simultaneously. DDAVP can cause fluid retention and therefore hyponatraemia.

Patients with type I disease may deliver vaginally. Patients with type II or III disease frequently have an elective caesarean section, with correction of their coagulopathy. In this situation, regional anaesthesia has been used if clotting is corrected. Where DDAVP is contraindicated, fresh frozen plasma (FFP), cryoprecipitate or infusions of vWF and factor VIII may be given.

In haemophilia, close monitoring of factor VIII or IX levels as appropriate is required. Administration of FFP, cryoprecipitate, DDAVP or purified clotting factors may be necessary to bring factor levels to the 30% considered adequate for vaginal delivery or the near 100% required for operative delivery. Regional analgesia and anaesthesia is generally contraindicated unless haematological advice suggests a fully corrected coagulation profile and the possible risks are outweighed by the benefits particular to the case concerned.

Key points

- Von Willebrand's disease is a heterogeneous condition that ranges in severity.
- The commonest form of von Willebrand's disease is improved by pregnancy.
- Coagulation may rapidly deteriorate after delivery in both von Willebrand's disease and haemophilia.
- In haemophilia, the fetus should be assumed to be affected.
- Specialist advice is necessary before, during and after delivery.

Further reading

Cata JP, Hanna A, Tetzlaff JE, Bishai A, Barsoum S. Spinal anesthesia for a cesarean delivery in a woman with type-2M von Willebrand disease: case report and mini-review. *Int J Obstet Anesth* 2009; **18**: 276–9.

Choi S, Brull R. Neuraxial techniques in obstetric and non-obstetric patients with common bleeding diatheses. *Anesth Analg* 2009; **109**: 648–60.

Kouides PA. Obstetric and gynaecological aspects of von Willebrand disease. *Best Pract Res Clin Haematol* 2001; **14**: 381–99.

Marrache D, Mercier FJ, Boyer-Neumann C. Epidural analgesia for parturients with type 1 von Willebrand disease. *Int J Obstet Anesth* 2007; **16**: 231–5.

Pacheco LD, Costantine MM, Saade GR, *et al.* von Willebrand disease and pregnancy: a practical approach for the diagnosis and treatment. *Am J Obstet Gynecol* 2010; **203**: 194–200.

Disseminated intravascular coagulation

In disseminated intravascular coagulation (DIC) the coagulation process is activated, resulting in consumption of clotting factors and platelets, with concomitant activation of the fibrinolytic pathway. Conventional treatment of this consumptive coagulopathy is removal of the underlying trigger and support of the patient with replacement of clotting factors and platelets. In many respects, DIC can be seen as the haematological manifestation of a multi-organ disease, e.g. sepsis, pre-eclampsia.

Problems/special considerations

- Diagnosis of DIC depends on clinical features and laboratory tests. Presentation may be of rapid collapse, with shock, respiratory failure, renal impairment, acidosis, hypoxaemia and bleeding from venepuncture sites and the respiratory, gastrointestinal and urogenital tracts (the last including the uteroplacental bed). Coagulation studies show prolonged coagulation times, decreased fibrinogen concentration and platelet count and raised titres of fibrin degradation products. Some authors favour thromboelastography because it demonstrates changes in both coagulation and thrombolysis.
- In some cases there may be a more insidious progression; initially, increased circulation of activated clotting factors may even shorten coagulation times.
- The common triggers for DIC in the obstetric population are listed in Table 101.1. Many of these conditions have their own particular implications for analgesia and anaesthesia. The coagulopathy usually precludes regional anaesthesia.
- Fibrin degradation products have an anticoagulant effect and reduce the efficiency of myometrial contraction, exacerbating blood loss.

Management options

Management of DIC should be to remove the cause. This usually involves delivering the fetus if antepartum.

In fulminant DIC there may be no time to wait for laboratory results in the face of massive blood loss, haemostatic failure and multi-organ failure. Patients often require empirical treatment with blood and blood products and surgical treatments such as hysterectomy. The successful management of fulminant DIC requires input from senior obstetricians, obstetric anaesthetists, haematologists, laboratory staff and intensivists (see Chapter 72, Major obstetric haemorrhage).

Conventional treatment of DIC is to correct the consumptive coagulopathy by administering exogenous clotting factors: fresh frozen plasma to treat prolongation of the activated

Table 101.1 Triggers of disseminated intravascular coagulation (DIC) in obstetrics

Placental abruption
Sepsis (particularly gram-negative)
Pre-eclampsia
HELLP (haemolysis, elevated liver enzymes and low platelet count) syndrome
Acute fatty liver of pregnancy
Intrauterine death (DIC may occur after 3–4 weeks)
Amniotic fluid embolism
Massive blood transfusion (produces a dilutional coagulopathy; however, tissue factors released from the cause of blood loss may induce DIC in a compromised circulation)
Transfusion reactions
Drug reactions
Placenta accreta
Hydatidiform mole

partial thromboplastin time or prothrombin time; cryoprecipitate to treat a low fibrinogen concentration (< 1–1.5 g/dl); and platelet concentrates.

Some authors have attempted to break the cycle of thrombosis and fibrinolysis by giving heparin, antithrombin or antifibrinolytic drugs. However, giving such agents to a bleeding patient is fraught with danger.

Transfer to an intensive care unit may be necessary to treat the multisystem dysfunction.

Key points

- Coagulopathy may co-exist with other organ failures.
- Treatment includes removing the cause of the coagulopathy.
- Aggressive treatment is required to treat fulminating disseminated intravascular coagulation.
- Management of massive obstetric haemorrhage requires coordinated care with haematologists, obstetricians, obstetric anaesthetists and intensivists.

Further reading

Levi M. Disseminated intravascular coagulation. *Crit Care Med* 2007; **35**: 2191–5.

Levi M. Disseminated intravascular coagulation (DIC) in pregnancy and the peri-partum period. *Thromb Res* 2009; **123**: S63–4.

Levi M, Toh CH, Thachil J, Watson HG. Guidelines for the diagnosis and management of disseminated intravascular coagulation. *Br J Haematol* 2009; **145**: 24–33.

Martí-Carvajal AJ, Comunián-Carrasco G, Peña-Martí GE. Haematological interventions for treating disseminated intravascular coagulation during pregnancy and postpartum. *Cochrane Database Syst Rev* 2011; (3): CD008577.

Chapter 102

Thrombocytopenia

A low platelet count ($< 150 \times 10^9$/l) may occur in pregnancy for a variety of reasons ranging from the relatively benign (gestational thrombocytopenia) to the frankly sinister (HELLP [haemolysis, elevated liver enzymes and low platelet count] syndrome, thrombotic thrombocytopenic purpura (TTP)). If the platelet count is low, a manual count is always advisable, as clumping of platelets is common in pregnancy.

Problems/special considerations

Conditions involving reduced platelet numbers or function include:

- *Gestational thrombocytopenia:* This is the most common cause of low platelet count in pregnancy, accounting for 70% of all cases. It is seen in around 5% of parturients, is probably caused by accelerated platelet destruction, and is rarely associated with a count of less than 75×10^9/l. In 75% of cases, the low platelet level is clinically unimportant and it has been suggested that levels between 75×10^9/l and 115×10^9/l do not need investigation. It does not appear to increase the risk of peripartum haemorrhage and is usually not regarded as a contraindication to regional analgesia.
- *Immune thrombocytic purpura (ITP):* This is seen in around 0.1% of pregnancies. It is characterised by the production of platelet autoantibodies that may cross the placenta, putting the fetus at risk of intracranial haemorrhage during delivery. Although the platelet count is often below 100×10^9/l, coagulation is rarely affected because the young platelets, which make up a higher than usual proportion of the platelet mass, are more aggressively haemostatic. ITP can be distinguished from gestational thrombocytopenia by the fact that the platelet count is already low in the early antenatal period. The mainstay of treatment is corticosteroid therapy, and this should be considered when the platelet count is $\leq 50 \times 10^9$/l; IgG administration has proved very effective in severe cases. Platelet transfusion may stimulate autoantibody production and should therefore be avoided. A number of drugs may induce thrombocytopenia (Table 102.1).
- *Thrombotic thrombocytopenic purpura (TTP) and haemolytic uraemic syndrome:* Thrombotic thrombocytopenic purpura is a rare condition comprising haemolytic anaemia and thrombocytopenia, which presents with widespread vascular occlusion, often resulting in neurological disturbance and renal failure. A deficiency in von Willebrand factor cleaving protease has been

Table 102.1 Drugs that may impair platelet function or cause thrombocytopenia

Impaired platelet function	Thrombocytopenia
Aspirin	Heparin
Non-steroidal anti-inflammatory drugs	Thiazide diuretics
Colloid plasma substitutes	Hydralazine
	H_2 blockers
	Digoxin
	Cocaine

identified as a causative factor. Unlike HELLP syndrome (see below), TTP usually presents in the second trimester. The high morbidity and mortality associated with this condition warrants aggressive intervention, and exchange transfusions and plasmapheresis may be employed. Haemolytic uraemic syndrome presents clinically in a similar way to TTP but the renal problems tend to be more severe.

- *Pre-eclampsia:* This is accompanied by a low platelet count in about 20% of cases. In its most malignant version, this manifests as HELLP syndrome. Mothers with evidence of pre-eclampsia must have their platelet count monitored frequently, and a fall should be regarded as evidence that the condition is worsening. The thrombocytopenia of pre-eclampsia is often accompanied by clotting defects; therefore, regular coagulation tests should also be done. Management should be targeted at treatment of the underlying condition, ultimately by delivery, but specific therapy may be needed, including platelet transfusion and fresh frozen plasma in severe cases.

- *Others:* Reduced platelet concentration may also result from other causes of impaired production, e.g. bone marrow depression, vitamin B_{12}/folate deficiency, hereditary defects, paroxysmal nocturnal haemoglobinuria, alcohol toxicity; or of shortened survival of platelets, e.g. malignancy, drugs (including heparin and α-methyldopa), disseminated intravascular coagulation.

Management options

The obstetric anaesthetist is often called upon to make a decision regarding the advisability of regional analgesia and anaesthesia in these cases. Several textbooks and articles offer guidance on this subject, and the general trend in recent years has been to lower the 'cut-off point' from a platelet count of $100 \times 10^9/l$ to 75–$80 \times 10^9/l$. Some authorities have even suggested that there is a very low risk of adverse outcomes following a neuraxial technique in women with platelet counts as low as $50 \times 10^9/l$; however, whether or not to perform a neuraxial technique in a patient with a platelet count of < 75–$80 \times 10^9/l$ should be the decision of a senior anaesthetist. Indeed, there is no evidence to support this sort of 'all-or-nothing' approach, and every case must therefore be considered on its merits, taking into account the underlying pathology, the general state of the patient, and the underlying trend in the platelet count (and how fast it has changed), with the risk of the procedure (epidural/spinal haematoma) balanced against the benefits (pain relief, better blood pressure control, avoidance of general anaesthesia).

The mother with a rapidly falling count should be regarded with more suspicion than the one with a low, but stable, platelet level. In general, patients with a platelet count of greater than $75 \times 10^9/l$ in the absence of pre-eclampsia are unlikely to have significantly altered platelet function.

Tests of platelet function, such as bleeding time, are very operator-dependent and therefore of limited predictive value. Thromboelastography/thromboelastometry and the platelet function analyser have received much attention but their roles in clinical practice have yet to be determined (see Chapter 99, Coagulopathy). Routine coagulation studies are usually indicated in thrombocytopenia, in case any other defect should be present. The mother should always be questioned about excessive bruising or bleeding since the presence of these may signify impaired platelet function in borderline cases.

Key points

- All patients with thrombocytopenia must be fully investigated.
- Trends in platelet count are more important than absolute values.
- There is no fixed 'cut-off point' for the platelet count when regional analgesia is being considered.
- Patients should be asked about excessive bruising or bleeding.

Further reading

Douglas MJ. Platelets, the parturient and regional anesthesia. *Int J Obstet Anesth* 2001; **10**: 113–20.

Kadir RA, McLintock C. Thrombocytopenia and disorders of platelet function in pregnancy. *Semin Thromb Hemost* 2011; **37**: 640–52.

Kam PCA, Thompson SA, Liew ACS. Thrombocytopenia in the parturient. *Anaesthesia* 2004; **59**: 225–64.

McCrae K. Thrombocytopenia in pregnancy. *American Society of Haematology Education Book* 2010; **2010**: 397–402.

Chapter 103

Lymphoma and leukaemia

Haematological malignancies are rare in pregnancy but nonetheless lymphomas are now the fourth most common malignancy in pregnancy. In the UK, this increase in prevalence is associated with pregnancy being delayed until later in life, whereas in the developing world it is associated with AIDS-related non-Hodgkin's lymphoma. Successful pregnancy has been described with chemotherapy for both acute and chronic leukaemia and lymphoma.

Increasing numbers of patients are surviving childhood or adult treatment of haematological malignancies. However, such treatment can leave both physical and psychological problems associated with chemotherapeutic treatment.

Problems/special considerations

- Treatment of haematological malignancies often involves intense periods of chemotherapy or radiotherapy followed by maintenance doses. The most aggressive forms of therapy result in permanent ablation of bone marrow. Bone marrow rescue is achieved by transplantation of stored autologous bone marrow or donated allogeneic bone marrow. Patients may require repeated lumbar punctures to test for disease and to administer chemotherapeutic agents (e.g. methotrexate).
- The limiting factor in administration of most chemotherapeutic agents is short- and long-term toxicity. Short-term problems include malaise, nausea and vomiting, anorexia and acute organ impairment, especially of the liver and kidneys (toxicity may also arise from drugs such as gentamicin and vancomycin, given to treat infections). Bone marrow depression may result in anaemia, neutropenia with increased risk of infection, and coagulopathy. Long-term toxicity of common chemotherapeutic agents includes neurotoxicity, neuropathies (e.g. vincristine) and arachnoiditis (e.g. methotrexate). Cardiomyopathy may occur as a dose-dependent result of anthracycline antibiotics such as danorubicin. Pulmonary toxicity and fibrosis may follow busulphan and bleomycin administration. Although sterility often occurs following high-dose chemotherapeutic treatments, many survivors do become pregnant spontaneously or following infertility treatments. Central and peripheral venous access may be a persisting problem.
- The long-term effects of chemotherapy on children exposed in utero is unknown. Although there are concerns regarding neurodevelopment, childhood malignancy and long-term fertility, the current data suggest that chemotherapy exposure in utero does not have significant impact.

- The psychological effects of a diagnosis of cancer in a young person followed by prolonged periods of toxic therapy, infection and isolation cannot be overlooked. They may have features of a post-traumatic stress syndrome with flashbacks, nightmares and phobias of hospitals, doctors and needles. Frequently, these psychological aspects influence management far more than physical aspects.

Management options

All such patients require a detailed assessment by a multidisciplinary antenatal team. Wherever possible, the treatment records should be obtained, preferably with a haematological summary. The patient may not (want to) remember details of their treatment, particularly if they received it as a child. In addition, repressed memories of unpleasant experiences such as general anaesthesia or lumbar puncture may induce unexpected irrational behaviour. A careful sensitive approach is required.

Commonly performed investigations include:

- Urea and electrolytes
- Full blood count
- Liver function tests
- Pulmonary function tests
- Echocardiography
- Chest radiography.

The spectrum of such patients varies from some that can be treated as normal to those with significant hepatic, renal and cardiorespiratory disease. In the last group, regional analgesia and anaesthesia is usually recommended, depending on the pattern of disease.

Key points

- Organ impairment may arise from the haematological malignancy itself or from its treatment.
- Survivors of leukaemia and lymphoma need support and sensitive, carefully planned care.

Further reading

Abadi U, Koren G, Lishner M. Leukemia and lymphoma in pregnancy. *Hematol Oncol Clin North Am* 2011; **25**: 277–91.

Brenner B, Avivi I, Lishner M. Haematological cancers in pregnancy. *Lancet* 2012; **379**: 580–7.

Pereg D, Koren G, Lishner M. The treatment of Hodgkin's and non-Hodgkin's lymphoma in pregnancy. *Haematologica* 2007; **92**: 1230–7.

Haemoglobinopathies

Haemoglobin abnormalities result from either synthesis of abnormal haemoglobin (e.g. sickle cell anaemia) or reduced rate of synthesis of normal haemoglobin chains (the thalassaemias).

Problems/special considerations
Sickle cell disease

Patients with sickle cell disease are homozygotes for an abnormal haemoglobin (haemoglobin S). Heterozygotes have a significantly attenuated form (sickle cell trait), which is not normally of clinical significance except when combined with another abnormal haemoglobin (e.g. haemoglobin C). Haemoglobin S is poorly soluble in its deoxygenated form and therefore crystallises at a variable oxygen concentration dependent on relative concentrations of normal and abnormal haemoglobin within the red cell. Haemoglobin S in heterozygotes appears to have some protective action against malaria and is therefore more common in Africa, Asia, Arabia and southern Europe, particularly coastal Greece/Turkey. Sickle cell disease is characterised by haemolysis, reticulocytosis, anaemia, recurrent sepsis, vaso-occlusive and sequestration crises and hypersplenism followed by splenic infarction. Diagnosis is based on demonstration of sickling (Sickledex test) followed by haemoglobin electrophoresis.

Sickle cell disease (homozygous SS) is a particularly aggressive disease. Affected patients may not survive into their third decade. Problems in pregnancy include vaso-occlusive and thromboembolic phenomena and infection. Placental infarction can occur and result in abortion, intrauterine growth retardation and pre-eclampsia. Maternal mortality rates of 30–40% and perinatal mortality rates of 50–70%, that were quoted 30–40 years ago, may be reduced to 1–2% and 1–5%, respectively, with careful management.

Despite earlier evidence to the contrary, recent work has demonstrated that sickle cell trait is not associated with a higher incidence of pre-eclampsia.

Thalassaemias

This disease is classified according to the haemoglobin chain affected (α or β). It is common in Mediterranean countries and also occurs in a narrow band distribution crossing Africa, the Middle East, India, Burma and South-East Asia. Its distribution therefore closely follows that of sickle cell disease, and both diseases are said to give some protection against falciparum malaria.

- α-*Thalassaemia:* The α haemoglobin gene is encoded twice on each chromosome 16, giving a total of four genes controlling its production. When all four genes are deleted, α

chain synthesis is completely suppressed and death occurs in utero (hydrops fetalis). Three α gene deletions lead to a moderately severe microcytic, hypochromic anaemia with splenomegaly (HbH disease). Precipitation of relatively insoluble HbH within cells induces mild haemolysis. Crises of haemolysis associated with infection may occur. Patients with two (thalassaemia trait) and one (silent carriers) α chain deletions are asymptomatic.

Pregnancies complicated by hydrops fetalis (Bart's hydrops) are associated with pre-eclampsia, retained placenta and ante- and postpartum haemorrhage.

• *β-Thalassaemia:* In contrast to α-thalassaemia, the β haemoglobin gene is coded by a single gene; thus patients can be homozygous or heterozygous for the faulty gene. However, about 125 individual mutations of the β gene have been described, which can markedly affect the clinical picture. Hence the terms thalassaemia major, intermedia and minor have been used to describe clinical pictures of varying severity. Furthermore, the geographical distribution of thalassaemia and sickle cell trait mean that it is possible to have a mixed sickle cell–thalassaemia genotype.

In thalassaemia major either no β haemoglobin chains are produced or small amounts are produced (5–30%). Anaemia results from ineffective erythropoiesis and haemolysis and inadequate supplies of haemoglobin for formed red cells. Features include skeletal abnormalities because of bone marrow hyperactivity and failure of many organ systems including the pancreas, liver and heart. Patients may be thrombocytopenic because of hypersplenism or thrombocythaemic following splenectomy. Thrombocythaemic patients require thromboembolic prophylaxis and may also develop arterial thrombosis including cerebral thrombosis. Frequent cannulation may make venous access difficult (many patients have permanent indwelling intravenous catheters). There is a high incidence of blood transfusion reactions and a small incidence of transfusion-related HIV and hepatitis C. Splenectomised patients are at risk of infection.

Treatment of β-thalassaemia includes frequent transfusion, with iron chelation therapy to reduce iron overload. Modern haematological management means that increasing numbers of women with thalassaemia major are becoming pregnant. There is an increased incidence of intrauterine growth retardation, fetal loss and obstetric intervention because of cephalopelvic disproportion resulting from skeletal abnormalities.

In thalassaemia intermedia there are usually few symptoms. Women may have chronic anaemia and require folate therapy in pregnancy. In severe cases, however, they may develop iron overload, with a clinical syndrome that lags behind the progression seen in thalassaemia major.

Thalassaemia minor behaves as a recessive condition, with few symptoms, although there appears to be higher incidence of intrauterine growth retardation.

Management options

In sickle cell disease, the haemoglobin concentration is usually maintained at 8 g/dl (optimum haematocrit 0.26) with blood transfusion. Exchange transfusion may decrease the rate of maternal complications in pregnancy but does not change fetal or obstetric outcome. A detailed plan is essential for delivery. In general, patients should be warm, well hydrated, not acidotic or hypercarbic and venous stasis should be avoided. An epidural provides analgesia without respiratory depression although mobility is beneficial. Regional anaesthesia is preferable for operative delivery. Oxygen administration is essential post-operatively especially after general anaesthesia. The safety of blood patch in sickle-cell disease has not been assessed, but colloid patches have been used successfully.

α-Thalassaemia rarely results in maternal disease sufficient to cause significant problems with anaesthesia. Related problems such as haemorrhage and pre-eclampsia are covered elsewhere.

In β-thalassaemia, haemoglobin should be kept greater than 10 g/dl with transfusion. Complications such as thrombocytopenia, diabetes, hypothyroidism, cardiomyopathy and facial and vertebral abnormalities mean that choice of anaesthesia and analgesia is assessed on an individual basis.

Key points

- Patients with sickle cell disease should be kept warm, well hydrated, mobile and well oxygenated.
- Haemoglobin should be kept at 8–9 g/dl in sickle cell disease.
- Exchange transfusion reduces maternal complications of sickle cell disease.
- Thalassaemia major causes significant multisystem compromise including cardiac, endocrine and skeletal abnormalities; it may cause intrauterine death and concomitant maternal disease.
- Non-fatal α-thalassaemias are of variable significance.

Further reading

American College of Obstetricians & Gynecologists. Hemoglobinopathies in pregnancy. Washington, DC: ACOG 2007 (ACOG practice bulletin; no. 78), http://www.guidelines.gov/content.aspx?id=10920.

Howard J, Oteng-Ntim E. The obstetric management of sickle cell disease. *Best Pract Res Clin Obstet Gynaecol* 2012; **26**: 25–36.

Royal College of Obstetricians and Gynaecologists. Management of sickle cell disease in pregnancy. *Green-top 61*. London: RCOG 2011, http://www.rcog.org.uk/womens-health/clinical-guidance/sickle-cell-disease-pregnancy-management-green-top-61.

Villers MS, Jamison MG, De Castro LM, James AH. Morbidity associated with sickle cell disease in pregnancy. *Am J Obstet Gynecol* 2008; **199**: 125.e1–5.

Connective tissue disorders

The connective tissue disorders are a diffuse group of diseases, which include the rheumatoid diseases (rheumatoid arthritis, ankylosing spondylitis), the collagen vascular diseases (systemic lupus erythematosus (SLE), scleroderma, the vasculitides), granulomatous diseases and inherited connective tissue disease (e.g. Ehlers–Danlos syndrome).

The factors of importance to the anaesthetist are firstly the widespread systemic nature of the diseases and secondly the drug treatment that is used.

Problems/special considerations

With the exception of the rheumatoid diseases, connective tissue disorders are rare in the antenatal population. The onset of significantly symptomatic disease is frequently towards the end of reproductive life. Both spontaneous abortion and late pregnancy loss are increased in women who do become pregnant.

Drug treatment

Drug treatment frequently includes long-term oral corticosteroids and may also include immunosuppressive agents such as azathioprine, chlorambucil, cyclophosphamide or methotrexate. Low-dose aspirin and subcutaneous heparin are often used in SLE. In arthritic conditions, non-steroidal anti-inflammatory drugs (NSAIDs) are invariably used. Monoclonal antibody therapy is used in severe forms of rheumatoid arthritis.

Cardiac involvement

Pericardial effusions are common, especially in rheumatoid and collagen disorders. A restrictive pericarditis may ensue. Valvular dysfunction can occur. A miscellany of electrocardiographic changes may be seen, and echocardiography is useful in assessing both valvular and ventricular function.

Pulmonary involvement

Pleural effusions are common. Impaired pulmonary function of both restrictive and obstructive patterns may occur, and pulmonary vasculitis can occur in both collagen and vasculitic disorders, rarely leading to spontaneous pulmonary haemorrhage.

Women with scleroderma may be at increased risk of chronic aspiration because of impaired gastrointestinal motility. These women may also have significant airway problems.

Multiple antibody formation

This is a significant problem in women with SLE and may also occur in other auto-immune connective tissue disorders. Maternal antibodies cause difficulty and delay in obtaining adequately cross-matched blood for transfusion. In severe cases there may be coagulation disorders in the mother that may be thrombotic or may increase risk of bleeding.

Anticardiolipin antibodies are associated with increased pregnancy loss and increased maternal morbidity. Treatment with aspirin combined with heparin has been associated with a decrease in miscarriage rate. Anti-Ro antibodies may cross the placenta and cause fetal cardiac conduction defects, rendering the fetus bradycardic and unable to mount a tachycardic response to stress. If present, Doppler echocardiography is recommended every 1–2 weeks between 16–28 weeks as this is considered the vulnerable stage for the fetus.

Musculoskeletal problems

Musculoskeletal involvement is a feature of a number of the connective tissue disorders. Women with scleroderma classically have very tight perioral skin and may also have involvement of the temporomandibular joints; both may limit mouth opening.

Cervical arthritis and consequent reduction of neck mobility is a feature of several connective tissue disorders.

Bullous diseases such as pemphigus and epidermolysis bullosa are characterised by formation of large bullae on the skin and mucous membranes in response to minor trauma. Although extremely rare, cases have been reported in pregnancy, and there are significant implications for the anaesthetist. Any airway instrumentation (including pressure from a facemask) can provoke bullous formation, and bullae may also form in the trachea. Regional anaesthesia is recommended in these cases.

Tissue fragility

Several conditions (e.g. certain forms of Ehlers–Danlos syndrome) may be associated with increased fragility of tissues including blood vessels, leading to an increased susceptibility to trauma and bleeding.

Management options

Early antenatal assessment is vital, and preconception counselling is ideal. If pregnancy has occurred unexpectedly, expert advice should be sought about the relative risks of terato-genicity of immunosuppressive drugs, and the patient counselled appropriately.

Many women with connective tissue disorder have multisystem involvement. Detailed history and examination is necessary, with particular reference to drug treatment and symptoms or signs suggestive of cardiac or pulmonary disease. The possibility of difficulty with airway management and cardiopulmonary involvement should be remembered if anaesthesia is required for termination of pregnancy. Maternal mobility may be limited by the underlying disease. The skin should be examined for fragility and ease of intravenous access. Investigations should include electro- and echocardiography, pulmonary function tests, chest radiography and full biochemical and haematological investigation.

Women who are continuing with a pregnancy should be regarded as high-risk and receive consultant obstetric care. Serial monitoring of the mother should include assessment of cardiac, pulmonary and renal reserve. Mothers needing maintenance NSAIDs throughout pregnancy will require fetal cardiac monitoring during the third trimester because of the risk of premature closure of the ductus arteriosus and potential fetal renal compromise.

An individualised, multidisciplinary plan is required, depending on the particular disorder with which a woman is presenting. There should be provision for high-dependency level of care during and after delivery. In the absence of coagulation disorder, regional analgesia is not contraindicated. Regional anaesthesia is considered unwise by some authorities because of the risk of major haemorrhage during surgery, but a risk–benefit analysis must be made for each patient. If difficulty with the airway is considered to be a major potential risk, relative contraindications to regional anaesthesia are usually outweighed by the benefits. There are no absolute contraindications to regional anaesthesia in these circumstances. Published case reports indicate successful management of individual cases with both general and regional techniques.

Key points

- Connective tissue disorders encompass a wide variety of clinical conditions. Each woman must be assessed on an individual basis.
- Many connective tissue disorders are associated with cardiac, pulmonary and renal dysfunction.
- Drug treatment frequently includes corticosteroids.
- Early and detailed antenatal assessment with serial monitoring during pregnancy are essential.
- Regional analgesia and anaesthesia are not contraindicated, but careful assessment of the balance of risks and benefits is necessary.

Further reading

Clowse MEB, Jamison M, Myers E, James AH. A national study of the complications of lupus in pregnancy. *Am J Obstet Gynecol* 2008; **199**: 127.e1–6.

Khamashta MA. Systemic lupus erythematosus and pregnancy. *Best Pract Res Clin Rheumatol* 2006; **20**: 685–94.

Märker-Hermann E, Fischer-Betz R. Rheumatic diseases and pregnancy. *Curr Opin Obstet Gynecol* 2010; **22**: 458–65.

Saar P, Hermann W, Muller-Ladner U. Connective tissue diseases and pregnancy. *Rheumatology* 2006; **45**: 30–2.

Chapter 106

Rheumatoid arthritis

Rheumatoid arthritis (RA) is three times more common in women than in men, and although the peak time of onset is not until the mid-thirties, it is reported to complicate approximately 0.1% of pregnancies. It is a non-specific autoimmune disease. A proportion of patients are seropositive for rheumatoid factor, an anti-IgG antibody.

RA tends to run a course of remissions and relapses. Pregnancy usually has a beneficial effect on disease progress though relapses during the puerperium are common but may be delayed by lactation. New onset rheumatoid arthritis is also more common in the post-partum period.

Problems/special considerations

The pregnant woman with RA poses several concerns for the anaesthetist:

- *Effects of the disease on the joints:* RA tends to affect primarily the small joints of the hands and wrists, and although this can be disabling for the patient, it is not usually a problem for the anaesthetist. In more severe cases there may be involvement of the hips, knees and lumbar spine, which may make positioning for regional analgesia or anaesthesia difficult. In very severe cases there may be kyphosis of the thoracic spine and fixed deformity of the ribs, causing restrictive lung disease.

  RA affects the cervical spine in up to 45% of cases and it is important to remember that the cervical spine may be unstable and prone to subluxation. The temporomandibular joints may also be affected and tracheal intubation may be difficult or impossible. Cricoarytenoid arthritis may be present, causing glottic constriction.

- *Systemic effects of the disease:* These are widespread. Both pericardial and pleural effusions may occur (often asymptomatically). Systemic granulomas can form in the lungs, myocardium, heart valves, aortic root and coronary arteries. Deposits in the cardiac conducting system may occur. A vasculitic process may rarely cause coronary or pulmonary arteritis.

  Syndromes associated with RA include Felty's and Sjogren's, in both of which peripheral neuropathies may occur.

- *Long-term medication:* The general principle of drug management during pregnancy is to reduce medication to a minimum and to restrict it to those drugs with the best safety record.

  Women with symptomatic RA are usually maintained on high-dose aspirin and non-steroidal anti-inflammatory drugs. Although both are relatively contraindicated during pregnancy it may be impossible to stop them. Serial ultrasound examination of the fetal heart helps to give early warning of closure of the fetal ductus arteriosus or of developing fetal pulmonary hypertension.

Gold, penicillamine and most immunosuppressive drugs are avoided during pregnancy where possible; the degree of risk from the newer immunomodulation preparations (e.g. tumour necrosis factor inhibitors) is unclear.

Management options

The mother with RA may have several anaesthetic risk factors and should be identified as early as possible during pregnancy and referred for anaesthetic assessment. History taking should include a drug history, and questioning about any previous anaesthetics, especially if these involved tracheal intubation. A detailed cardiorespiratory history is essential. The neck and jaw should be examined to assess potential difficulty with tracheal intubation and where appropriate cervical spine x-rays should be taken in extension and flexion. Pulmonary function tests may be considered, and electrocardiography should be performed to exclude conduction defects. If there is suspicion of a rheumatoid cardiomyopathy, echocardiography should be requested. The extent of any peripheral neuropathy must be documented.

The mother should be advised to accept early epidural analgesia. If this is precluded by coagulopathy or absolute maternal refusal, patient-controlled opioid analgesia may be offered. If caesarean section is necessary, a graduated epidural top-up or combined spinal–epidural (CSE) is often recommended in preference to single-shot spinal anaesthesia, in order to reduce the risk of an unexpectedly high motor or sensory block compromising the airway, and to provide greater haemodynamic stability in the event of undiagnosed cardiac problems.

If there are known cervical spine problems and general anaesthesia is essential, the anaesthetist must have access to fibreoptic equipment and awake intubation. Even if there is severe fetal distress, general anaesthesia should not be induced without additional aids for difficult intubation (and the presence of an anaesthetist who is familiar with their use).

Key points

- Rheumatoid arthritis is a multisystem autoimmune disease.
- Pregnancy tends to be associated with remission of the disease.
- The anaesthetist should expect difficulty with tracheal intubation.
- Cardiac and respiratory manifestations of the disease may be present.
- Peripheral neuropathy may infrequently occur.
- The mainstay of drug treatment is non-steroidal anti-inflammatory drugs, which the mother may need to continue throughout pregnancy.

Further reading

Elliott AB, Chakravarty EF. Management of rheumatic diseases during pregnancy. *Postgrad Med* 2010; **122**: 213–21.

Marker-Hermanna E, Fischer-Betz R. Rheumatic diseases and pregnancy. *Curr Opin Obstet Gynecol* 2010; **22**: 458–65.

Cervical spine disorders

Women may have limited cervical spine movement because of rheumatoid arthritis, ankylosing spondylitis, cervical disc disease, trauma, accessory cervical ribs and cervical spondylosis, although the last is extremely uncommon in women of childbearing age.

A rare but important cause of cervical kyphoscoliosis is the Klippel Feil syndrome. In extreme cases the patient may present with severe webbing of the neck, marked scoliosis and virtually no neck movement, but milder cases may pass unnoticed until the woman presents to the anaesthetist in the obstetric theatre.

Problems/special considerations

The major concern of the obstetric anaesthetist is reduced flexibility of the neck and the likelihood of difficulty with tracheal intubation. In addition, there may be other features of the underlying cause of the neck problems (e.g. rheumatoid arthritis).

Management options

Whenever possible, antenatal identification and assessment should be performed. The woman with limited cervical spine movement should be advised of the potential hazards associated with general anaesthesia and advised to accept epidural analgesia for labour and regional anaesthesia for any proposed operative procedure.

Obstetric and midwifery staff must be aware that patients with potentially difficult airways represent increased anaesthetic risk, and that the anaesthetist should be involved early in any decision that might lead to operative delivery.

If general anaesthesia is essential, the anaesthetist must fully assess the patient pre-operatively (including women presenting for emergency surgery). Basic assessment must include neck movement and mouth opening. If difficulty with intubation is anticipated, senior assistance must be sought before proceeding with induction of general anaesthesia. Local protocols should be followed in the event of unexpected failed intubation.

All obstetric theatres should have a difficult intubation trolley readily available, with a variety of laryngoscopes, including McCoy and polio blades, and in most units a videolaryngoscope, e.g. GlideScope or Airtraq. Awake fibreoptic intubation is now thought by many to be the management of choice when general anaesthesia is required in a woman who is known to have significant cervical spine abnormality, although elective preoperative tracheostomy has also been suggested.

Key points

- The main problem posed by cervical spine disorders is potentially difficult tracheal intubation.
- Regional techniques are usually considered best.

Kyphoscoliosis

Kyphoscoliosis may be congenital, associated with neuromuscular disorders (muscular dystrophies, neurofibromatosis, poliomyelitis or cerebral palsy) or idiopathic. Idiopathic kyphoscoliosis is much more common in females than males (ratio of 4:1) and accounts for 80% of all cases of kyphoscoliosis.

Progressive kyphoscoliosis is almost invariably accompanied by progressive symptoms and signs of restrictive pulmonary disease and ultimately, if left uncorrected, leads to pulmonary hypertension and death.

Severe uncorrected kyphoscoliosis is extremely uncommon in the UK, and most women presenting to the antenatal clinic will either have mild deformity or will have had corrective orthopaedic surgery.

Problems/special considerations

Although kyphoscoliosis in pregnant women is likely to be idiopathic, alternative causes are important to eliminate. Neurofibromatosis is associated with other serious complications (intracranial tumours, congenital heart disease), and familial dysautonomia, characterised by massive swings in blood pressure and generalised autonomic dysfunction, is associated with kyphoscoliosis in 90% of cases.

The bony pelvis is normal in women with idiopathic scoliosis and the likelihood of vaginal delivery is not usually reduced. However, if spinal instrumentation extends near the lumbosacral junction this may impair sacral movement and interfere with descent of the fetus within the pelvis.

Women who have had corrective surgery have two major sources of potential morbidity, firstly residual cardiorespiratory disease and secondly limited access to the thoracolumbar spine.

Management options

Antenatal assessment is important, and access to previous medical records, x-ray films and MRI scans, where available, should be sought as early as possible in the pregnancy. Respiratory function tests can readily be performed on an outpatient basis and may be repeated later in the pregnancy to assess any deterioration. It has been suggested that correction of scoliosis improves respiratory function, whereas in women with uncorrected scoliosis, cardiorespiratory function is likely to deteriorate further as a result of pregnancy.

In women with corrected scoliosis, the major problem for the anaesthetist is provision of regional analgesia and anaesthesia. The most common means of correction of kyphoscoliosis is with Harrington rods or with the newer adaptations, Luque and Cofrel–Duousset instrumentation. Each technique involves metal instrumentation and bone grafting. Thoracoplasty is sometimes also offered as an additional surgical procedure in order to reduce the rib 'hump' that affects some patients. This is also used to obtain bone grafts from the ribs instead of the pelvis. Although preservation of the L5/S1 interspace is a cardinal orthopaedic rule, instrumentation and grafting may extend down to L4/5 in up to 20% of cases. The level of skin scar is a poor guide to the level of fixation, and therefore operation notes and/or imaging results are extremely helpful during antenatal assessment. If there is no pre-pregnancy imaging available, and there is doubt about the extent of instrumentation of the lumbar spine, relevant radiography may be performed during the third trimester of pregnancy.

Assessment and written documentation of any existing neurological deficit and any pre-existing back pain is important.

Successful insertion of both epidural and spinal needles is well described in women with Harrington rod fixation, but women should be warned that the procedure may be technically difficult. False loss of resistance has been described, and the risk of accidental dural puncture is increased. There is an increased risk of patchy analgesia or anaesthesia with epidural techniques, thought to be caused by epidural adhesions and scarring following disruption of the ligamentum flavum.

Owing to the potential problems of epidural analgesia and anaesthesia, spinal techniques may offer significant advantages. Spinal needle insertion at the L5/S1 interspace is more likely to be successful, even in very low fusions. There is a definite endpoint, which overcomes the problem of false loss of resistance, and deliberate dural puncture with an appropriate needle avoids the risks of accidental dural puncture with an epidural needle. Spread of local anaesthetic within the cerebrospinal fluid is unlikely to be affected by previous surgery, and therefore anaesthesia for operative delivery is more reliable with spinal than with epidural techniques. There are theoretical reasons to recommend continuous spinal catheter analgesia for labour as an alternative to epidural analgesia, depending on local expertise and familiarity with the technique.

It is important to discuss in advance alternative methods of analgesia and the potential need for general anaesthesia in case regional techniques fail.

Key points

- Although at least 80% of kyphoscoliosis is idiopathic, association with other diseases such as neurofibromatosis and familial dysautonomia should not be forgotten.
- Uncorrected progressive kyphoscoliosis leads to severe restrictive pulmonary disease and pulmonary hypertension.

- The major anaesthetic problem in pregnant women with corrected kyphoscoliosis is provision of regional anaesthesia and analgesia. Spinal techniques offer several advantages over epidural.
- Lumbar fusions are unlikely to involve the L5/S1 interspace.
- Radiography of the lumbar spine may be performed during the third trimester to aid management of regional analgesia.

Further reading

Ko JY, Leffert L. Clinical implications of neuraxial anesthesia in the parturient with scoliosis. *Anesth Analg* 2009; **109**; 1930–4.

Smith PS, Wilson RC, Robinson AP, Lyons GR. Regional blockade for delivery in women with scoliosis or previous spinal surgery. *Int J Obstet Anesth* 2003; **12**: 17–22.

Chapter

Low back pain

109

Low back pain, sacroiliac pain and sciatic pain are common during pregnancy, affecting between 50% and 90% of women. Symptoms vary from mild 'normal' backache to severe pain that may render the woman bed bound and necessitate early delivery.

The prevalence of low back pain during pregnancy increases with increasing maternal age. Numerous other risk factors have been investigated, but reports are contradictory about the relevance of maternal weight, socioeconomic class, number of pregnancies and previous history of back pain, although it is thought that women with a previous history of spinal surgery are not necessarily at increased risk of back pain during pregnancy.

Retrospective studies significantly under-report low back pain, usually quoting an incidence of 20–25%. This accounts for the conflicting data concerning any putative relationship between epidural analgesia and backache. Several prospective studies have now confirmed the absence of any causal relationship between epidural analgesia and the development of new long-term backache.

Problems/special considerations

- *Non-specific back pain:* The majority of back pain in pregnancy is directly attributable to the physiological changes that occur. The influence of relaxin, which is produced by the corpus luteum, leads to generalised ligamentous laxity. Serum levels of relaxin are highest during the first trimester of pregnancy. The pelvis widens, which may lead to sacroiliac joint instability. This may in turn allow anterior displacement of the sacrum, causing stretching of the lumbosacral plexus and subsequent pain. The expanding uterus alters the woman's centre of gravity and causes an increased lumbar lordosis and pelvic tilt, and this, combined with the additional weight carried as pregnancy progresses, contributes to development of back pain. Some women complain of night-time back pain, for which a vascular mechanism has been proposed. It is suggested that inferior vena caval compression and increased intravascular volume occurring during recumbency may lead to distension in the vertebral venous plexus and subsequent stagnant hypoxia in the nerve roots and vertebral bodies, producing radicular and low back pain.

- *Pelvic girdle pain:* Some women have symptoms relating specifically to the sacroiliac joints or the symphysis pubis. These women complain of pain localised to the pelvis and pubic symphysis, with radiation to the buttocks and thighs but not to the calf or foot, and commonly complain of pain when turning over in bed at night. In extreme cases there may be separation of the pubic symphysis, in which case the woman may become unable to walk or weight bear at all. Abduction of the legs and external rotation of the hips may be difficult, and women may have anxieties about their ability to cope with labour and vaginal delivery.

- *Acute disc prolapse:* Central disc herniation occurs in about 1 in 10 000 pregnancies and may require surgical decompression. Large central disc herniations can occur during pregnancy and at the time of delivery, and if there is an associated significant neurological deficit, surgical decompression is indicated. If magnetic resonance imaging is used, disc bulges and herniations can be demonstrated in approximately half of all pregnant women, which is the same incidence as in asymptomatic non-pregnant women. Low back pain with sciatic radiation is common in pregnancy, and careful history taking and examination are needed to ensure that the availability of magnetic resonance imaging does not lead to unnecessary surgical intervention.

- *Other causes:* Less common causes of back pain should not be overlooked. Spinal cord tumours are extremely rare and most reported during pregnancy are angiomas, presumed to be present before pregnancy. The increased vascularity of pregnancy is assumed to cause the tumours to become symptomatic. Secondary metastasis to the spine of primary malignancies such as breast can occur during pregnancy.

Management options

General management

Back care advice early in pregnancy has been reported to reduce the incidence and severity of low back pain during pregnancy. This may be particularly important for women with a history of pre-pregnancy back pain, who may be at increased risk of worsening pain during pregnancy. Simple physiotherapy, exercise programmes and the use of lumbosacral corsets have all been reported to provide symptomatic pain relief during pregnancy.

Use of simple analgesics such as paracetamol and codeine-based preparations is acceptable during pregnancy but non-steroidal anti-inflammatory drugs should be avoided whenever possible. If their use is considered essential, treatment should be agreed with the obstetrician and fetal cardiac ultrasound monitoring arranged because of the risk of premature closure of the ductus arteriosus. Amitriptyline may be prescribed as a co-analgesic, especially if pain is disrupting normal sleep patterns. In cases of severe back pain, strong opioid analgesia may be required.

Transcutaneous electrical nerve stimulation for back pain during the second half of pregnancy is not recommended by the manufacturers of the machines but is used in clinical practice, frequently with good effect. Injection of local anaesthetic and steroid into the epidural space, the sacroiliac joints or the symphysis pubis may be considered necessary if symptomatic control of pain cannot be achieved by other methods. The safety of such procedures during pregnancy is unknown, and a risk–benefit analysis must be undertaken for each woman.

Delivery before term may be considered when pain control is difficult to achieve.

Anaesthetic management

Women with pre-existing musculoskeletal pathology should be fully assessed during the antenatal period. Previous spinal surgery is not a contraindication to regional analgesia and anaesthesia, although women may have been told by their midwife, general practitioner or orthopaedic surgeon that they will be unable to have epidural analgesia. There may be respiratory impairment following significant corrective surgery, and some postoperative neurological deficit, and if so these must be documented antenatally. Women should be told that epidural analgesia for labour does not increase the likelihood of experiencing postnatal backache.

There is no contraindication to vaginal delivery nor to the use of regional analgesia in women with pregnancy-related back pain, although many women request (and some obstetricians suggest) delivery by elective caesarean section to avoid any risk of exacerbating existing back symptoms.

Previous hospital records are helpful in women who have had surgery, since the position of the scar on the woman's back is not a reliable guide to the level of surgery. Most women will know whether they have had metal instrumentation of the spine or merely bony fusion. Those who have had instrumentation should be warned about possible technical difficulties in correctly positioning an epidural needle; it may be easier to perform spinal anaesthesia or analgesia. If successful epidural catheterisation is achieved, it may be difficult to obtain reliable spread of local anaesthetic, and this should be explained before starting the procedure.

Regional anaesthesia and analgesia in women who have had discectomy or laminectomy is not usually technically difficult, but there may be a slightly increased risk of accidental dural puncture, and patients should be warned about this.

Key points

- Low back pain is common in pregnancy; it is usually mechanical and should be treated symptomatically.
- Although rare, acute disc prolapse with neurological deficit may occur and require surgical treatment.
- There is no contraindication to epidural or spinal analgesia or anaesthesia in women with low back pain.
- Serious spinal and neurological pathology may, rarely, present during pregnancy and should always be considered in the differential diagnosis of new back pain.

Further reading

Orlikowski CE, Dickinson JE, Paech MJ, McDonald SJ, Nathan E. Intrapartum analgesia and its association with post-partum back pain and headache in nulliparous women. *Aust N Z J Obstet Gynaecol* 2006; **46**: 395–401.

Pennick VE, Young G. Interventions for preventing and treating pelvic and back pain in pregnancy. *Cochrane Database Syst Rev* 2007; (2): CD001139.

Vermani E. Mittal R, Weeks A. Pelvic girdle pain and low back pain in pregnancy: a review. *Pain Practice* 2010; **10**: 60–71.

Chapter

110

Neurological disease

The pregnant woman may have suffered ($\pm$ recovered) from a neurological condition before she becomes pregnant or she may develop neurological disease while pregnant (Table 110.1).

Problems/special considerations

- Traditionally, regional analgesia and anaesthesia have been avoided in most chronic neurological disease because of the fear of making the woman's condition worse or being blamed should a worsening occur. Since randomised controlled trials are lacking for most of these conditions, traditional prejudices persist, although such evidence that there is supports regional techniques in many cases.
- Acute neurological conditions may put both the mother and the fetus at risk. Anaesthetic input may be required for peripartum analgesia or anaesthesia, acute medical management of critically ill patients, or surgery indicated by the neurological condition.

Management options

The management of both groups of women depends on the nature of the disease, its effects on pregnancy and delivery and the implications of the physiological changes of pregnancy.

Ideally, women who have a diagnosed neurological disease should be counselled before conception, so that they are aware of the possible problems that may be associated with their disease during pregnancy and delivery. In practice, the majority of women are seen after conception, and the aim should be early antenatal assessment. The effect of maintenance therapy and the necessity to change treatment to avoid teratogenic effects must also be

Table 110.1 Neurological conditions that may be seen in pregnancy

Pre-existing		
Previous history	Trauma	Head injury
		Spinal cord injury
	Infection	Meningitis
		Acute post-infective neuropathy
	Tumour	
	Cerebrovascular accident	
Established neurological disease	Migraine	
	Myasthenia gravis	
	Spina bifida	
	Epilepsy	
	Multiple sclerosis	
	Benign intracranial hypertension	
Arising during pregnancy	Trauma	Acute head injury
		Acute spinal cord injury
	Infection	Meningitis
		Acute post-infective neuropathy
	Tumour	
	Cerebrovascular accident	

considered. Good communication between the clinicians involved is essential in the management of these women. Clear guidelines for care should be written in the medical record and should be revised and updated as necessary.

Key points

- Neurological conditions may already be present before pregnancy or may arise acutely during pregnancy.
- Management depends on the condition, the effects on pregnancy and the effects of pregnancy on the condition.
- Early assessment and drawing up of management plans should take place whenever possible.

Further reading

Chang LY, Carabuena JM, Camann W. Neurologic issues and obstetric anesthesia. *Semin Neurol* 2011; **31**: 374–84.

Karnad DR, Guntupalli KK. Neurologic disorders in pregnancy. *Crit Care Med* 2005; **33** (10 Suppl): S362–71.

Ng J, Kitchen N. Neurosurgery and pregnancy. *J Neurol Neurosurg Psychiatry* 2008; **79**: 745–52.

Wang LP, Paech MJ. Neuroanesthesia for the pregnant woman. *Anesth Analg* 2008; **107**: 193–200.

Meningitis

Acute infections of the nervous system may occur at any time during pregnancy or the peripartum period. The most important infection for the anaesthetist to consider is meningitis, as this can (rarely) occur as a sequel to spinal anaesthesia and confuse the differential diagnosis of a postdural puncture headache.

Women may also present having previously had meningitis.

Problems/special considerations

- Meningitis may be:
    (i) Infective, caused by bacteria, viruses and, rarely, others, e.g. tuberculosis, fungal infections.
    (ii) Aseptic, caused by topical chemical agents (e.g. disinfectants) and rarely, systemic drugs, e.g. H_2-blockers, non-steroidal anti-inflammatory drugs and antibiotics.
- Meningitis that occurs as a complication of regional anaesthesia may be either of the above, and in each case prevention is better than cure. Meticulous attention to aseptic technique (this includes the use of a facemask to prevent droplet spread) is an essential part of minimising the risk of introducing infection or chemical contamination at the time of performing the regional block.
- The classic signs of meningitis are headache, neck stiffness, photophobia, vomiting, fever and raised white cell count. Many of these symptoms are also produced by an accidental dural puncture, and so the exclusion of meningitis is essential in the differential diagnosis of any headache that develops after a regional anaesthetic.
- Almost all women with a history of previous meningitis have had a diagnostic lumbar puncture that may have been a frightening experience, leading to apprehension of any further similar procedures. Some may have residual neurological impairment although this is uncommon with modern management.

Management options

Meningitis should be considered as a possible diagnosis in any patient who has a raised temperature or white cell count associated with a headache. Differentiation between meningitis and accidental dural puncture as the cause of the headache may be difficult.

Table 111.1 Typical cerebrospinal fluid (CSF) findings in meningitis

	Postdural puncture headache	Viral meningitis	Bacterial meningitis	Aseptic meningitis
CSF	Clear, normal	Clear, normal	May be cloudy	May be cloudy
CSF protein	–	↑	↑	↑
WBC in CSF	–	↑ Lymphocytes	↑	↑*
Glucose	Normal	↓	↓	Normal
Culture	Negative	Negative	May be positive	Negative

WBC: white blood cells. *Variable, usually leucocytes.

When there is any doubt, a neurological consultation is essential, and where appropriate a diagnostic lumbar puncture should be performed (Table 111.1). Antibiotics are usually prescribed empirically whilst awaiting the results of microbiological investigation.

Ideally, women with a previous history of meningitis should be seen antenatally by the obstetric anaesthetist for assessment and reassurance. In general, most women can be reassured that they are not at extra risk from regional analgesia and anaesthesia.

Key points

- Meningitis is the most important acute neurological infection in obstetrics.
- Meningitis should always be considered in a woman with severe postpartum headache.
- Analysis of cerebrospinal fluid may aid the diagnosis.

Further reading

Loo CC, Dahlgren G, Irestedt L. Neurological complications in obstetric regional anaesthesia. *Int J Obstet Anesth* 2000; **9**: 99–124.

van de Beek D, de Gans J, Spanjaard L, *et al.* Clinical features and prognostic factors in adults with bacterial meningitis. *N Engl J Med* 2004; **351**: 1849–59.

Wong CA. Nerve injuries after neuraxial anaesthesia and their medicolegal implications. *Best Pract Res Clin Obstet Gynaecol* 2010; **24**: 367–81.

Chapter

112

Acute post-infective peripheral neuropathy (Guillain–Barré syndrome)

Acute post-infective peripheral neuropathy (Guillain–Barré syndrome; Landry's paralysis) is a rare condition that usually follows an acute respiratory infection, although it may follow clostridial diarrhoea or surgery. There may be a slight increase in incidence in the early postpartum period. The symptoms usually commence some days after the infection, which triggers an autoimmune acute demyelinating neuropathy. The first symptoms are peripheral sensory paraesthesiae followed by a loss of motor power. The neuropathy ascends and may affect respiratory muscles. Generally, the disease is short lived, and full recovery is usual over a period of weeks or months.

Problems/special considerations

- Rarely, an acute episode of Guillain–Barré syndrome may occur during pregnancy, when the course may be very rapid. As a result of the physiological changes of pregnancy, the respiratory reserve is less than normal, making patients especially prone to respiratory impairment.
- Women with a past history of Guillain–Barré syndrome may present for obstetric analgesia and anaesthesia. The most common clinical problems are:
  (i) There may be concerns about whether regional analgesia or anaesthesia will cause a recurrence of the disease.
  (ii) Women are often very frightened about having a needle in their back as they may have had a bad experience with a lumbar puncture during investigation of the acute episode.
  (iii) Regional anaesthesia or analgesia causing a significant motor block (e.g. when a caesarean section is performed) may provoke a panic reaction.
  Residual neurological impairment is rare after an acute episode.

Management options

Management of the acute illness should take into account the physiological changes of pregnancy and the wellbeing of the growing fetus. Careful monitoring of respiratory function is required, with ventilatory support when necessary. If the mother becomes immobilised, it is important to avoid aortocaval compression and to give thromboprophylaxis.

There is no contraindication to regional analgesia or anaesthesia, when there is a past history of Guillain–Barré syndrome, and the woman can be reassured that it will not cause a recurrence of the acute episode. The risks and benefits of regional blocks should be discussed before the woman is in pain and preferably at an antenatal consultation. The woman's fears of a motor block need to be considered by the anaesthetist, particularly if she has required ventilation for her acute illness. If there is any neurological deficit, this should be assessed and documented before a regional anaesthetic is performed.

Considerable reassurance by the anaesthetist may be required.

Key points

- Acute Guillain–Barré syndrome is rare in pregnancy.
- Antenatal assessment of women with a previous history of Guillain–Barré syndrome is advisable since they may be very worried about regional analgesia and anaesthesia.
- Regional analgesia and anaesthesia is not contraindicated.

Further reading

Chan LY, Tsui MH, Leung TN. Guillain–Barré syndrome in pregnancy. *Acta Obstet Gynecol Scand* 2004; **83**: 319–25.

Dua K, Banerjee A. Guillain-Barré syndrome: a review. *Br J Hosp Med* 2010; **71**: 495–8.

Karnad DR, Guntupalli KK. Neurologic disorders in pregnancy. *Crit Care Med* 2005; **33** (10 Suppl): S362–71.

Chapter

113 Past history of neurological trauma

It is not uncommon for patients with previous head or spinal cord injury to become pregnant. Many of these women will seek preconceptual advice, but others will present in the antenatal period.

Problems/special considerations

The extent of the problems depends on the neurological deficit. For head-injured patients, the main concerns are related to:

- The presence of upper motor neurone lesions (causing difficulties with positioning and mobility; possible hyperkalaemic response to suxamethonium).
- Immobility (increasing the risk of thromboembolism, pressure sores and atelectasis following general anaesthesia).
- Any associated injuries, especially neck (affecting the airway) and pelvis or vertebral column (affecting mode of delivery and regional analgesia/anaesthesia).
- Difficulties in communication.

For spinal-cord injured patients, the above concerns may also exist. The level of the neurological deficit is the most important issue; the major considerations are:

- *Pulmonary function and the effect of pregnancy and delivery:* If the level is above T4, there is likely to be some reduction in respiratory reserve. The phrenic nerve supply to the diaphragm arises from cervical roots 3–5 so this is usually spared in paraplegics; however, the intercostal nerves which contribute to ventilation and which may be particularly important in pregnancy will be affected.
- *Risk of autonomic hyperreflexia:* This is associated with injuries above T4–6 and results in increased sensitivity of sympathetic reflexes in response to cutaneous or visceral stimulation below the level of the lesion. There is resultant labile blood pressure, typically causing massive vasoconstriction and hypertension associated with high levels of circulating catecholamines; there may be a compensatory bradycardia. Susceptibility usually develops within a few weeks of injury.
- *Mode of delivery:* A sensory level above T10 is usually associated with a painless labour and these women are also more likely to deliver prematurely. This may result in a painless precipitate delivery. Some of these women will suffer from muscle spasms and many will need an assisted delivery.

Management options

These women should be seen antenatally and any neurological deficit carefully assessed. When the delivery is planned, the above points should be taken into consideration, with epidural analgesia part of the management in most cases.

Epidural analgesia has been shown to be effective in prophylaxis and treatment of autonomic hyperreflexia. The epidural should be carefully managed to minimise any cardiovascular changes, and a low concentration of local anaesthetic combined with an opioid is usually considered the method of choice although the need for more concentrated local anaesthetic has been suggested in order to block the powerful afferent triggers of autonomic hyperreflexia. Autonomic hyperreflexia is difficult to treat pharmacologically, and the use of α- and β-blocking drugs and nifedipine are of limited value. The use of magnesium sulphate has been described although experience is limited.

Regional anaesthesia is the anaesthetic of choice for operative delivery in most cases. If general anaesthesia is used, alternatives to suxamethonium should be considered if within the period of risk of hyperkalaemia (10 days to 6–7 months). Care must be taken to avoid autonomic hyperreflexia, and deep anaesthesia is needed.

Key points

- Each patient requires individual assessment of her neurological deficit and associated injuries in order to estimate her risk factors.
- Regional analgesia and anaesthesia is indicated in most cases.
- Autonomic hyperreflexia is best prevented or controlled by epidural block.

Further reading

Vercauteren M, Waets P, Pitkanen M. Neuraxial techniques in patients with pre-existing back impairment or prior spine interventions: a topical review with special reference to obstetrics. *Acta Anaesthesiol Scand* 2011; **55**: 910–17.

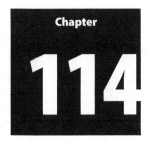

Benign intracranial hypertension

Benign intracranial hypertension (pseudotumour cerebri) is defined as raised intracranial pressure that is not associated with intracranial pathology. It is a rare but well-recognised syndrome that typically affects young to middle-aged overweight females, causing headache and visual disturbances. The aetiology is unclear and there are no focal neurological signs.

Problems/special considerations

- There may be fear of puncturing the dura in someone with increased cerebrospinal fluid (CSF) pressure. However, dural puncture (deliberate or accidental) will not lead to coning in this group of patients and it may even be temporarily beneficial in relieving CSF pressure.
- Concerns have been raised over the possibility that injection of epidural solutions might cause excessive increases in intracranial pressure, and slow injections or the use of infusions have been suggested. Spinal anaesthesia may be potentially difficult as the CSF is under pressure, and drainage of some CSF may be needed before injection of the local anaesthetic. If there has been recent CSF drainage, a block that is higher than expected may occur. Both epidural and spinal techniques have been successfully used for labour and caesarean section, including in women with lumboperitoneal shunts.
- Headache and visual disturbances may also occur in pre-eclampsia and postdural puncture headache, possibly causing confusion.

Management options

General treatment is to advise weight loss and if necessary to prescribe diuretics. In more severe cases, lumbar puncture and the removal of CSF may be recommended. Insertion of lumboperitoneal shunts and optic nerve sheath decompression have been performed in very severe cases.

There is no reason that these women should not be given appropriate regional analgesia or anaesthesia. There need be no anxiety about accidental dural puncture. Because of the relatively benign nature of the disease, general anaesthesia is not contraindicated, although peaks of raised intracranial pressure are to be avoided.

Key points

- Benign intracranial hypertension may present with severe headache and visual disturbances.
- Regional analgesia and anaesthesia (including spinal block) are not contraindicated.

Further reading

Chang LY, Carabuena JM, Camann W. Neurologic issues and obstetric anesthesia. *Semin Neurol* 2011; **31**: 374–84.

Karmaniolou I, Petropoulos G, Theodoraki, K. Management of idiopathic intracranial hypertension in parturients: anesthetic considerations. *Can J Anesth* 2011; **58**: 650–7.

Karnad DR, Guntupalli KK. Neurologic disorders in pregnancy. *Crit Care Med* 2005; **33** (10 Suppl): S362–71.

Chapter

115

Intracranial tumour

A tumour may present during pregnancy or labour; the obstetric anaesthetist may be involved in looking after a woman with acutely raised intracranial pressure (ICP) or in the diagnosis of the tumour in the peripartum period. Women may also present with a previous history of intracranial tumour.

Problems/special considerations

Tumour diagnosed during pregnancy

Particular problems may be related to:

- The nature of the tumour.
- The treatment the patient is receiving, e.g. steroids.
- Whether there is raised ICP, how severe it is and whether there is an associated risk of coning.
- The effect of pushing in the second stage of labour on ICP and the tumour.
- The presence of any other medical problems.
- The risks of regional analgesia or anaesthesia and general anaesthesia.

Tumour manifesting itself in the peripartum period

The woman may present with neurological signs or symptoms that may be related to the position of the tumour or to the development of raised ICP. The obstetric anaesthetist may be asked to see the woman, particularly if she had a regional anaesthetic and the symptoms arose in the postpartum period.

The patient may present with altered consciousness, focal signs, a convulsion or a headache. The differential diagnosis will include eclampsia, epilepsy, meningitis, posterior reversible encephalopathy syndrome and postdural puncture headache. The headache associated with raised ICP is usually present when the patient is supine and does not have the same postural changes as a postdural puncture headache. The headache will be made worse by stooping, coughing or straining. The associated symptoms and signs of photophobia, vomiting and neck stiffness may be present both in raised ICP and following dural puncture.

Previous history of tumour

There may be residual neurological impairment, as for a past history of neurological trauma. A small number of women have residual tumour left and this may be affected by the pregnancy. There may be a shunt to maintain normal cerebrospinal fluid (CSF) pressures. Generally, these shunts drain from the brain into the peritoneal cavity; however, some drain CSF around the spinal cord into the peritoneum. The latter may be placed in the lumbar region and thus cause a problem if regional block is to be considered. The risk of introducing infection at the time of a regional block is very small but may be a deterrent to regional block in these women. Many patients will be particularly anxious about the effects of both regional and general anaesthesia on their neurological function.

Management options

If a tumour has been diagnosed during pregnancy, the obstetric anaesthetist should be consulted about the management of the labour. It is generally accepted that the delivery should be as stress free as possible, and normally regional analgesia would be part of the management. The benefits of regional analgesia/anaesthesia for these patients must be balanced against an accidental dural puncture causing coning. If epidural analgesia is considered to be the best management, a senior anaesthetist should be involved. Pushing in the second stage should be minimised to reduce the possibility of bleeding into the tumour. If the patient is suffering from a significant increase in ICP and the obstetrician advises urgent delivery, caesarean section under general anaesthesia may be the technique of choice. General anaesthesia may need to be modified to give a 'neuro' anaesthetic that would minimise raised ICP at the time of induction of anaesthesia. It is important to remember that decreased arterial partial pressure of carbon dioxide from the normal value in pregnancy (approximately 4 kPa) in the mother will reduce placental perfusion and this may compromise the fetus.

When new headaches, convulsions or other neurological symptoms and signs present in the peripartum period, it is easy to assume more common conditions such as postdural puncture headache and eclampsia, rather than think of intracranial tumour. A careful history and examination (where appropriate by a neurologist) is important in reaching the correct diagnosis. Magnetic resonance imaging and/or computerised tomography should be considered. Once diagnosed, treatment is as for any non-pregnant patient.

The majority of women who have had previous intracranial tumours are entirely normal and have no residual problems. Neurological advice will be necessary to know if the pregnancy will affect any residual tumour. Examination of the medical records and discussion with the neurosurgeon is wise.

Key points

- Regional analgesia is usually indicated during labour, but an accidental dural puncture may be catastrophic; thus the decision should depend on the individual features of each case.
- Underlying intracerebral pathology should always be considered when new symptoms or signs present postpartum.
- A neurologist should be consulted if in doubt.

Further reading

Cohen-Gadol AA, Friedman JA, Friedman JD, *et al.* Neurosurgical management of intracranial lesions in the pregnant patient: a 36-year institutional experience and review of the literature. *J Neurosurg* 2009; **111**: 1150–7.

Lynch JC, Gouvêa F, Emmerich JC, *et al.* Management strategy for brain tumour diagnosed during pregnancy. *Br J Neurosurg* 2011; **25**: 225–30.

Ng J, Kitchen N. Neurosurgery and pregnancy. *J Neurol Neurosurg Psychiatry* 2008; **79**: 745–52.

Wang LP, Paech MJ. Neuroanesthesia for the pregnant woman. *Anesth Analg* 2008; **107**: 193–200.

Chapter

116

Cerebrovascular accident

Cerebrovascular accidents (CVAs) may occur during pregnancy and delivery and may be caused by intracranial haemorrhage or thrombosis. The incidence varies but is thought to be between 11 and 26 per 100 000 deliveries.

Problems/special considerations

CVA presenting during pregnancy or peripartum

Pregnancy and labour increase the risk of CVAs. This risk will be further increased if there is associated obesity, smoking or hypertensive disease of pregnancy.

- *Intracerebral haemorrhage:* This may occur at any stage during the pregnancy, including the peripartum period. The most common problem is subarachnoid haemorrhage (SAH), which presents as an acute onset of severe headache, often with associated neck stiffness, photophobia and vomiting. There may be loss of consciousness. SAH is often associated with an underlying berry aneurysm or arteriovenous malformation and is also a cause of death associated with pre-eclampsia.

- *Cerebral thrombosis:* Pregnancy predisposes to cerebral thrombosis, including cortical vein thrombosis. Other predisposing factors include dehydration and other hypercoagulable states (e.g. thrombophilias). Although cortical vein thrombosis is rare, it is important to the obstetric anaesthetist in the differential diagnosis of postdural puncture headache. The patient may present with focal neurological signs or signs of raised intracranial pressure.

Sudden collapse carries the risk of airway obstruction and hypoxaemia, aspiration of gastric contents, aortocaval compression and fetal compromise. As for many acute medical emergencies in the maternity suite, staff may be unfamiliar with basic resuscitative measures unless these are regularly practised.

Previous history of CVA

The most common presentation in the childbearing age group is a previous history of SAH. Some of these women will have made a complete recovery and others will have a neurological deficit of which the anaesthetist should be aware. They may be very frightened by the thought of a needle in their back after a bad experience with lumbar puncture. There may be an exaggerated hyperkalaemic response to suxamethonium 10 days to 6–7 months after CVA. Women with a previous cerebral thrombosis may be taking heparin or aspirin.

Management options

If there is loss of consciousness, basic resuscitation must be performed, with particular attention to uterine displacement and avoidance of aspiration. There is a significant risk of rebleeding following SAH; therefore, assessment by neurosurgeons with a view to surgical treatment is essential. The indication for surgical intervention should not be altered by the fact that the woman is pregnant. The risk of SAH is one reason for ensuring adequate blood pressure control in pre-eclampsia, particularly in the peripartum period.

Management of delivery depends on the clinical condition of the patient, who may still have a significant neurological deficit. If the patient is well recovered, a stress-free vaginal delivery with epidural analgesia is the management of choice, taking care to avoid significant fluctuations in blood pressure. The indications for caesarean section should only be obstetric. However, if the patient is confused or has a problem with cognitive function, the wisest course of action may be delivery by caesarean section under general anaesthesia. General anaesthesia should be carefully managed to minimise the hypertensive response to tracheal intubation. Each patient will need to be considered individually in consultation with the obstetrician and neurosurgeons and other disciplines where appropriate. Combined caesarean section and neurosurgery has been performed.

Diagnosis of CVA is by computerised tomography or magnetic resonance imaging of the brain; if the diagnosis is suspected, it is wise to involve the neurologists early. Although the use of lumbar puncture has largely been superseded by imaging techniques for the diagnosis of SAH, partly because of the risk of coning if intracranial pressure is increased, lumbar puncture may still have a place in selected cases.

The management of women with previous SAH depends on whether the underlying pathology has been surgically treated. If so, the woman can be regarded as relatively normal. The risk of a further bleed is increased if there is hypertension and in particular if there are sudden surges in blood pressure. The control of blood pressure and the avoidance of stress during labour or delivery are therefore important. Generally, regional analgesia should be recommended for labour. If a caesarean section is required, regional anaesthesia is appropriate. No regional technique should be performed without a detailed discussion with the woman, and this ideally should take place in the antenatal period, when a plan for the management of analgesia and anaesthesia should be written in her notes. If general anaesthesia is necessary, the hypertensive response to intubation should be modified and alternatives to suxamethonium used if within the period of risk.

Rarely, CVA (usually subdural or subarachnoid haemorrhage) has followed spinal anaesthesia or accidental dural puncture.

Key points

- Control of blood pressure in hypertension is important in pregnancy, whether or not it is pregnancy related.
- Headaches are not always caused by dural puncture.
- Pregnancy is not a contraindication to neurosurgery.
- Regional analgesia or anaesthesia is usually indicated unless there is significant neurological impairment.

Further reading

Davie CA, O'Brien P. Stroke and pregnancy. *J Neurol Neurosurg Psychiatry* 2008; **79**: 240–5.

James AH, Bushnell CD, Jamison MG, Myers ER. Incidence and risk factors for stroke in pregnancy and the puerperium. *Obstet Gynecol* 2005; **106**: 509–16.

Lockhart E, Baysinger CL. Intracranial venous thrombosis in the parturient. *Anesthesiology* 2007; **107**: 652–8.

Treadwell SD, Thanvi B, Robinson TG. Stroke in pregnancy and the puerperium. *Postgrad Med J* 2008; **84**: 238–45.

Epilepsy

Epilepsy is the most common neurological disease: it is estimated that 2–5% of the population have suffered a convulsion in the past and around 0.5–1% of the population suffer from epilepsy. Therefore, pregnancy and epilepsy may commonly co-exist. However, convulsions may develop for the first time in pregnancy and cause a problem in differential diagnosis.

Problems/special considerations

- *Pre-existing epilepsy:* It is generally thought that epilepsy is affected by the hormonal changes of pregnancy and that the frequency of fits may increase in 15–30% of women during pregnancy. However, in an equal proportion of women, the symptoms improve. If the woman has not sought advice before conception, it is possible that she may stop her medication as she may be worried about teratogenic effects on the fetus. In addition, the pharmacodynamics and pharmacokinetics of antiepileptic drugs may be affected by the physiological changes of pregnancy. Both hyperventilation and the pain and stress of labour may lower the threshold for convulsions.
- In recent Reports on Confidential Enquiries into Maternal Deaths, epilepsy (especially poorly controlled) has been a major factor in deaths from neurological disease, frequently associated with drowning in the bath.
- *Convulsions occurring in pregnancy:* Delivery and labour are particularly hazardous periods. Immediate problems include aortocaval compression, hypoxaemia, cerebrovascular accident and aspiration of gastric contents. In addition, differential diagnosis may include a number of conditions both related and unrelated to pregnancy.

Management options

Ideally, the woman with diagnosed epilepsy should have had counselling before pregnancy to discuss the management of her epilepsy during pregnancy. Pre-conception planning aims to simplify the drug regimen, and medication may be stopped in a woman who has been convulsion-free for a long time.

During pregnancy, normal medication should be maintained. This may necessitate alternative routes of administration when gastric absorption is affected. The risks and benefits of changing the treatment requires specialist advice for each individual. It is important to remember the effects of pregnancy on the pharmacodynamics and pharmacokinetics of the antiepileptic drugs, and the regular monitoring of drug levels during pregnancy is useful.

When carefully managed, women with epilepsy do not usually experience problems during pregnancy and most can be offered any form of pain relief that they wish. The poorly controlled epileptic will benefit from epidural analgesia to reduce the stress of labour and hyperventilation. General anaesthesia is not a greater problem in these women, and thiopental remains a good anticonvulsant.

Convulsions are managed in the normal way, taking into account the risk of aortocaval compression and aspiration of gastric contents (see Chapter 118, Convulsions).

Key points

- Epilepsy is the commonest neurological disease.
- Eclampsia is not the only cause of convulsions in pregnancy.
- Epilepsy may become poorly controlled in pregnancy.
- Management of the well-controlled epileptic is as for normal women.

Further reading

Tomson T. Epilepsy in pregnancy. *BMJ* 2007; **335**: 769.

Walker SP, Permezel M, Berkovic SF. The management of epilepsy in pregnancy. *BJOG* 2009; **116**: 758–67.

Chapter

118

Convulsions

Convulsions occurring ante-, peri- or postpartum are uncommon but important causes of collapse on labour ward; they may herald significant maternal disease or reflect a transient disturbance, but in either case management must be prompt and appropriate. Although petit mal (absence seizures) and focal seizures may occur, they are less common in the maternity suite than grand mal (tonic–clonic seizures).

Problems/special considerations

- The diagnosis may be uncertain if not witnessed by an experienced observer; e.g. a simple faint may be labelled as a 'fit'. A history of a tonic–clonic seizure may not always be obtained. Furthermore, collapse from non-neurological causes may themselves lead to convulsions if severe hypotension or hypoxaemia occurs.
- Physiological effects include increased cerebral and whole body oxygen requirements, with increased carbon dioxide production. Together with hypoventilation arising from airway obstruction and chest wall rigidity, this may result in hypoxaemia, acidosis, hypercapnia and increased sympathetic activity. These effects may be exacerbated by the increased cardiac output and metabolic requirements of the pregnant woman compared with the non-pregnant one.

Table 118.1 Causes of convulsions on the labour ward

Neurological disease	Pre-existing epilepsy
	Stroke
	Cerebral vein thrombosis
	Infection
	Migraine
	Posterior reversible encephalopathy syndrome
	Incidental disease, e.g. tumours
Hypoxaemia	Cardiovascular collapse, e.g. haemorrhage
	Pulmonary embolus
Obstetric	Eclampsia
	Amniotic fluid embolism
Metabolic	Hypoglycaemia
	Hypocalcaemia
	Hyponatraemia*
	Uraemia
Drugs	Anaesthetic, e.g. local anaesthetics
	Others, e.g. cocaine intoxication, overdoses, acute withdrawal (including alcohol)

*Hyponatraemia is especially important in the delivery suite, where it may follow prolonged infusion of oxytocin diluted in dextrose solutions.

Convulsions in pregnancy may be more likely to lead to stroke than in the non-pregnant state. Aortocaval compression further exacerbates the situation before delivery. If inadequately treated, convulsions may merge into each other without breaks in-between (status epilepticus).

• As for collapse generally, the labour ward staff may be less familiar with emergency equipment and drugs than staff elsewhere. Although most of the possible causes of convulsions are the same as outside of the maternity suite (Table 118.1), the emphasis is different in this setting.

Management options

Initial management includes avoidance of aortocaval compression, protection of the airway (remembering the risk of aspiration) and support of the ventilation and circulation.

The differential diagnosis (Table 118.1) is usually one of exclusion; the initial task is to distinguish between a primary convulsion and one resulting from hypoxaemia and/or cardiovascular collapse, hence the importance of a careful history from the patient and observer(s). Since eclampsia is such an important and relatively common cause in the peripartum period, it should be assumed until proven otherwise. Although 'pre-eclampsia screening' investigations are commonly performed, eclampsia may precede other evidence of pre-eclampsia. Baseline laboratory investigations should be done and computerised tomography/magnetic resonance imaging scan of the head is generally advised unless a clear history of epilepsy is obtained. Blood gas analysis may be useful in guiding management but not in the differential diagnosis; it may reveal marked metabolic and respiratory acidosis resulting from the seizure itself, although this may also represent cardiorespiratory collapse preceding the convulsion. Hypoxaemia may be apparent if aspiration has occurred. Further investigations are guided by the results of preliminary testing and the clinical course.

Drug treatment is with standard anticonvulsant drugs (e.g. diazepam 5–10 mg boluses intravenously; phenytoin 10–15 mg/kg slowly intravenously preferably with electrocardiographic monitoring), although magnesium sulphate has been shown to be more effective in preventing recurrent eclamptic seizures and should be the first choice unless eclampsia can be excluded. Thiopental, tracheal intubation and controlled ventilation may be required if convulsions are severe and continuous; however, this does prevent further neurological assessment.

Fetal monitoring should not be forgotten. Once control of the convulsion has been achieved and the mother is stabilised, delivery should be considered, depending on the aetiology of the convulsions, the gestation and the state of the mother and fetus. In eclampsia, delivery is usually expedited as soon as the stability of the mother allows.

Key points

- Convulsions on the labour ward should be considered as eclampsia until proven otherwise, although other causes should not be forgotten.
- Immediate management is with support of the airway, breathing and circulation, and avoidance of aortocaval compression; magnesium sulphate is the treatment of choice in eclampsia to prevent further convulsions.

Chapter

119

Migraine

The classic presentation of migraine is with a paroxysmal unilateral headache preceded by visual and sensory phenomena, accompanied by or followed by nausea and vomiting. Migraine may present for the first time in or shortly after pregnancy.

Problems/special considerations

- Migraine often improves in pregnancy. However, many women are anxious about how labour and the pain-relieving drugs given in labour will affect them and may seek advice as to whether regional analgesia is a problem.
- Many drugs used for migraine cross the placenta, and drug therapy may need altering during pregnancy.
- Stress, including pain and starvation, can precipitate an attack of migraine.

- An acute migraine attack presenting with severe headache and visual disturbances may be confused with pre-eclampsia. Rarely, migraine may be associated with other neurological symptoms.
- In the postpartum period, migraine may be confused with postdural puncture headache (PDPH); indeed, the cerebral vasodilatation that is thought to cause the headache of migraine may in part be responsible for the headache that follows dural puncture.

Management options

There is no contraindication to epidural or spinal analgesia or anaesthesia.

Migraine can usually be easily distinguished from PDPH. In migraine, the headache is usually unilateral and frontal, whereas in PDPH the headache is usually bilateral, occipital and frontal. The dramatic improvement in PDPH on lying down is not present with migraine. New onset severe headache should always alert medical staff to the possibility of other underlying conditions (see Chapter 42, Postdural puncture headache).

Key points

- Migraine is common but often improves during pregnancy.
- Migraine may resemble pre-eclampsia and postdural puncture headache.
- Anaesthetic management is routine.

Further reading

Contag SA, Bushnell C. Contemporary management of migrainous disorders in pregnancy. *Curr Opin Obstet Gynecol* 2010; **22**: 437–45.

Goadsby PJ, Goldberg J, Silberstein SD. Migraine in pregnancy. *BMJ* 2008; **336**: 1502–4.

Klein AM, Loder E. Postpartum headache. *Int J Obstet Anesth* 2010; **19**: 422–30.

Chapter

120

Multiple sclerosis

Multiple sclerosis is a disease of unknown aetiology in which the clinical symptoms are caused by patches of damage to the myelin sheath of the central, but not peripheral, neurones. The onset of the disease is generally between the ages of 20 and 40 years and it is usually a disease of relapse and remission.

The prevalence of the disease is around 110 per 100 000 in the UK and it is more common in females (two out of three patients will be female). Therefore, it is not uncommon in women who present for obstetric care. The rate of relapse may decrease during pregnancy, especially in the third trimester, and pregnancy is usually well tolerated, although the rate of relapse may increase in the first three months postpartum before returning to the basal rate.

Problems/special considerations

- Anaesthetists might feel reluctant to perform regional analgesia in these women since a relapse may occur after a stressful event such as delivery of a baby. The regional anaesthetic may then erroneously be blamed. Previous studies have suggested an increased incidence of relapse if higher concentrations of bupivacaine are used, although subsequent evidence has not confirmed this.
- Women who are very disabled may have impairment of laryngeal reflexes and ventilation. They also may be unable to position themselves for regional blockade and may be physically unable to achieve a vaginal delivery without assistance.
- Women will be concerned about any possible effect of regional analgesia and anaesthesia on their disease.

Management options

Antenatal counselling is advised if possible, to enable a plan for analgesia and anaesthesia to be drawn up and documented in the mother's notes. Time should be taken to discuss the risks and benefits of regional techniques so that the woman may give informed consent where appropriate.

There is no logical reason why these women should not have regional analgesia and there may be benefits in reducing the stress of labour caused by pain. Where practical, it is good practice to assess the neurological deficit before performing a regional block and to maintain as much motor power as possible. Similarly, both spinal and epidural anaesthesia are suitable if caesarean section is necessary. If general anaesthesia is used, standard techniques are used.

Key points

- Epidural analgesia should not be denied in labour.
- Relapse is not more common with regional anaesthesia than without.
- Routine techniques are used, taking into account any pre-existing neurological deficit.

Further reading

Drake E, Drake M, Bird J, Russell R. Obstetric regional blocks for women with multiple sclerosis: a survey of UK experience. *Int J Obstet Anesth* 2006; **15**: 115–23.

Lee M, O'Brien P. Pregnancy and multiple sclerosis. *J Neurol Neurosurg Psychiatry* 2008; **79**: 1308–11.

May AE, Fombon FN, Francis S. UK registry of high-risk obstetric anaesthesia: report on neurological disease. *Int J Obstet Anesth* 2008; **17**: 31–6.

Tsui A, Lee MA. Multiple sclerosis and pregnancy. *Curr Opin Obstet Gynecol* 2011; **23**: 435–9.

Chapter

121

Myasthenia gravis

Myasthenia gravis is an autoimmune disease affecting the neuromuscular junction, at which circulating antibodies compete with acetylcholine. It has an incidence of around 1 per 100 000. It is more common in females, with an onset at any age. The muscles that are most commonly involved are the oculomotor, facial, pharyngeal and respiratory. The weakness of the muscles is improved by rest. The effect of pregnancy on the disease is variable.

The disease is treated with acetylcholinesterase inhibitor therapy. The treatment of choice is pyridostigmine in a dose range of 30–120 mg orally at regular intervals through the day. The side effects of treatment may include bradycardia, sweating and increased salivary secretion.

Problems/special considerations

- As with many neurological diseases, women with myasthenia gravis may be very worried about regional analgesia and anaesthesia and any adverse effect on their disease.
- Myasthenia gravis is generally made worse by stress, physical exertion, minor infections and fatigue. During labour an increase in weakness can be expected. In severe disease there is a risk of respiratory insufficiency and aspiration of gastric contents, which may thus increase as labour progresses.
- Maternal expulsive efforts may be markedly reduced at the end of labour, increasing the need for instrumental delivery.
- Requirements for acetylcholinesterase inhibitors may be difficult to estimate during labour because of worsening weakness and possibly reduced gastric absorption of oral pyridostigmine (especially if opioids have been administered). Inadequate dosage may lead to severe weakness (myasthenic crisis), whereas overdosage with acetylcholinesterase inhibitors may lead to a cholinergic crisis (muscle weakness and fasciculation, sweating, miosis, lacrimation, abdominal colic, etc.).
- There is increased sensitivity to non-depolarising neuromuscular blocking drugs, with the risk of prolonged neuromuscular blockade during and after general anaesthesia. Resistance to suxamethonium has been reported, although most authorities recommend a normal dose. Magnesium sulphate worsens muscle weakness.
- Placental transfer of maternal antibodies may cause neonatal myasthenia.

Management options

There should be a team approach to the management of women with myasthenia gravis during the antenatal period. The extent of her muscle weakness and whether this affects the bulbar and respiratory muscles should be carefully assessed. The variable effect of pregnancy on the disease means that the mother will need constant monitoring of her disease.

Table 121.1 Oral and parenteral acetylcholinesterase inhibitors
(all the following dosages are equivalent in clinical effect)

Neostigmine	15 mg orally 0.7–1.0 mg i.m. 0.5 mg i.v.
Pyridostigmine	60 mg orally 3–4 mg i.m. 2 mg i.v.

Treatment will need to be adjusted to maintain muscle strength, and pulmonary function tests may be useful in assessing the strength of the respiratory muscles.

The mode of delivery should be decided on obstetric grounds, taking into account the severity of the illness and the ability of the woman to tolerate the work of labour.

Regional analgesia is advisable, to minimise the stress of labour and to avoid the sedative effects of pethidine or Entonox. If opioids have not been given, gastric function can be considered to be near-normal and oral medication continued. If in doubt in severe cases, equivalent doses of parenteral acetylcholinesterase inhibitors can be given (Table 121.1). Atropine should also be given to reduce unwanted cholinergic effects. If in doubt over whether worsening weakness represents a myasthenic or cholinergic crisis, edrophonium 2 mg intravenously will improve the former but worsen or have no effect on the latter.

In well-controlled myasthenia gravis, caesarean section may be performed under regional anaesthesia. If the disease is not well controlled, the risk of aspiration and respiratory impairment with a high regional block must be weighed against the risks of respiratory impairment following general anaesthesia. Non-depolarising neuromuscular blocking drugs are usually not necessary. Following general anaesthesia, mothers may require postoperative ventilation whilst their medication is reintroduced and their muscle power has returned to normal.

Key points

- Team management is essential.
- Regular monitoring of muscle strength throughout pregnancy is essential.
- Oral medication can be continued throughout labour unless the disease is very severe and gastric function is in doubt, when parenteral medication may be substituted.
- Both myasthenic and cholinergic crises may occur.
- Regional analgesia and anaesthesia is indicated in most cases.

Further reading

Almeida C, Coutinho E, Moreira D, Santos E, Aguiar J. Myasthenia gravis and pregnancy: anaesthetic management – a series of cases. *Eur J Anaesthesiol* 2010; 27: 985–90.

Hoff JM, Daltveit AK, Gilhus NE. Myasthenia gravis: consequences for pregnancy, delivery, and the newborn. *Neurology* 2003; 61: 1362–6.

Chapter

122

Spina bifida

Spina bifida is a congenital neural tube defect with a spectrum of severity. Neural tube defects in survivable form are estimated to occur in 1–3 in 1000 live births; with modern management 25-year survival is over 80%. Many of these survivors will have a significant neurological deficit, in spite of which they will strive to achieve as normal a lifestyle as possible; for women this includes pregnancy and childbirth. Spina bifida is generally categorised as occulta and cystica:

- *Spina bifida occulta:* Its reported incidence is between 5% and 20% of the population and it is not associated with a neurological deficit. It may only be discovered incidentally on radiography or when a woman presents for regional analgesia. It is a vertebral defect and occurs when the two halves of the vertebral arch fail to fuse.
- *Spina bifida cystica:* This is a collective term for the more severe forms of spina bifida. Common to all these malformations is a sac-like protrusion through the defect in the vertebral arch. The neurological deficit depends on the severity and level of the defect and, to an extent, on the effect of subsequent surgery.

Problems/special considerations

Pregnancy in women with spina bifida can prove to be a serious challenge to both obstetric and anaesthetic staff, depending on both the severity of the neurological deficit and any associated skeletal abnormality:

- Kyphoscoliosis and distortion of the pelvis may make vaginal delivery difficult.
- There may be an intraventricular shunt to maintain normal cerebrospinal fluid pressure.
- There is an increased risk of accidental dural puncture, particularly when the needle is inserted at the level of the defect. The spinal cord may be tethered.
- There is a risk of abnormal spread of local anaesthetic resulting in either excessive cranial spread or inadequate sacral spread.
- There is often anxiety regarding the conduct of regional anaesthesia, particularly in patients with an established neural deficit.
- If caesarean section is required, surgery may be difficult because of previous urological surgery, such as ileal conduit.
- Latex allergy is more common in patients with spina bifida cystica.

Management options

Ideally, women should be seen by the anaesthetist in the antenatal period when the risks of regional anaesthesia can be assessed and explained. Women who have spina bifida occulta usually have no neurological deficit and may be offered regional analgesia or anaesthesia when appropriate. The lesions are usually in the low lumbar or sacral areas and so the impact of regional techniques is minimal. The patient should be warned that there may be an increased risk of inadequate/failed blocks, and also of dural puncture as the supporting ligaments (interspinous and ligamentum flavum) may be abnormal at the level of the lesion. It should be remembered that spinal cord tethering may be present in these patients, especially if they give a history of neurological abnormalities and cutaneous manifestations. Cord tethering is unlikely in the absence of any neurological symptoms, in which case imaging is of little value. Occasionally, spina bifida occulta may only be discovered incidentally during siting the epidural/spinal, but this is not a reason to deny appropriate analgesia or anaesthesia.

In spina bifida cystica, there may be significant neurological deficit including skeletal abnormalities and impairment of bladder and bowel function. Some women may be wheelchair bound. The aim is to achieve as normal a pregnancy and labour as possible for the individual; for this, effective antenatal consultation and team planning is essential in order that all the options for delivery are discussed and documented. Before regional analgesia is contemplated, baseline clinical findings should be documented in the records, including neurological assessment and where possible pre-existing spinal and pelvic x-ray films (pelvic radiography in pregnancy may not be advisable). The neurological examination is helpful in assessing whether the pain pathways of labour are intact and how regional analgesia can be used to help in labour and delivery. Women may have been told that they will not feel the pain of labour because of their pre-existing sensory deficit. However, this ignores the fact that most are neurologically intact above the lower lumber segments and therefore they will experience the normal pain of the first stage of labour, although it is true that the pain of the second stage may be modified. The increased risk of failed regional analgesia/anaesthesia and dural tap must be explained.

For analgesia in labour, epidural analgesia is generally not contraindicated. However, siting the epidural may be difficult and it is advisable to insert it above the defect and/or the scar from previous surgery. For caesarean section, regional anaesthesia is acceptable. Spinal anaesthesia may be more predictable than epidural anaesthesia, particularly for spread of the block to the sacral roots. Normal volumes of subarachnoid injectate may be used. However, depending on the complexity of the previous surgery and the wishes of the women, some may opt for general anaesthesia. This usually poses no particular problems, although tracheal intubation may be difficult in some patients with kyphoscoliosis. These patients have a normal response to suxamethonium.

Key points

- Antenatal assessment of women with spina bifida is important.
- Regional analgesia or anaesthesia may be difficult but should not be denied.
- Women should be warned of the risks of accidental dural tap and inadequate block.
- Spinal anaesthesia may be preferable to epidural anaesthesia for caesarean section.

Further reading

Kreeger RN, Hilvano A. Anesthetic options for the parturient with a neural tube defect. *Int Anesth Clin* 2005; **43**: 65–80.

May AE, Fombon FN, Francis S. UK registry of high-risk obstetric anaesthesia: report on neurological disease. *Int J Obstet Anesth* 2008; **17**: 31–6.

Respiratory disease

Women with respiratory disease are becoming pregnant in increasing numbers: the incidence of asthma is increasing, and more women with chronic conditions such as cystic fibrosis are surviving into reproductive life.

Problems/special considerations

Both primarily obstructive and primarily restrictive disease may be exacerbated by the increased respiratory demands of pregnancy (although asthma often improves in pregnancy), with further worsening in labour. In addition, the physiological changes of pregnancy may further hinder respiratory function, in particular airway oedema, upward displacement of the diaphragm and reduced functional residual capacity. It is also important to remember the increased risk factors associated with obesity, smoking and kyphoscoliosis, any of which may complicate the underlying respiratory condition.

Management options

The clinician must be familiar with the physiological changes of pregnancy in the respiratory system in order to understand the relevant pathophysiology. Early antenatal assessment of the woman, including pulmonary function tests when appropriate, is essential. Ideally, this should be in the first trimester. If the condition is severe, preconception counselling may be advisable. The effect of the pregnancy and delivery may then be assessed in light of the physiological changes of pregnancy and the respiratory stresses of delivery. Specifically, pulmonary function tests will give an idea of how the mother might cope with labour.

Women with mild disease can be treated as normal. In more severe disease, regional analgesia and anaesthesia is usually indicated to reduce the stress and demands of labour. Continuous pulse oximetry is advisable throughout labour in severe disease. If operative delivery is required, regional techniques avoid the depressant effects of general anaesthetic drugs, but care must be taken in case of high regional blocks.

Key points

- Respiratory disease may be exacerbated by the physiological changes of pregnancy and the increased demands of the fetus.
- Careful antenatal assessment is important.
- Regional analgesia and anaesthesia is usually indicated.

Chapter 124

Asthma

Asthma is defined as reversible airways obstruction characterised by the narrowing of the small and large airways. This is caused by spasm in the smooth muscle, oedema of the bronchial wall, inflammation in the mucosa and mucous plugging. Patients with asthma have hyperreactive bronchi and are sensitive to a variety of external and internal stimuli.

Asthma is one of the most common diseases in the UK, with a prevalence of 15% in children and 10% in adults. Its incidence is increasing. Asthma is thus the most common respiratory condition seen in pregnancy, occurring in approximately 10% of pregnant women. Of these, around 10% will need hospital admission for an acute exacerbation.

Anaesthetists may be involved in looking after women who have an exacerbation of their asthma during pregnancy or when on the delivery suite.

Problems/special considerations

- In pregnancy, asthma remains stable in approximately one third of patients, worsens in one third, and improves in another third of patients, an effect thought to be caused by progesterone and cortisol.
- In severe cases, patients may be taking a number of bronchodilator and anti-inflammatory drugs, including steroids.
- Stress, especially pain and anxiety, may precipitate an acute exacerbation, although viral infections are thought to be the most common cause of an acute exacerbation.
- The increased demands of pregnancy make mothers more vulnerable to acute exacerbations of asthma. During an acute attack, physicians not accustomed to the assessment of pregnant patients may misinterpret blood gas results, e.g. by not appreciating that an arterial partial pressure of carbon dioxide of 5.5–6.0 is grossly abnormal.
- Both maternal and neonatal (low birth weight, intrauterine growth retardation) complications are more common in mothers with asthma, especially if poorly controlled.
- Pethidine has been implicated in worsening asthma because of its histamine-releasing action, though it is thought to be better than other opioids as it has a smooth muscle relaxant effect.
- General anaesthesia in an asthmatic pregnant patient may provoke severe bronchospasm, especially when the airway is instrumented. Thiopental has been implicated in causing bronchospasm although this is disputed. Non-steroidal anti-inflammatory drugs are well known to induce bronchospasm in susceptible patients.

Management options

Ideally, moderate and severe asthmatics should be counselled in the antenatal period and a plan set out for their management in labour. The primary aim of treatment is the maintenance of oxygenation. As asthmatics often play down their symptoms, direct questioning about their exercise tolerance and their current treatment, including steroids, is required for the antenatal record. Acute exacerbations should be treated aggressively. Current advice is that influenza vaccinations should not be given until after 12 weeks' gestation.

Basic techniques for analgesia and anaesthesia are as for non-asthmatic mothers, bearing the above points in mind. Bronchospasm in labour may interfere with effective self-administration of Entonox. The woman should be fully alert and in control during her labour as much as possible, and therefore able to manage her asthma treatment with her inhalers. Epidural analgesia should be generally recommended.

Regional anaesthesia is indicated for operative deliveries, although a high block may reduce the ability to cough.

There is no contraindication to the standard treatments for an asthmatic attack in pregnancy or labour, including the use of inhaled or systemic steroids. It is important to remember that peak flow measurements are useful for monitoring the condition and that respiratory reserve is less during pregnancy, particularly if the mother's attack is precipitated by a respiratory tract infection.

Key points

- Both maternal and neonatal complications are more common in mothers with asthma, especially if poorly controlled.
- Epidural analgesia should be encouraged in labour.
- Regional anaesthesia is indicated for operative delivery.
- Acute exacerbations should be treated as for non-pregnant patients.

Further reading

Boulet LP, Rey E. Asthma in pregnancy. *BMJ* 2007; **334**: 582–5.

Kwon HL, Belanger K, Bracken MB. Effect of pregnancy and stage of pregnancy on asthma severity: a systematic review. *Am J Obstet Gynecol* 2004; **190**: 1201–10.

Schatz M, Dombrowski MP. Asthma in pregnancy. *N Engl J Med* 2009; **360**: 1862–9.

Cystic fibrosis

Cystic fibrosis is an autosomal recessive genetic disorder with a frequency of approximately 1 in 2000 births. It is primarily a disease of exocrine gland function. As a result of improved medical care, women with cystic fibrosis are increasingly reaching childbearing age and presenting in pregnancy. Pregnancy itself is not thought to increase mortality in women unless pre-pregnancy forced expiratory volume in one second (FEV_1) is less than 50–60% of predicted, there is respiratory colonisation with *Burkholderia cepacia*, or she has pancreatic insufficiency. Overall mortality has been reported as 5% within two years of pregnancy and 10–20% within 5–10 years.

Problems/special considerations

- Depending on their pre-pregnant state, women with cystic fibrosis may tolerate the physiological changes of pregnancy poorly.
- The main anaesthetic consideration is limited pulmonary reserve. These patients have tenacious secretions and they suffer multiple respiratory infections. They may also develop bronchiectasis for which regular postural drainage is required. Regional blockade may further impair respiratory function, especially if extensive.
- Pulmonary hypertension with right heart failure may also occur; it carries with it a poor outcome for both mother and baby.
- Diabetes, renal impairment and obstructive jaundice may occur.

Management options

The outcome of the pregnancy will depend on the woman's nutritional status and the degree of pulmonary insufficiency. The latter is best assessed by performing pulmonary function tests in the first and third trimesters. Careful cardiac assessment is also required to exclude the co-existence of right heart failure.

Vaginal delivery

Oxygenation should be optimal at all times. Stress and pain during labour will increase the respiratory demands and it is thus important to reduce these. The respiratory depressant effect of drugs and in particular opioids should be considered. Mobility is important to facilitate postural drainage. Low-dose epidural analgesia is the management of choice in most cases in order to satisfy these conditions.

Caesarean section

In addition to obstetric indications, caesarean section may also be required for worsening maternal respiratory function. Regional anaesthesia is recommended, although it may be difficult for women with severe respiratory impairment to lie flat. Care should be taken to avoid a high block and an incremental technique, e.g. using combined spinal–epidural anaesthesia, may be best if impairment is already severe. If general anaesthesia is undertaken, bronchial secretions will need regular suction, particularly before extubation. Postoperative analgesia is particularly important and is best provided by neuraxial opioids. During the recovery period, high-dependency care is essential and should include regular physiotherapy.

Key points

- Antenatal planning is essential.
- Maintenance of oxygenation should be given high priority at all times.
- Regional analgesia and anaesthesia is usually indicated but care should be taken to avoid high blocks.

Further reading

Cameron AJ, Skinner TA. Management of a parturient with respiratory failure secondary to cystic fibrosis. *Anaesthesia* 2005; **60**: 77–80.

Huffmyer JL, Littlewood KE, Nemergut EC. Perioperative management of the adult with cystic fibrosis. *Anesth Analg* 2009; **109**: 1949–61.

McArdle J. Cystic fibrosis in pregnancy. *Clin Chest Med* 2011; **32**: 111–20.

Whitty JE. Cystic fibrosis in pregnancy. *Clin Obstet Gynecol* 2010; **53**: 369–76.

Chapter

126

Pulmonary fibrosis

The most common fibrotic pulmonary lesion in young women is pulmonary fibrosis secondary to radiotherapy. The progressive alveolar and pulmonary fibrotic conditions tend to occur in later life; the general principles are the same, although these conditions are potentially life threatening.

Problems/special considerations

Many women who have had a successfully treated malignancy expect to have children. Many of them are unaware that their pulmonary function is not normal as they have no symptoms during ordinary activities, and they may not have been told that there has been any pulmonary damage as a result of treatment of their malignancy. Pulmonary function tests show a reduction in the vital capacity and forced expiratory volume. They show no evidence of restrictive lung disease unless they have other pathology. Most of these women tolerate the pregnancy with little or no problem, although they need a plan for their delivery. Patients who have had a treated malignancy have usually had chemotherapy and may have had drugs that cause myocardial damage, e.g. bleomycin. It is therefore important that these women have echocardiography to assess their cardiac function.

Management options

It is important to assess these women antenatally so that they may understand their restrictions and how these may affect the management of labour and delivery. The delivery plan will depend on the degree of pulmonary damage. Some women may be treated as entirely normal, whereas others require a clear plan comprising avoidance of general anaesthesia and sedative drugs, epidural analgesia during labour and regional anaesthesia for operative delivery.

Key points

- Antenatal assessment is essential, including pulmonary function tests and echocardiography when appropriate.
- Intrapartum management is as for respiratory disease in general.

Further reading

Budev MM, Arroliga AC, Emery S. Exacerbation of underlying pulmonary disease in pregnancy. *Crit Care Med* 2005; **33** (10 Suppl): S313–18.

Wexler ID, Johannesson M, Edenborough FP, Sufian BS, Kerem E. Pregnancy and chronic progressive pulmonary disease. *Am J Respir Crit Care Med* 2007; **175**: 300–5.

Chapter

127

Sarcoidosis

Sarcoidosis is a systemic granulomatous reaction affecting many organs. The main effects of the disease are seen in the peripheral and central nervous systems and the pulmonary and cardiac systems. An important aspect of the disease for the anaesthetist is the pulmonary infiltration, which occurs in up to 80% of cases and produces a restrictive type of lung disease; therefore it is considered with the respiratory diseases.

The disease is treated with steroids and is not made worse by pregnancy.

Problems/special considerations

- Sarcoidosis produces a restriction of the lungs, causing a reduction in the vital capacity and functional residual capacity. These changes, compounded by the physiological changes of pregnancy, mean that these patients may have little or no significant pulmonary reserve and may tolerate pregnancy (and especially labour) poorly.
- Cardiac impairment may be related to the primary disease (e.g. causing heart block or heart failure) or secondary to pulmonary involvement (causing pulmonary hypertension and right sided failure).
- There may also be renal impairment and central nervous system involvement, including isolated cranial nerve lesions.

Management options

The main consideration is to assess the pulmonary and cardiac functions of the woman, and the effect of pregnancy and delivery on function. All these women should have pulmonary function tests performed in the first and third trimester of their pregnancy unless mildly affected, and the management of the labour should be guided by the results. Electrocardiography should also be performed, with echocardiography in selected cases.

In labour, the respiratory challenge of the work of labour and the ventilatory response to pain may be poorly tolerated; therefore epidural analgesia is recommended.

For caesarean section, general anaesthesia is best avoided, regional anaesthesia being the technique of choice.

Key points

- It is important to be aware of the generalised nature of the disease.
- Pulmonary involvement occurs in up to 80% of cases.
- Pulmonary and cardiac function should be assessed carefully in the antenatal period.
- Regional analgesia and anaesthesia is usually indicated in severe cases.

Further reading

Freymond N, Cottin V, Cordier JF. Infiltrative lung diseases in pregnancy. *Clin Chest Med* 2011; **32**: 133–46.

Chapter 128

Acute lung injury (acute respiratory distress syndrome)

The syndrome of lung inflammation and increased permeability that is not explained by left atrial or pulmonary capillary hypertension (although they may co-exist) is now called acute lung injury (ALI). The previous term, adult (now acute) respiratory distress syndrome (ARDS), is now reserved for the most severe form of ALI. Both conditions are characterised by their acute onset, bilateral diffuse infiltrates on chest radiography, pulmonary artery wedge pressure < 18 mmHg or absence of clinical evidence of left atrial hypertension, and arterial hypoxaemia resistant to oxygen therapy alone (ratio of arterial partial pressure: inspired fractional concentration of oxygen < 39.9 kPa [300 mmHg] for ALI; < 26.6 kPa [200 mmHg] for ARDS). Other features include reduced respiratory compliance and lung volumes, increased work of breathing, ventilation/perfusion mismatch and increased shunt. ALI or ARDS associated with pulmonary oedema is a common feature of deaths associated with pregnancy, and has received special attention in past Reports on Confidential Enquiries into Maternal Deaths. It has been suggested that ALI may be more likely in the pregnant state, possibly as result of the physiological changes of pregnancy, especially the increased cardiac output, lower colloid osmotic pressure and leaky capillaries. It is also suspected that aggressive fluid therapy, especially in obstetric haemorrhage and pre-eclampsia, has led to many cases of ALI. In the case of haemorrhage, this may be related to rapid transfusion in the presence of high circulating levels of catecholamines and a relatively constricted pulmonary circulation; in pre-eclampsia, over-emphasis on treating oliguria by 'pushing fluids' may lead to pulmonary oedema and ALI.

Problems/special considerations

The causes of ALI in pregnancy are generally the same as those in the non-pregnant state, although pre-eclampsia, haemorrhage, sepsis, aspiration of gastric contents, presence of a dead fetus and amniotic fluid embolism are particularly important. Use of β_2-agonists in premature labour may also contribute by causing pulmonary oedema (although whether this in itself leads to ALI and ARDS is uncertain). It is important to consider other causes of respiratory failure, especially peripartum cardiomyopathy, as this is more common than ARDS.

The increased demands on the maternal cardiovascular and respiratory systems make the obstetric patient with ALI less able to cope with hypoxaemia, especially in the third trimester. The decreased functional residual capacity increases the likelihood of airway closure and ventilation/perfusion mismatch. However, established ALI has a similar mortality in both pregnant and non-pregnant women. The fetus is particularly at risk from hypoxaemia and this is compounded by any associated cardiovascular instability and the risk of aortocaval compression.

Management options

Management requires early referral to the intensive care unit and involves increasing levels of respiratory support as ALI increases in severity. Management of the predisposing condition should continue as for any acutely ill patient. The physiological changes of pregnancy pose particular problems for the critically ill obstetric patient (see Chapter 145, Critical care in pregnancy).

Key points

- Obstetric patients may be especially prone to acute lung injury.
- Acute lung injury is a common feature in deaths caused by pre-eclampsia, sepsis and massive obstetric haemorrhage.
- The increased physiological demands of pregnancy make obstetric patients especially susceptible to hypoxaemia.

Further reading

Bandi VD, Munnur U, Matthay MA. Acute lung injury and acute respiratory distress syndrome in pregnancy. *Crit Care Clin* 2004; **20**: 577–607.

Catanzarite V, Willms D, Wong D, *et al.* Acute respiratory distress syndrome in pregnancy and the puerperium: causes, courses, and outcomes. *Obstet Gynecol* 2001; **97**: 760–4.

Cole DE, Taylor TL, McCullough DM, *et al.* Acute respiratory distress syndrome in pregnancy. *Crit Care Med* 2005; **33**: S269–78.

Chapter

Pneumonia

The incidence of pneumonia in pregnant women overall is thought to be similar to that in the non-obstetric population, although it is more common in women with underlying respiratory disease, anaemia, immunosuppression (e.g. HIV infection, corticosteroids) and advanced pregnancy. Respiratory infection is a consistent but relatively uncommon cause of death in Confidential Enquiry into Maternal Deaths reports, although the full impact of the H1N1 influenza ('swine flu') pandemic of 2009–10 on UK maternal mortality statistics has yet to be ascertained (12 deaths in the UK, and one in Ireland, were reported to the Centre for Maternal and Child Enquiries, between April 2009 and January 2010). The increased mortality from certain pneumonias in pregnancy, compared with the non-pregnant, is thought to arise from the altered immune responses, combined with the decreased functional residual capacity, decreased residual volume and increased oxygen consumption, that are part of the normal physiological changes of pregnancy. Anaesthetists are likely to be involved in women with chest infection through the need for analgesia/anaesthesia around delivery, or for supportive/intensive care should a parturient become critically ill.

Problems/special considerations

- Signs and symptoms may be similar to the changes of respiratory physiology in pregnancy and may be non-specific, e.g. fever, rigors, nausea/vomiting, chest discomfort/pain and shortness of breath. Thus, diagnosis may be delayed.
- Medical staff are often reluctant to perform a chest x-ray to confirm a diagnosis in pregnant women, because of anxiety over fetal exposure to radiation. However, the risks from a single x-ray are small and usually considered to be outweighed by the advantages if pneumonia is suspected.
- The usefulness of sputum and blood cultures has been debated, and in a significant proportion of patients the aetiological agent may not be identified.
- Pneumonia in the mother is associated with significant fetal morbidity, e.g. premature labour, growth retardation and premature birth.
- Viral pneumonia may be associated with a high risk of infecting staff, increasing spread and hampering the ability of healthcare services to cope in an epidemic or pandemic. The severe acute respiratory syndrome (SARS) epidemic of 2002–03 and the H1N1 pandemic of 2009–10, in particular, carried significant risk to staff.

Bacterial pneumonia

This is usually community-acquired. Common bacterial agents include *Streptococcus pneumoniae* and *Haemophilus influenzae*, but others, e.g. *Mycoplasma, Staphylococcus, Legionella, Klebsiella* and *Pseudomonas,* may also be responsible. Management involves supportive therapy with the appropriate antibiotics. Guidelines from the American Thoracic Society suggest administering a macrolide antibiotic for mild disease and adding a beta-lactam if the pneumonia is more severe. These antibiotics are safe for use in pregnancy and have coverage for most of the microorganisms associated with bacterial pneumonia in pregnancy.

Viral pneumonia

The most common causative agents in pregnancy are the influenza A (the strain most commonly affecting humans) and varicella (chickenpox) viruses. Viral pneumonia may lead to severe acute respiratory failure, secondary bacterial infection and acute lung injury.

- *Influenza:* Seasonal flu is more likely to cause severe illness in pregnant women than in non-pregnant women, and annual vaccination is recommended unless there are contraindications. Recently, a number of newer influenza viral strains have been identified, all of which have been associated with significant maternal and perinatal morbidity. In 2009, the World Health Organization declared a pandemic of H1N1 that caused over 18 000 deaths worldwide (over 450 in the UK). Severe disease was notably more common in young people, unlike seasonal influenza, with other risk factors being diabetes, obesity, immunosuppression and particularly pregnancy, with an estimated increased mortality risk of 4–6 times that in the non-pregnant population. Signs and symptoms are similar to those in non-obstetric women and range from mild illness, typically with high fever, to severe and progressive hypoxaemia. Diagnosis is by nasal/pharyngeal swabs. The mortality rate for those admitted to the intensive care unit is approximately 20–25%, and is thought to be greater in those not receiving antiviral therapy within two days of the onset of symptoms. There is an increased risk of premature delivery (times three) and stillbirth/early neonatal death (times five) in pregnant women admitted to hospital.

- *Varicella:* Chickenpox is an illness usually seen in childhood, but primary varicella may also occur in adults, 16% of whom develop complications – one of which is varicella pneumonia. The diagnosis is usually clinical, based on the history, rash and/or previous contact, but may be helped by the presence of granular infiltrates seen on chest x-ray combined with the presence of serum antibodies, although these may not be seen for two weeks. Pneumonia occurs in up to 10% of pregnant women with chickenpox; risk factors include smoking, pre-existing lung disease, immunosuppression, e.g. with steroid therapy, and late pregnancy. With appropriate modern therapy (antiviral drugs and intensive care), mortality is thought to be under 1% (approximately five times the rate in non-pregnant adults), though historical rates of up to 45% have been reported.

Fungal pneumonia

This is not commonly seen in pregnancy but if it is, may be associated with immunosuppression. Signs and symptoms are as in the non-obstetric population, but as for viral infection, severe respiratory disease may ensue. The diagnosis may be made with sputum culture or serum antigens and chest x-ray changes (usually a nodular pattern is seen on the x-ray). Treatment is with intravenous amphotericin in the peripartum period and flucanozole in the postpartum period, as there has been an association with flucanozole and fetal malformations.

Management options

Several strategies exist to prevent pneumonia in this high-risk population. Risk factors should be identified and modified where possible; if the mother has a co-existing respiratory disease, this should be optimised. Vaccinations are available for influenza, varicella and pneumococcus and are associated with fewer complications including pneumonia and mortality.

Management of pneumonia in pregnancy includes admission, appropriate investigation (including white blood cell count, C-reactive protein, arterial blood gas analysis and chest x-ray), initiation of antimicrobial/antiviral/antifungal therapy, fetal evaluation and respiratory support when required. Supplemental oxygen is usually required, to improve both maternal and fetal oxygenation.

In swine flu, antivirals such as oseltamivir and zanamivir have been used in pregnancy with success, provided that they are administered early. In chickenpox, aciclovir is usually the treatment of choice. Delivery during varicella viraemia may be associated with maternal coagulopathy and hepatitis and severe neonatal infection, and should be delayed if possible.

Respiratory failure may require tracheal intubation and ventilation, although non-invasive methods (e.g. mask-delivered continuous positive airway pressure) may be effective, at least in the short term. Respiratory failure is a result of intrapulmonary shunting rather that hypoventilation, and so ventilation with positive end-expiratory pressure (PEEP) may be beneficial. Hypoxia may not be responsive to therapies such as PEEP, nitric oxide or use of the prone position. High-frequency ventilation/oscillation, extracorporeal membrane oxygenation (ECMO) and intravenacaval membrane oxygenation has been described for refractory cases but experience in pregnancy is limited.

Delivery of the fetus may be necessary to improve the functional status of the mother, but whether improvement in clinical status really results is debatable; some advocate that delivery should be only for obstetric reasons. If caesarean section is required, the choice of regional or general anaesthesia requires careful consideration of the relative risks and benefits, including the likelihood that the mother's condition may worsen after delivery.

Units should have a clear policy for caring for women with potentially contagious respiratory infections, including the provision of, and training in, protective masks etc.

Key points

- Respiratory disease may be exacerbated by the physiological changes of pregnancy and the increased demands of the fetus.
- Careful antenatal assessment is important.
- Regional analgesia and anaesthesia is usually indicated.

Further reading

Brito V, Niederman MS. Pneumonia complicating pregnancy. *Clin Chest Med* 2011; **32**: 121–32.

Centre for Maternal and Child Enquiries. Review of maternal deaths in the United Kingdom related to A/H1N1 2009 Influenza. London: CMACE 2010, http://www.rcog.org.uk/files/rcog-corp/CMACE %20swine%20flu%20and%20pregnancy%20report%202010_10_21_H1N1_final.pdf.

Graves CR. Pneumonia in pregnancy. *Clin Obstet Gynecol* 2010; **53**: 329–36.

Lamont RF, Sobel JD, Carrington D, *et al.* Varicella-zoster virus (chickenpox) infection in pregnancy. *BJOG* 2011; **118**: 1155–62.

Lapinsky S. H1N1 novel influenza A in pregnant and immunocompromised patients. *Crit Care Med* 2010; **38**: S52–6.

Mosby LG, Rasmussen SA, Jamieson DJ. Pandemic influenza A (H1N1) in pregnancy: a systematic review of the literature. *Am J Obstet Gynecol* 2011; **205**: 10–18.

Shariatzadeh MR, Marrie TJ. Pneumonia during pregnancy. *Am J Med* 2006; **119**: 872–6.

Chapter 130

Sepsis

The incidence of sepsis in the obstetric population is thought to have increased in recent years and in the 2006–08 Confidential Enquiry into Maternal Deaths (CEMD) report, it was the most common direct cause of maternal mortality (the rate of deaths caused by sepsis increasing in each of the last three triennial reports). Sepsis in the pregnant population may occur at any time; it may arise from a number of sources and not just the genital tract; and it may range from mild sepsis to severe systemic infection leading to multi-organ failure and maternal or fetal demise. Sepsis in non-pregnant patients is a clinical syndrome manifested by infection and a systemic inflammatory response defined by the presence of at least two of the following: temperature $< 36\,^{\circ}$C or $> 38\,^{\circ}$C; heart rate > 90 bpm; respiration rate > 20/min or a PCO_2 < 4.3 kPa (32 mmHg); and a white blood cell count < 4 or $> 12 \times 10^9$/l. Applying these criteria to pregnant patients is difficult, as these parameters change in pregnancy.

Pregnancy is associated with certain risk factors for sepsis that may be divided into: patient factors, e.g. diabetes, obesity, history of streptococcal B infection or of pelvic infection; and obstetric factors, e.g. prolonged rupture of membranes, caesarean section, retained products. The most common organisms associated with bacteraemia or sepsis in pregnancy include *E. coli*, enterococci, *Klebsiella*, *Staphylococcus aureus* and beta-haemolytic streptococci.

The recognition and aggressive management of developing sepsis, involving a multi-disciplinary approach, is thought to be key in preventing morbidity and mortality from a potentially very rapidly evolving condition.

Problems/special considerations

- Severe sepsis in obstetrics is usually associated with bacterial infection. Rather than the traditional view that pregnant women are more predisposed to infection owing to a general reduction in immunity during pregnancy, it is now thought that pregnancy may exhibit a modified response to infection owing to an altered reactivity of the immune system, that serves to protect both the mother and the baby.

- The physiological changes that occur in pregnancy mean that the signs and symptoms of sepsis are often masked; thus, diagnosis and management may be delayed. Severe sepsis associated with bacteraemia may present with non-specific signs such as abdominal pain and diarrhoea, with or without pyrexia; typically, it is rapidly progressive and when death occurs it may do so within hours of presentation.

- A raised white blood cell count, that might support a diagnosis of infection in the non-pregnant population, is less useful in the obstetric setting, since the white cell count is commonly increased by labour and by steroids given to aid fetal lung maturation in prematurity. Thus counts of up to 30×10^9/l are not uncommon in the absence of infection.

- Institution of an epidural or spinal block in the presence of systemic infection is potentially very hazardous since cardiovascular compensation, which may be just adequate to maintain blood pressure etc. within normal limits, may be abolished, with catastrophic results as sympathetic blockade develops. In addition, there is a risk of epidural/meningeal infection arising from blood-borne organisms. A more common occurrence is a request for regional analgesia in an otherwise asymptomatic woman with pyrexia (see Chapter 135, Pyrexia during labour).
- The fetus is at increased risk from many infections during pregnancy, whether manifested by increased incidence of congenital malformations, premature delivery, the consequences of general maternal illness or neonatal infection. Chorioamnionitis itself has been implicated in causing premature labour; thus prophylactic antibiotics have been studied as a means of delaying onset of labour in premature rupture of membranes.

Management options

Prophylactic intraoperative antibiotic therapy has been shown to reduce the incidence of sepsis following caesarean section and should be routine. Usually this is given by the anaesthetist; administration has traditionally been delayed until after delivery to avoid passage of drugs to the fetus, and because should an allergic reaction occur, the baby will already have been delivered. However, recent guidance from the National Institute for Health and Clinical Excellence (NICE) recommends administration before skin incision, on the basis of greater efficacy. Great care must be taken when following this advice, since thiopental/antibiotic syringe-swap drug errors are easily made, especially in emergencies.

Developing sepsis is easily missed, even by experienced medical staff. A high index of suspicion is therefore important.

It is recommended that the management of septic obstetric patients follows the guidelines of the Surviving Sepsis Campaign, a collaboration between the European Society of Intensive Care Medicine, the Society of Critical Care Medicine and the International Sepsis Forum. These aim to standardise care and improve the outcome in sepsis generally; the main points of care are aggressive resuscitation, adequate oxygenation and appropriate antibiotic treatment.

Resuscitation with fluids and vasopressors is necessary to ensure oxygenation and prevent tissue hypoxia. Appropriate resuscitation before organ failure occurs is thought to improve survival by approximately 20%. Fluid overload is always a concern in obstetric patients because of the haemodynamic changes of pregnancy, especially those that occur in the peripartum period, and because of the use of uterotonic drugs, which are associated with fluid retention (e.g. Syntocinon). Thus, some clinicians advocate invasive monitoring with central venous lines, but these are not without hazard (see Chapter 146, Invasive monitoring). Successive CEMD reports have stressed the importance of involving intensivists early in the care of critically ill women, and that 'intensive care' can be provided outside the intensive care unit.

Blood culture samples should be taken and intravenous antibiotics administered within the first hour of diagnosis, which is considered the 'golden hour' – this is thought to be key to improving maternal and fetal outcome. It is good practice to seek advice from the microbiology department regarding the most appropriate choice of antibiotics. If there is a focus of infection that can be removed surgically, then this should be done.

When and how to deliver the baby is an obstetric decision, but the discussion should involve the anaesthetist with regard to timing and whether the mother's clinical condition has or can be stabilised. The choice of anaesthetic is dependent on each individual case; the presence of systemic infection and a developing coagulopathy secondary to sepsis may preclude the use of a neuraxial technique. Moreover, the risk of cardiovascular block secondary to sympathetic blockade caused by a regional technique should also be considered. General anaesthesia may be the preferred choice of anaesthesia for delivery; however, it must be remembered that general anaesthesia may also result in cardiovascular instability.

Transfer of the patient to a more appropriate environment, such as the high-dependency or intensive care unit, should be discussed between the obstetrician, anaesthetist and intensivist.

Key points

- Sepsis is the main direct cause of death in pregnancy.
- Diagnosis is not always immediate because of the physiological changes in pregnancy and so clinical deterioration may not be recognised until too late.
- Management involves aggressive treatment with fluid resuscitation/cardiovascular support, appropriate antibiotic treatment and adequate oxygenation.
- Transfer to HDU/ITU facilities early rather than later may be advisable.

Further reading

Centre for Maternal and Child Enquiries (CMACE). Saving mothers' lives: reviewing maternal deaths to make motherhood safer: 2006–2008. The eighth report of the Confidential Enquiries into Maternal Deaths in the United Kingdom. *BJOG* 2011; **118** (Suppl 1): 1–203.

Galvagno SM Jr, Camann W. Sepsis and acute renal failure in pregnancy. *Anesth Analg* 2009; **108**: 572–5.

Levy MM, Dellinger RP, Townsend SR, *et al.* Surviving Sepsis Campaign. The Surviving Sepsis Campaign: results of an international guideline-based performance improvement program targeting severe sepsis. *Crit Care Med* 2010; **38**: 364–74.

Lucas DN, Robinson N, Nel MR. Sepsis in obstetrics and the role of the anaesthetist. *Int J Obstet Anesth* 2012; **21**: 56–67.

Paruk F. Infection in obstetric critical care. *Best Pract Res Clin Obstet Gynaecol* 2008; **22**: 865–83.

Chapter 131

Hepatitis

Hepatitis may predate pregnancy or may occur coincidentally during pregnancy. The diagnosis of acute viral hepatitis is made from the history and from blood tests of liver function (increased conjugated bilirubin, markedly increased transaminases, and slightly increased alkaline phosphatase). Chronic hepatitis (active, persistent, drug- or alcohol-induced) also causes abnormality of liver function tests, but definitive diagnosis is made by liver biopsy.

Problems/special considerations

Viral hepatitis

Viral hepatitis accounts for 40% of all liver disease associated with pregnancy. It is thought that pregnant women might be more susceptible to viral hepatitis because of their relatively immunosuppressed state.

- Hepatitis A is highly contagious and spread by the faecal–oral route. The incidence in pregnancy is unknown since many infections are mild, but is thought to be low in the UK.
- Hepatitis B is thought to infect up to 1:50 pregnant women in UK inner cities, in which there is a large immigrant population. It is readily spread by contact with blood and body fluids. Women who are known to have been exposed to intravenous drug use or to have had multiple sexual partners, should be assumed to be at high risk of having hepatitis B, and appropriate precautions should be taken. Prostitutes are at particularly high risk, since many are working as prostitutes to fund an illegal drug habit. There is a ~10% risk of developing chronic liver disease; this may be increased by co-infection with hepatitis D. The risk of transmission to the fetus is 10–20% if the mother is positive for the hepatitis B surface antigen and so pregnant women have been screened for hepatitis B in the UK since 2000. If a pregnant woman tests positive for hepatitis B, she should receive hepatitis B immune globulin and the baby should receive it at birth, and be vaccinated 1 week, 1 month and 6 months after birth. This reduces the risk that the infant will become infected with hepatitis B.
- Hepatitis C is unusual in pregnancy in the UK; it is thought to be prevalent in 0.5–1% of parturients in inner cities. It is spread mainly by contact with blood although sexual transmission may also occur. There is a ~5% risk of transmission to the baby during pregnancy/delivery and a 50–80% risk of developing chronic liver disease. There is currently no preventive treatment to decrease the risk of transmission to the fetus.
- Hepatitis E is similar to hepatitis A. It may cause serious infection during the last trimester and may also cause miscarriage. It is unusual in the UK.

Symptoms are non-specific, and include fatigue, general malaise, loss of appetite, nausea, vomiting, headache and pyrexia. There may be some abdominal discomfort. Overt jaundice only occurs in about a quarter of cases. Treatment is symptomatic, and in the majority of cases there is complete resolution of all signs and symptoms over the course of a few weeks. Women with significantly impaired liver function may be thrombocytopenic or have abnormal clotting studies. Renal function may also be impaired. In end-stage hepatitis, alteration in mental state may occur as a result of hepatic encephalopathy. There is no evidence that pregnancy affects the course of the disease nor that hepatitis has any significant effect on pregnancy in the majority of cases. For the small number of pregnant women who develop hepatitis C, it has been suggested that maternal morbidity and mortality is higher than in non-pregnant women. However, this increased risk may be apparent, due to misdiagnosis of conditions such as fatty liver of pregnancy, rather than a genuine risk.

Chronic hepatitis

Chronic persistent hepatitis is usually unaffected by pregnancy. Chronic active hepatitis is associated with impaired fertility; if pregnancy does occur it may be associated with accelerated deterioration in liver function. Treatment includes corticosteroids and antiviral drugs including interferon. The risk of interferon to the fetus is unknown. Lupus antibodies may occur in up to 20% of women with chronic active hepatitis. Chronic active hepatitis may be complicated by arthritis, impaired renal function, myocarditis and neuropathies. Diabetes, hypertension and osteoporosis may also occur as a result of long-term steroid therapy.

Management options

Regional analgesia and anaesthesia is not contraindicated if coagulation studies are normal. If there is chronic impairment of liver function, invasive venous pressure monitoring may assist fluid management, especially if regional anaesthesia is performed. Although fluid overload must be avoided, hypotension will aggravate any reduction in liver blood flow.

There may be impaired clearance of lidocaine; dose reduction is advisable.

Patients with severe liver disease may have oesophageal varices and often have severely impaired liver function and coagulopathy. Avoidance of pushing during vaginal delivery is recommended, but frequently superimposed obstetric complications (pre-eclampsia, intrauterine growth retardation) will necessitate operative delivery. Rapid sequence induction of general anaesthesia for caesarean section should be used. Suxamethonium can be used safely, despite the greater than normal reduction in plasma cholinesterase levels that is likely to be present. Use of a peripheral nerve stimulator is mandatory, since the action of non-depolarising neuromuscular blockers is variable, though usually prolonged.

Standard infection control precautions should be used if women with viral hepatitis are hospitalised.

Key points

- Viral hepatitis is highly contagious.
- Regional analgesia and anaesthesia are not contraindicated, but impaired liver function may be associated with disorders of coagulation.

Further reading

Joshi D, James A, Quaglia A, Westbrook RH, Heneghan MA. Liver disease in pregnancy. *Lancet* 2010; **375**: 594–605.

Mackillop L, Williamson C. Liver disease in pregnancy. *Postgrad Med J* 2010; **86**: 160–4.

Chapter

132

Herpes simplex infection

The herpes simplex virus (HSV) is a common infective agent during both childhood and adult life. Although HSV-1 is traditionally considered to be responsible for orolabial herpes and HSV-2 for genital herpes, there is considerable overlap. HSV is important in pregnancy because of the adverse effects of primary infection on maternal health and premature labour and also because of the risks of primary neonatal infection, which may be severe.

Problems/special considerations

Primary infection may result in local lesions and viraemia with systemic effects, e.g. malaise, myalgia, meningitis, encephalitis and hepatitis. Local lesions may reappear weeks to years later, often following emotional or physical stress. Primary infection is associated with a ~40% incidence of neonatal transmission. Secondary infection is not associated with viraemia and the risk of neonatal transmission is < 3%.

Women with severe primary infection may present in premature labour or with acute systemic manifestations, whereas those with active genital lesions may present for caesarean section, performed to reduce neonatal transmission.

It is not known whether epidural or spinal anaesthesia increases the likelihood of central nervous system involvement if there is a history of secondary HSV infection, although there are published series of successful obstetric regional anaesthesia performed without problems. Epidural morphine is associated with up to 11 times the risk of recurrence of oral lesions compared with parenteral morphine; the mechanism is unclear but may be related to direct activation of the dormant virus in cranial nerve nuclei.

Fentanyl has been implicated in a single report. However, there are other confounding factors such as emotional and physical stress that may also account for recurrence. Avoidance of regional anaesthesia in primary infection is often advised but less is known about the risks since primary infection at the time of delivery is rare. There are series of successful regional blocks in the presence of primary infection but numbers are very small.

Management options

Aciclovir is generally avoided during pregnancy because of fears of interfering with fetal thymidine metabolism. However, aciclovir is indicated in cases of severe disseminated infection. In recurrent HSV infection, routine genital culturing is no longer recommended as an indicator of the need for caesarean section, since the presence of visible genital lesions has been shown to be more reliable and easier to ascertain. Thus vaginal delivery is generally advised unless genital lesions are present, in which case caesarean section is performed (unless the membranes have been ruptured for more than 4 hours, since caesarean section makes no difference to neonatal transmission).

Mothers should be fully informed of the theoretical risks and benefits of regional anaesthesia, especially before caesarean section when the alternative (i.e. general anaesthesia) is generally perceived as being more hazardous. The neonate born of a mother with HSV should be carefully evaluated for evidence of infection.

Key points

- Primary herpes simplex virus (HSV) infection may cause severe systemic illness and premature labour.
- Neonatal infection may occur if there are active genital lesions.
- The risk of central neural infection following regional anaesthesia in secondary HSV infection is thought to be theoretical only.
- Epidural morphine may cause recurrence of orolabial HSV lesions.

Further reading

Chen YH, Rau RH, Keller JJ, Lin HC. Possible effects of anaesthetic management on the 1 yr followed-up risk of herpes zoster after Caesarean deliveries. *Br J Anaesth* 2012; **108**: 278–82.

Corey L, Wald A. Maternal and neonatal herpes simplex virus infections. *N Engl J Med* 2009; **361**: 1376–85.

Chapter 133

HIV infection

The prevalence of human immunodeficiency virus (HIV) has been found on population screening to be present in about 0.2% of women giving birth in England (0.04–0.05% in those born in the UK and 3–4% in those born in sub-Saharan Africa), and 0.03% of those in Scotland in 2003. In inner London the prevalence is ~0.4%, a figure similar to that in New York. In parts of central and east Africa, the incidence may reach 20–30% in the larger cities. The natural course of infection is an acute viral-type illness, followed on average 3 months later by seroconversion when the patient becomes 'HIV-positive'; progression to the acquired immunodeficiency syndrome (AIDS; characterised by lymphadenopathy and conditions indicating reduced cell-mediated immunity, e.g. chronic opportunistic/invasive infections, chronic diarrhoea, malignancies, neurological involvement) occurs in about two thirds of cases over the next 10 years although up to 20% of cases survive for 20 years without progression to AIDS. Median survival once AIDS is diagnosed is about 3–4 years; in Africa, survival is shorter, with about one third of cases progressing to death without developing AIDS itself.

HIV infection has altered the way in which contaminated materials are handled in labour ward, and the way in which blood and blood products are administered. It is now recommended that all pregnant women undergo routine antenatal HIV testing as neonatal transmission occurs in 25–30% of cases, with a further 14% increase if the mother breastfeeds; with appropriate medical management of known cases (see below) this can be reduced to under 3%. Since this recommendation by the Department of Health in 1999, the proportion of HIV-infected women diagnosed before delivery has risen to > 90%. Human T cell leukaemia/lymphoma virus (HTLV) types I and II have been found to have a similar prevalence to that of HIV in pregnancy, and screening of blood donations and/or pregnant women is performed in some countries.

Since the target of infection is primarily the lymphocyte, plasma counts of the CD4-positive cells (mainly helper T-lymphocytes) have been used to monitor the course of infection and guide treatment. The CD4:CD8 ratio and plasma viral load (amount of viral RNA measurable in the plasma, representing degree of viral replication) are also used.

Problems/special considerations

Problems may be related to:

- The acute viral illness of initial HIV infection.
- Impaired organ function and immunodepression of AIDS.
- The risk of transmission of HIV to the neonate.
- The risk of transmission of HIV to medical and midwifery staff and to other patients.

Management options

All units should offer counselling and testing for at-risk women prenatally or even pre-pregnancy, and this should continue during pregnancy. Many units have protocols in place for joint management of HIV-positive women by obstetricians and HIV specialists.

Acute HIV infection is rarely a known problem on labour ward and in general is managed as for any acute viral illness. For those with acute organ dysfunction, supportive management is directed at the organ system affected.

Patients with chronic HIV infection are managed according to their degree of organ impairment, which in most cases presenting to labour ward will not be severe. All systems may be affected, either by primary HIV infection or secondary infection, e.g. with fungi or other atypical organisms. Neurological manifestations are especially important to anaesthetists and include neuropathy, encephalopathy, meningitis, focal brain lesions, dementia, myelopathy and myopathy. In addition, HIV-positive subjects' life expectancy is increased by taking prophylactic highly active antiretroviral therapy (HAART). These drugs may cause blood dyscrasias, gastrointestinal disturbances, neurological and hepatic impairment and increased drug metabolism via hepatic enzyme indication. Before any anaesthetic intervention, all patients must therefore be assessed carefully for evidence of organ system impairment.

In general, patients with HIV infection are managed as for any obstetric patient, unless specific contraindications exist. Particular care with invasive techniques has been suggested, to reduce the risk of introducing infection, but standard aseptic methods should be adequate if they are followed. The use of epidural or spinal anaesthesia has been questioned for fear of seeding the virus into the cerebrospinal fluid (CSF), thus accelerating the central nervous system (CNS) progression of the infection; because of a theoretical risk of seeding opportunistic infective organisms into the CNS; and because there may be complications related to underlying and undiagnosed CNS pathology. Since CSF involvement occurs very early in HIV infection, however, no further risk is generally felt to exist, and this is supported by clinical experience, albeit limited. Epidural blood patching has also been performed in HIV-positive patients without apparent adverse consequences. There has been no report of secondary CNS infection introduced during administration of regional anaesthesia in the HIV-infected mother and this risk is generally felt to be theoretical only. Further, if no evidence of CNS involvement exists then most authorities recommend regional anaesthesia as routine. If CNS abnormalities do exist then management is dependent on their severity and other considerations such as the presence of other complications.

Most units now treat HIV-positive mothers with antiviral drugs, e.g. zidovudine, which has been shown to reduce transmission to the neonate by up to two thirds. Combination with elective caesarean section reduces the risk further, to about 1%, although if the mother is well-controlled on HAART and the viral load is under 400 copies/ml, vaginal delivery is associated with a similar risk of vertical transmission. There is wide consensus that breastfeeding should be discouraged.

Owing to the implications of testing for HIV, most health authorities advocate the approach of 'universal precautions' to potentially at-risk patients; thus routine management of all women on labour ward should involve the use of protective clothing where appropriate (gloves, goggles, etc., according to individual choice), use of disposable equipment and/or appropriate sterilisation techniques and careful handling and disposal of contaminated sharps. If these practices are routinely followed, the known HIV-positive patient should need no extra measures. Units that have policies such as this have accepted the cost implications of such all-inclusive guidelines, especially given the high cost and high profile of legal proceedings against establishments where cross-infection has occurred. If an accidental needlestick injury or similar event occurs, local protocols and specialists should be consulted for guidance about prophylactic zidovudine therapy, since this is a controversial area. The risk of seroconversion after needlestick is about 0.3%.

Key points

- HIV infection affects 0.04–4% of UK obstetric patients, depending on their place of birth and the unit's location.
- HIV-positive mothers may have many systems affected and may be taking several drugs.
- General anaesthetic management is according to standard criteria for indications and contraindications.
- Universal precautions should apply to all patients to reduce contamination of staff.

Further reading

Gray GE, McIntyre JA. HIV and pregnancy. *BMJ* 2007; **334**: 950–3.

Health Protection Agency. *HIV in the United Kingdom: 2010 Report*. London: HPA 2010.

Hignett R, Fernando R. Anesthesia for the pregnant HIV patient. *Anesthesiol Clin* 2008; **26**: 127–43.

Royal College of Obstetricians and Gynaecologists. Management of HIV in pregnancy. *Green-top 39*. London: RCOG 2010, http://www.rcog.org.uk/womens-health/clinical-guidance/management-hiv-pregnancy-green-top-39.

Chapter

134 Malaria in pregnancy

Malaria is a major cause of maternal and fetal morbidity and mortality across the world, especially tropical/sub-tropical regions, and though not indigenous to the UK it may present in women who have recently returned from infected areas. Pregnant women are more susceptible to infection (especially if HIV-infected), and are more likely to suffer a recurrence and develop severe complications, with increased risk of death.

Malaria is caused by one of predominantly four plasmodium species: *P. falciparum*, *P. vivax*, *P. ovale* and *P. malariae*. In the UK, malaria is more commonly associated with *P. falciparum* and less so with *P. vivax*. Infection with *P. falciparum* is more insidious and associated with a higher mortality than the other species. In Asia, particularly India, infection with *P. vivax* is more likely and this can cause a relapsing type of malaria. The infection is transmitted via the female Anopheles mosquito, each bite inoculating 10–15 sporozoites. These sporozoites pass via the bloodstream to the liver and develop into schizonts containing thousands of merozoites, that are released into the circulation when the schizont bursts, accounting for the typical cyclical nature of symptoms. The merozoites infect red blood cells and once inside the red blood cell can multiply over 2–3 days. These parasites are then responsible for infecting new red blood cells. In falciparum malaria, large numbers of parasites may be sequestered in the placenta.

Problems/special considerations

- *Prevention:* Women who are pregnant or planning to become pregnant should be advised not to travel to an endemic area unless necessary. Prevention advice is the same as for the non-pregnant population, though certain antimalarials are relatively contraindicated at certain stages of pregnancy and specialist advice is required.
- *Presentation:* Typically, symptoms develop within 1–3 weeks of infection. Presentation may be atypical in pregnant women, who may present with symptoms of anaemia, fever (which may be very variable or even absent) or complications, e.g. seizures, coma (that may suggest cerebral malaria and may be the only presenting symptom). Splenomegaly may be present.
- *Diagnosis:* Thick and thin films for malarial parasites should be examined but parasites may not be visible on peripheral blood films. Other more rapid diagnostic tests, based on malaria antigens, are available but the accuracy of some is debated; polymerase chain reaction methods may be more accurate.
- *Maternal issues:* Haemolytic anaemia may be exacerbated by decreased iron and folate levels, leading to severe anaemia. Disseminated intravascular coagulopathy may occur. Hypoglycaemia is common and may be aggravated by certain antimalarials. More severe complications such as acute lung injury and cerebral malaria are associated with a high mortality rate.
- *Fetal issues:* Fetal mortality associated with malaria is high and in the region of 15% for *P. vivax* and 30% for *P. falciparum*. Problems for the fetus include prematurity, anaemia, growth retardation and congenital malaria, the latter resulting from transfer of parasites across the placenta. Treatment of the mother may not always prevent congenital malaria; affected neonates may feed poorly and be pyrexial, irritable or jaundiced (this may be confused with jaundice of the newborn), and long-term developmental problems such as short stature and metabolic disturbances have been described.

Management options

A high index of suspicion is required since presentation may be atypical. If malaria is suspected, then the patient should be referred to a tertiary centre where full facilities are available, including input from specialists in infectious diseases. The diagnosis of malaria is considered to be a medical emergency, and early admission to the intensive care unit is recommended for all but the mildest disease. Quinine and clindamycin are the standard drugs used for falciparum malaria, and chloroquine for the other types; intravenous artesunate or quinine is recommended for severe falciparum malaria (see RCOG guidelines for dosage). Careful monitoring of both mother and fetus is required because of the high mortality associated with the disease. Management of severe complications is largely supportive.

Although regional anaesthetic techniques have been described in mothers with malaria, the presence of complications often precludes their use.

Key points

- Pregnant women are more susceptible to malaria because of their decreased immunity.
- Malaria may present with atypical symptoms and mortality is high for both fetus and mother.
- Senior staff should be involved in obstetric and anaesthetic management, and advice should be sought from clinicians experienced in the management of malaria.
- The choice of anaesthetic technique should be based on each individual situation.

Further reading

Chiodini P, Hill D, Lalloo D, *et al.* Guidelines for malaria prevention in travellers from the UK. London: Health Protection Agency 2007, http://www.hpa.org.uk/Publications/InfectiousDiseases/TravelHealth/0701MalariapreventionfortravellersfromtheUK/.

Lalloo DG, Shingadia D, Pasvol G, *et al.* UK malaria treatment guidelines. *J Infect* 2007; **54**: 111–21.

Mathew DC, Loveridge R, Solomon AW. Anaesthetic management of caesarean delivery in a parturient with malaria. *Int J Obstet Anesth* 2011; **20**: 341–58.

Royal College of Obstetricians and Gynaecologists. The prevention of malaria in pregnancy. *Green-top 54A.* London: RCOG 2010, http://www.rcog.org.uk/prevention-malaria-pregnancy-green-top-54a.

Royal College of Obstetricians and Gynaecologists. Malaria in pregnancy diagnosis & treatment. *Green-top 54B.* London: RCOG 2010, http://www.rcog.org.uk/diagnosis-and-treatment-malaria-pregnancy-green-top-54b.

Chapter

135

Pyrexia during labour

Variously defined as core temperature exceeding 37.5 °C or 38 °C, pyrexia in labour has traditionally been taken to be a marker of infection requiring investigation and antibiotic therapy. However, there are many other medical causes of pyrexia (e.g. inflammatory disease, thyrotoxicosis, pulmonary embolism, malignancy) that should not be forgotten. In addition, it has recently been recognised that epidural analgesia itself may be associated with a gradual increase in maternal (and thus fetal) temperature after about 6–8 hours, of up to 0.5–1 °C, although most studies are poorly controlled and the phenomenon is controversial (for example, women with predisposing factors for infection are often those who request epidural analgesia). Fetal heart rate may increase as a direct consequence of maternal pyrexia. Suggested mechanisms include alteration of afferent temperature-related neural input to the hypothalamus, impaired thermoregulatory mechanisms in the lower body (such as absent shivering in the legs) and a re-setting of the central 'thermostat'.

The fetal temperature is $\sim 1\,^\circ$C higher than the maternal core, and follows maternal oral readings more closely than tympanic.

Problems/special considerations

Pyrexia itself has been implicated in causing premature labour and may stress an at-risk fetus. Neonatal encephalopathy is more common if mothers are pyrexial during labour, although whether this is related to the increased temperature itself or to any underlying cause (particularly infection) is uncertain.

Infection causing pyrexia is a potentially serious problem since severe sepsis may affect both the mother and the fetus. Thus, most protocols call for screening tests and possibly antibiotic therapy if infection is suspected.

It has been claimed that huge amounts of money are spent each year investigating neonates born of pyrexial mothers in whom the only cause of pyrexia was epidural analgesia, although the epidural's role in causing the pyrexia is disputed. Nevertheless, it is thus important that all anaesthetists, obstetricians, midwives and paediatricians are aware that the phenomenon may exist. In protocols and guidelines for the management of pyrexia during labour, provision should be made for the effect of epidurals; separate instructions may be required for mothers with epidurals and those without.

Management options

In most cases, mild pyrexia is not in itself troublesome. Fanning, sponging or treatment with paracetamol may be used, although the possibility of masking underlying sepsis should not be forgotten. Pyrexia above $38.5\,^\circ$C, especially if it occurs within 6 hours of siting the epidural, is unlikely to be related to epidural analgesia. If infection is suspected, screening should include blood cultures, high vaginal swabs and mid-stream urine sampling. Infection may not be accompanied by localising signs, at least initially; in addition, white cell count may increase during normal labour to as high as 30×10^9/l.

Mothers who are pyrexial and who request epidural analgesia present a separate dilemma since regional blockade may be complicated by severe cardiovascular compromise or epidural/meningeal infection in the presence of sepsis, which is therefore a relative contraindication to regional anaesthesia. For mild localised infection, such as chorioamnionitis (which may be associated with subclinical bacteraemia), regional analgesia is generally felt to be safe if covered with antibiotic therapy.

Set procedures should exist for monitoring of maternal temperature and management of pyrexia, including provision of regional blockade in pyrexial mothers and neonatal screening. A high level of general awareness and education is important since staff of all disciplines may be unaware of the relationship between epidural analgesia and pyrexia.

Key points

- There are many causes of fever, including infection.
- Epidural analgesia exceeding 6–8 hours has been associated with pyrexia.
- Protocols should exist for monitoring of temperature during labour and screening ± treatment of pyrexial mothers.

Further reading

Apantaku O, Mulik V. Maternal intra-partum fever. *J Obstet Gynaecol* 2007; **27**: 12–15.

Riley LE, Celi AC, Onderdonk AB, *et al.* Association of epidural-related fever and noninfectious inflammation in term labor. *Obstet Gynecol* 2011; **117**: 588–95.

Segal S. Labor epidural analgesia and maternal fever. *Anesth Analg* 2010; **111**: 1467–75.

Wedel DJ, Horlocker TT. Regional anesthesia in the febrile or infected patient. *Reg Anesth Pain Med* 2006; **31**: 324–33.

Chapter

136

Migrants/disadvantaged women

Migration into the European Union (EU) has risen over the last decade, with approximately half of the migrants being under 30 years old. It is thought that over a third of live births in the EU occur to mothers who are immigrants. About 500 000–600 000 people have come to live in the UK each year in the last decade, with 300 000–400 000 leaving each year. There is evidence from the Confidential Enquiries into Maternal Deaths, the UK Obstetric Surveillance System (UKOSS) and other national reports that the morbidity and mortality is higher in migrant mothers. This is not just limited to international migration; migration from rural to inner city areas is also increasing, and it is thought that mothers who move in this way have similar risks to those who migrate internationally.

Many of the problems exhibited by migrant parturients are not exclusive to migrants; thus there are other vulnerable and disadvantaged groups of women who should also be considered high-risk, e.g. the homeless, the destitute, drug addicts and prostitutes. Many will have mental health issues and many of these groups overlap.

Problems/special considerations

The management of pregnancy and safe delivery of the baby in migrant or disadvantaged women provides a challenge to both obstetric and anaesthetic staff for a number of reasons:

- Some mothers may present with poor general health, poor nutrition and co-existing diseases, e.g. tuberculosis, rheumatic heart disease and HIV infection, that may impact on maternal and neonatal outcome. In certain parts of Asia, Africa and the Middle East, female genital mutilation is commonly practised, and this has implications for their delivery options.
- Migrant mothers may not be entitled to healthcare, or they may be unaware that they are entitled to healthcare during pregnancy. They may therefore seek antenatal care late, if at all, and they may be poor attenders of appointments, making it easy for them to be

lost to the system. Thus, any pre-existing medical conditions may go untreated or not optimised until late in pregnancy. Similarly, conditions that develop during pregnancy, e.g. pre-eclampsia or intrauterine growth retardation, may not be detected.

- Language may pose a barrier to women seeking antenatal care and this has been identified as a major contributory factor to maternal morbidity.
- Certain cultures or religions believe that obstetric intervention, e.g. caesarean section, is linked to death. The mother and/or father may therefore be reluctant to follow the advice of obstetric staff when any sort of operative delivery is suggested, leading to delay and even fetal demise.

Management options

A multimodal approach is necessary. As in all cases of good obstetric practice, communication is paramount – both within the team (which should include other specialists and social services as appropriate), and with the patient and her partner (and if necessary, elder members of her family). If language prevents this, then interpreter services must be provided; it is no longer acceptable to use family or staff members to interpret, as they themselves may have limited English skills. Proper explanation of antenatal care and the plan for delivery is necessary. It may be prudent antenatally to put forward the analgesic options available for labour and, if necessary, a separate appointment may be organised with an anaesthetist and an interpreter. If these are not available, other translation aids may be used. The Obstetric Anaesthetists' Association has leaflets available that may be downloaded, explaining the analgesic options.

Antenatal care should identify any co-existing disease in order that this is optimally managed and the patient should be advised where to seek help if her symptoms change.

Interpreter services should be available during labour and delivery.

Key points

- The migrant obstetric population is increasing in number.
- There is a higher morbidity and mortality associated with this group of women, and with other disadvantaged groups.
- Good communication and early antenatal care is paramount in identifying high-risk patients.
- Interpreter services should be available to all women where language is a barrier.

Further reading

Ameh CA, Van den Broek N. Increased risk of maternal death among ethnic minority women in the UK. *Obstetrician Gynaecologist* 2008; **10**: 177–82.

Centre for Maternal and Child Enquiries (CMACE). Saving mothers' lives: reviewing maternal deaths to make motherhood safer: 2006–2008. The eighth report of the Confidential Enquiries into Maternal Deaths in the United Kingdom. *BJOG* 2011; **118** (Suppl 1): 1–203.

Hayes I, Enohumah K, McCaul C. Care of the migrant obstetric population. *Int J Obstet Anesth* 2011; **20**: 321–9.

Knight M, Kurinczuk JJ, Spark P, Brocklehurst P; UKOSS. Inequalities in maternal health: national cohort study of ethnic variation in severe maternal morbidities. *BMJ* 2009; **338**: b542.

Royal College of Obstetricians and Gynaecologists. Female genital mutilation and its management. *Green-top 53*. London: RCOG 2009, http://www.rcog.org.uk/female-genital-mutilation-and-its-management-green-top-53.

Chapter 137

Psychiatric disease

Suicide and psychiatric disease are a common cause of maternal death in the Reports on Confidential Enquiries into Maternal Deaths in the United Kingdom. As well as women with pre-existing psychiatric disease, it is estimated that 10–15% of women suffer from postnatal depression, and as many as 60% experience postnatal 'blues'. The risk of admission to hospital with psychosis in the first three months after childbirth is more than 300 times greater than at other times.

Much of the challenge in providing effective care to women with psychiatric disease relates to the organisation and funding of services, and the identification of women at risk. Thus there is emphasis on attempting to identify women with a past history of mental illness antenatally, and routine screening questions on booking should include past history and risk factors, e.g. family history. Anaesthetists' involvement is usually restricted to care for women who present peripartum or who have attempted suicide.

Problems/special considerations

- *Pre-existing disease:* Patients may be taking drugs that are affected by pregnancy, that have important maternal or fetal effects, or that affect anaesthesia. Women with bipolar disorder may be maintained on lithium or, less commonly, carbamazepine. Serial monitoring of plasma drug levels is particularly important for these drugs. Lithium may potentiate neuromuscular blockade (with both suxamethonium and non-depolarising neuromuscular blocking drugs). Women with schizophrenia are likely to be taking a variety of antipsychotic drugs, high doses of which can cause sedation and postural hypotension due to α-blockade. The latter is likely to be exacerbated by the physiological changes of pregnancy. Monoamine oxidase inhibitors (MAOIs) have a number of potential interactions, the most important of which concern pethidine and vasopressors.

  Women who have been psychiatrically well and taking maintenance drugs may stop their medication when they become pregnant and present with recurrence of symptoms. Many of the psychotropic drugs are relatively contraindicated during pregnancy, but a risk–benefit analysis must be made before changing or stopping such medication.

  Women with psychiatric disease may lack capacity to give consent to treatment (see below). In acute mental states, they may also refuse treatments, disrupt the care of other patients and not follow feeding policies.

- *Postnatal psychiatric disease:* Women who develop postnatal depression may not have had any warning symptoms or signs. Women with a past history of psychiatric disease or drug dependence may conceal this from obstetricians and midwives because of the perceived stigma of these conditions. Those with a previous history of postnatal depressive psychosis run a 50% risk of recurrence, classically at the same time postnatally as before. It is important for all healthcare professionals to maintain a high level of awareness of such disorders, and ask all women at booking about previous psychiatric illness.
- *Substance abuse:* Drug abuse is more common in North America than in the UK but nevertheless is an important cause of morbidity and mortality in the UK (see Chapter 138, Substance abuse). Mothers may conceal their use of recreational drugs as they may feel that they are being judged, or for fear of being reported to the police or of child protection issues. Liaison between the general practitioner, social services and the maternity services is required.

Management options
Antenatal care
Women with poorly controlled psychiatric disease may default from antenatal care and may thus be at increased risk from undetected complications of pregnancy. They may exhibit hospital phobia and may lack insight into the need for medical care if pregnancy-related problems occur. Continuity of care, which enables a trusting relationship to be developed with one or two healthcare professionals, is vital. Antenatal discussion about the options for analgesia in labour and the possibility of needing anaesthesia for operative delivery is particularly important, and such discussions should be documented and witnessed by the woman's partner, and a third party if possible. There must be discussion between the psychiatrist, obstetrician, general practitioner and the woman herself about continuing drug therapy throughout pregnancy.

Women who are maintained on drug therapy should be monitored regularly to ensure that the pregnancy-related increase in blood and plasma volume does not result in subtherapeutic drug levels.

Labour and delivery
Regional analgesia and anaesthesia are not contraindicated for women with psychiatric disease.

Women taking a MAOI can receive ephedrine or phenylephrine to correct hypotension caused by regional anaesthesia, but smaller doses than usual should be used as pressor responses may be exaggerated. Pethidine should be avoided, but fentanyl and morphine have both been used uneventfully. Postoperatively, use of patient-controlled intravenous analgesia is preferable to intramuscular analgesia.

There is a need for a high level of awareness amongst all healthcare professionals involved in intrapartum and postnatal care. Symptoms and signs suggestive of depressive illness must be treated promptly. Tri- and tetracyclic antidepressants, the selective serotonin reuptake inhibitor group of antidepressants and MAOIs may all be necessary in the treatment of both non-pregnancy-related and postnatal depression. Electroconvulsive therapy may also be indicated.

Women known to abuse illegal drugs should be treated with particular care. There are numerous interactions with medical drugs, and women frequently abuse multiple drugs.

Consent

A psychiatrist's input may be invaluable in characterising a psychiatric patient's illness and advising on her state of mind, though the decision on whether she has capacity should be made by the treating doctor, after considering such advice (see Chapter 158, Consent). The doctrine of necessity allows treatment to be administered without consent if this is in the patient's best interests, but it cannot be assumed that what the obstetric team would wish to do always reflects the mother's 'best interests', and a psychiatrist's advice may be useful here too. In the UK, the unborn fetus has no legal status or rights (though it may have moral ones). If the mother is held in hospital under the Mental Health Act (1983), this only covers treatment of the primary mental condition and does not allow other treatments to be enforced unless they are considered to affect it directly.

Patients in whom consent may be problematic require multidisciplinary discussion antenatally in order to formulate a management plan. Often there is extensive discussion but the obstetric anaesthetist is not invited, so that the first contact he/she has may be when analgesia or anaesthesia is required.

Key points

- Psychiatric disease is common in pregnancy.
- A patient's drug therapy requires careful monitoring during and after pregnancy.
- The possibility of substance abuse should always be considered.
- Difficulties with consent should be anticipated and plans made in good time.

Further reading

Brockington I. Postpartum psychiatric disorders. *Lancet* 2004; **363**: 303–10.

Jablensky AV, Morgan V, Zubrick SR, Bower C, Yellachich LA. Pregnancy, delivery, and neonatal complications in a population cohort of women with schizophrenia and major affective disorders. *Am J Psychiatry* 2005; **162**: 79–91.

National Institute for Health and Clinical Excellence. Antenatal and postnatal mental health. *Clinical Guideline 5*. London: NICE 2007, http://guidance.nice.org.uk/CG45.

Royal College of Obstetricians and Gynaecologists. Management of women with mental health issues during pregnancy and the postnatal period. *Good Practice No. 14*. London: RCOG 2011, http://www.rcog.org.uk/management-women-mental-health-issues-during-pregnancy-and-postnatal-period.

Substance abuse

The definition of this term is difficult, since use of non-medically indicated substances ranges from socially acceptable activities such as smoking and moderate alcohol intake to abuse of intravenous drugs. Many types of abuse co-exist.

Drug abuse is an increasing problem in inner city units. Most experience is from the USA, where up to 20% of pregnant women are thought to have abused illicit substances (usually marijuana or cannabis) at some point during their pregnancy.

Problems/special considerations

Problems may be related to the maternal effects of drug use, including acute intoxication, chronic organ impairment and the risk of HIV infection and endocarditis for intravenous drug users; the control of drug use and withdrawal during pregnancy and labour; and the effects of drug abuse on the fetus and neonate. Because delivery is seen as a 'normal' process and the mothers may not consider themselves as unwell, they may continue taking the drug up to and through the peripartum period, thus presenting with the acute effects of intoxication, including altered mental state. This may make communication, and especially consent, difficult or impossible. Many addicts present for the first time in labour, with poor antenatal care. There is a greater incidence of sexually transmitted disease in addicts.

Alcohol

Alcohol abuse is a more widespread problem than abuse of many recreational drugs, with well known manifestations including malnutrition, hepatic and cardiac impairment, etc. Acutely intoxicated mothers may be aggressive and may have taken other drugs as well. If the stomach is full there may be increased risk of aspiration. Acute withdrawal typically reaches its worst about 24–36 hours after cessation of intake. A particular feature of alcohol abuse in pregnancy is the fetal alcohol syndrome, which comprises craniofacial, neurological, cardiac, urological and musculoskeletal abnormalities. The upper safe limit of alcohol consumption in pregnancy has not been determined, but recent evidence suggests that even minimal intake may be associated with behavioural difficulties.

Tobacco

Smoking is a common problem worldwide; in the UK its prevalence is about 20% in women of childbearing age. Maternal effects are well known; in the neonate it has been long associated with low birthweight although the precise mechanism is unclear.

Cocaine

Cocaine, or its water-insoluble derivative crack, causes central and peripheral dopaminergic and adrenergic stimulation resulting in euphoria, increased alertness, vasoconstriction and hypertension. Myocardial ischaemia and arrhythmias may occur, and convulsions, intracranial haemorrhages and renal, hepatic and haematological impairment (including thrombocytopenia) have been reported. Cocaine abuse has been associated with increased incidence of spontaneous abortion, placental abruption, premature labour and fetal morbidity and mortality. Prolonged action of suxamethonium has also been reported. Diagnosis may be difficult since its use is often denied and the presentation may resemble that of pre-eclampsia and phaeochromocytoma. Urine remains positive for cocaine metabolites up to 3 days after use, and testing has been suggested in all at-risk groups (e.g. known users of other drugs, unbooked pregnancies, etc.).

Opioids

Opioid abuse is associated with hepatic, renal, pulmonary and cardiovascular impairment. Gastric emptying is impaired. The incidence of pre-eclampsia is reportedly increased. Addicts may require central venous cannulation because of their poor peripheral veins. Apart from these considerations, opioid withdrawal may complicate labour and delivery, and postoperative analgesia may be dificult to provide. Withdrawal typically occurs 8–16 hours after cessation of intake, with features increasing over 1–3 days. Opioid antagonists may precipitate acute withdrawal (including neonatal). Neonatal withdrawal may occur several days postpartum. Other neonatal effects of opioid addiction include increased fetal loss and growth retardation.

Cannabis

Cannabis has been associated with increased incidence of peripartum complications, including arrest of labour and fetal morbidity. Cardiac arrhythmias, especially tachycardia, and myocardial depression have also been reported.

Amphetamines

Although less commonly abused than the above drugs, amphetamines acutely cause similar effects to cocaine including hypertension, arrhythmias, agitation, fever and confusion. Fetal effects include growth retardation, premature labour and abruption. Acute ingestion may increase the requirement for anaesthetic drugs, whereas chronic abuse may result in central depression and depletion of catecholamine stores. Both regional and general anaesthesia may be accompanied by severe hypotension in chronically abusing patients.

Others

Experience with methylenedioxymethylamphetamine (MDMA; 'ecstasy') and solvent abuse in obstetrics is limited but the same maternal manifestations may occur as is seen in non-pregnant subjects. Barbiturate abuse is less common now; its main problems are acute intoxication and chronic addiction/withdrawal.

Management options

General management is directed at any specific organ impairment (including central nervous system depression) and providing appropriate nutrition and psychological support and counselling. Substance abuse should always be considered in the differential diagnosis of any atypical case, e.g. unexplained collapse or acute confusion.

Management of acute alcohol withdrawal includes oral chlormethiazole or benzodiazepines. Alcohol infusion may also be used (10–150 ml/h of a 5–10% solution) although it may suppress uterine contractions.

If abusers of cocaine require general anaesthesia, pretreatment with antihypertensive drugs should be considered, since severe hypertension and arrhythmias may follow tracheal intubation. Labetalol has been suggested as the drug of choice since pure β-blockade may precipitate severe hypertension via unopposed α-stimulation. Glyceryl trinitrate has also been used. Benzodiazepines have been recommended to reduce sympathetic activity. Drugs causing sympathetic stimulation (e.g. ketamine) should be avoided. During regional anaesthesia, haemodynamic instability may be greater than normal and resistance to ephedrine has been reported, possibly related to noradrenaline depletion (directly acting vasopressors such as phenylephrine may be preferable). Increased requirement for analgesic supplementation during caesarean section has also been described.

Management of opioid addicts is often simplified if opioids are avoided altogether and local anaesthetic alone is used for regional analgesia and anaesthesia.

Key points

- Problems of substance abuse in pregnancy/labour include the maternal effects of chronic abuse, acute effects on presentation and fetal/neonatal effects.
- A high index of suspicion is required in all atypical cases on the labour ward.

Further reading

Kuczkowski KM. Peripartum care of the cocaine-abusing parturient: are we ready? *Acta Obstet Gynecol Scand* 2005; **84**: 108–16.

Kuczkowski KM. The effects of drug abuse on pregnancy. *Curr Opin Obstet Gynecol* 2007; **19**: 578–85.

Ludlow J, Christmas T, Paech MJ, Orr B. Drug abuse and dependency during pregnancy: anaesthetic issues. *Anaesth Intensive Care* 2007; **35**: 881–93.

Wong S, Ordean A, Kahan M; Society of Obstetricians and Gynecologists of Canada. SOGC clinical practice guidelines: Substance use in pregnancy, no. 256. *Int J Gynaecol Obstet* 2011; **114**: 190–202.

Obesity

The World Health Organization has classified obesity according to body mass index (Table 139.1). By this definition, 22% of men and 24% of women were obese in the UK in 2009; this number has trebled in the last 20 years. The obese mother presents significant challenges to the obstetric anaesthetist, and obesity has been highlighted as an important contributory factor to maternal mortality.

Problems/special considerations

- The physiological changes that occur in pregnancy already put the parturient at risk and obesity puts further stress on the limited physiological reserve of the pregnant mother.
- The risks of diabetes, hypertension and coronary artery disease are all increased. Airway closure may occur within tidal volume, especially in supine and semi-supine positions. A small number of morbidly obese women may develop secondary pulmonary hypertension and chronic right ventricular failure.
- Antenatal assessment, including accurate estimation of gestation, may be difficult.
- Symptomatic reflux occurs in nearly all obese pregnant women.
- Aortocaval compression will occur in all but the full upright and full lateral positions, owing to the large pannus.
- Fetal growth retardation is possible, as well as the more commonly occurring macrosomic fetus. There is also a higher incidence of birth defects and stillbirth. Furthermore, monitoring the fetus antenatally and during labour is more difficult in the obese patient.
- The obese mother has an increased likelihood of developing pre-eclampsia, of requiring operative delivery (a risk of caesarean section of 30–50% has been reported) and of developing thromboembolic disease and infective postoperative complications.

Table 139.1 World Health Organization classification of obesity

Underweight	$< 18.5 \text{ kg/m}^2$
Normal	$18.5–24.99 \text{ kg/m}^2$
Overweight	$25.0–29.9 \text{ kg/m}^2$
Obese: class 1	$30.0–34.9 \text{ kg/m}^2$
class 2	$35.0–39.9 \text{ kg/m}^2$
class 3	$\geq 40.0 \text{ kg/m}^2$

- The massively obese woman may not fit on a standard operating table and she may exceed the weight limit of a standard hospital lift.
- Intravenous access and non-invasive monitoring of the mother may be difficult. The use of invasive arterial monitoring has been suggested where it is thought that the blood pressure cuff may not give accurate blood pressure measurements.
- The risk of epidural failure and dislodgement of the epidural catheter is higher in obese patients.

Management options

Thromboprophylaxis should be used, preferably with low-dose heparin (in increased doses; Table 139.2), and graduated compression stockings should be worn for the entire hospital admission – this alone needs special consideration since it may be difficult or even impossible to find stockings that fit effectively. H_2-antagonists and antacids should be used throughout labour.

Difficulty in securing intravenous access should be anticipated as should difficult tracheal intubation. For labour, the benefits of regional analgesia usually outweigh the risks of epidural haematoma resulting from heparin prophylaxis. Early use of epidural analgesia should be recommended, since the risk of obstetric intervention is greater, and epidural insertion may be difficult, and the failure rate higher, than in non-obese women. Although identification of landmarks is difficult, standard length needles can be used for the majority of women. The use of ultrasound may help to identify the midline. The lowest effective concentrations of local anaesthetic combined with an opioid should be used; combined spinal–epidural analgesia offers a suitable alternative. The aim should be to minimise any motor blockade whilst providing effective analgesia. There is some circumstantial evidence suggesting that the incidence and severity of postdural puncture headache is reduced in obesity, perhaps because of increased intra-abdominal pressure. Once an epidural has been sited, these patients should be reviewed regularly during labour and there should be a low threshold to re-site a non-functioning epidural early.

For caesarean section, regional anaesthesia is usually recommended in preference to general, and an existing epidural can be usually be extended for emergency delivery. Where a *de novo* block is required, combined spinal–epidural anaesthesia may be preferable to single-shot spinal anaesthesia, because it allows better control over the final height of the block and surgical difficulty may lead to prolonged operating time. It is important to pay meticulous attention to avoidance of aortocaval compression.

If general anaesthesia is necessary, the risks of hypoxia and regurgitation of gastric contents should be assumed to be higher than in the non-obese pregnant woman. Adequate preoxygenation is essential and tipping the operating table head-up may help to reduce the

Table 139.2 CMACE/RCOG recommended daily doses of low molecular weight heparin in obese parturients

	Enoxaparin	Dalteparin	Tinzaparin
91–130 kg	60 mg	7500 units	7000 units
131–170 kg	80 mg	10 000 units	9000 units
> 170 kg	0.6 mg/kg	75 units/kg	75 units/kg

functional residual capacity and improve the efficiency of preoxygenation. Difficulty with tracheal intubation should be anticipated and suitable aids to intubation should be readily available. Often, extra pillows are required under the patient's shoulders and neck to position the mother optimally. The so called 'ramped' position has been advocated in obese patients as this is thought to be associated with the optimal position for intubation; it may be achieved using ordinary pillows/blankets or specific wedge-shaped pillows, ± altering the configuration of the operating table.

Trained and experienced anaesthetic assistance is essential, and the presence of a second anaesthetist is desirable.

In order to ensure good oxygenation, higher tidal volumes, the use of PEEP and a higher inspired oxygen concentration have been recommended. Residual neuromuscular blockade has been implicated in maternal death and is a particular hazard in the obese woman. A peripheral nerve stimulator should be used to confirm reversal of neuromuscular blockade, and the trachea should be extubated with the patient in a slightly head-up position. Recovery from general anaesthesia should take place in a well lit recovery area under the supervision of trained recovery staff.

Good postoperative analgesia, e.g. with epidural or spinal opioids, is important to allow early mobilisation. Intravenous patient-controlled opioid analgesia is recommended for women in whom the central neuraxial route is unavailable. Postoperative physiotherapy should be provided, and high-dependency midwifery care should also be available.

Key points

- The obese mother has an increased risk of obstetric and anaesthetic complications.
- Early regional analgesia for labour should be encouraged.
- Difficulty with tracheal intubation should be anticipated.
- Thromboprophylaxis should be used in appropriate dosage.

Further reading

Centre for Maternal and Child Enquiries/Royal College of Obstetricians and Gynaecologists. Management of women with obesity in pregnancy. London: CMACE/RCOG 2010, http://www.rcog.org.uk/womens-health/clinical-guidance/management-women-obesity-pregnancy.

Gunatilake RP, Perlow JH. Obesity and pregnancy: clinical management of the obese gravida. *Am J Obstet Gynecol* 2011; **204**: 106–19.

Mace HS, Paech MJ, McDonnell NJ. Obesity and obstetric anaesthesia. *Anaesth Intensive Care* 2011; **39**: 559–70.

Saravanakumar K, Rao SG, Cooper GM. Obesity and obstetric anaesthesia. *Anaesthesia* 2006; **61**: 36–48.

Soens MA, Birnbach DJ, Ranasinghe JS, Zundert AV. Obstetric anaesthesia for the obese and morbidly obese patient: an ounce of prevention is worth more than a pound of treatment. *Acta Anaesthesiol Scand* 2007; **52**: 6–19.

Tsoi E, Shaikh H, Robinson S, Ghee T. Obesity in pregnancy: a major healthcare issue. *Postgrad Med J* 2010; **86**: 617–23.

Renal failure

Renal failure may be present before the patient becomes pregnant or it may develop during (or following) pregnancy, perhaps as a complication of a pregnancy-related problem. Either way, it has implications for the obstetric anaesthetist.

Although pregnancy was uncommon in patients with renal failure in the past, improvements in the care of patients requiring renal replacement means that women on dialysis programmes or having received renal transplants are increasingly likely to present to the maternity department. Conversely, acute renal failure (ARF) related to an obstetric complication should be becoming less common as care of the sick mother (in both the maternity suite and the intensive care unit) improves, although there are few data relating to this.

It should be remembered that the normal physiological changes of pregnancy result in an increased glomerular filtration rate and a lowering of the 'normal' blood indices of renal function. Thus, the usual blood urea concentration in pregnancy is 3.0–4.0 mmol/l and the creatinine concentration 55–65 µmol/l. An increase in blood urea concentration from, say, 4.0 mmol/l to 9.0 mmol/l may represent significant renal impairment, which may not be the case in non-pregnant subjects.

Problems/special considerations

Pre-existing disease

In terms of general anaesthetic management, the problems of pre-existing renal disease are the same as in the non-pregnant population. These include the underlying cause of renal impairment, systemic manifestations of renal failure (in particular hypertension and ischaemic heart disease, thrombocytopenia and anaemia), the patient's medication, altered handling of drugs and fluid management, including the nature and timing of dialysis.

Obstetric management may be influenced by the above factors and any history of previous abdominal surgery, including the presence of a transplanted kidney. There is an increased risk of pre-eclampsia in mothers with renal impairment. The fetus may be at risk from the underlying disease that caused renal impairment or from the above complications.

Acute renal failure related to pregnancy

Typically, pregnancy-related ARF is especially associated with pre-eclampsia, HELLP (haemolysis, elevated liver enzymes and low platelet count) syndrome, septic abortion and massive haemorrhage (traditionally caused by placental abruption, although any cause of hypovolaemia may be followed by renal failure). Other important causes include pyelonephritis, drug reactions (especially non-steroidal anti-inflammatory drugs (NSAIDs)), acute fatty liver and incompatible blood transfusion. In most cases, ARF is caused by acute tubular necrosis although cortical necrosis has been seen after abruption and pre-eclampsia. Problems are those of ARF generally, especially related to fluid balance and the apparently increased susceptibility of pregnant women to developing pulmonary oedema.

Management options

Pre-existing disease

Standard anaesthetic and analgesic techniques are suitable, given the above considerations. Renal function and blood pressure should be closely monitored during pregnancy. Discussion with the renal physicians and obstetricians is required regarding the timing of dialysis and method of delivery. Any arteriovenous shunt should be noted and steps taken to protect it during labour and/or delivery. Drugs excreted renally should be used with caution, and those known to impair renal blood flow or function (especially NSAIDs) should be avoided.

Acute renal failure related to pregnancy

Management of renal failure is along standard lines. Careful fluid balance is especially important given the propensity of obstetric patients to pulmonary oedema. Individual predisposing conditions are considered under their own headings. Most mothers regain normal renal function, depending on the underlying cause, although a degree of renal impairment may persist.

Key points

- Mothers with pre-existing renal failure require careful monitoring and an interdisciplinary approach.
- Obstetric anaesthetic management uses standard techniques, taking into account the underlying cause and systemic effects of renal failure, use of drugs and problems relating to fluid management.
- Renal failure may develop during or after obstetric catastrophes; management is along standard lines, and recovery of function is usual.

Further reading

Galvagno SM, Camann W. Sepsis and acute renal failure in pregnancy. *Anesth Analg* 2009; **108**: 572–5.

Gammill HS, Jeyabalan A. Acute renal failure in pregnancy. *Crit Care Med* 2005; **33** (10 Suppl): S372–84.

Ramin SM, Vidaeff AC, Yeomans ER, Gilstrap LC 3rd. Chronic renal disease in pregnancy. *Obstet Gynecol* 2006; **108**: 1531–9.

Royal College of Obstetricians and Gynaecologists. Renal Disease in Pregnancy: Consensus views arising from the 54th Study Group. London: RCOG 2008, http://www.rcog.org.uk/womens-health/clinical-guidance/renal-disease-pregnancy.

Williams D, Davison J. Chronic kidney disease in pregnancy. *BMJ* 2008; **336**: 211–15.

Steroid therapy

In pregnancy, steroids are used for the same conditions as in the non-pregnant state, i.e. inflammatory conditions such as sarcoidosis, rheumatoid arthritis, etc. They may also be used for obstetric medical conditions, e.g. antiphospholipid syndrome. Finally, maternal administration of glucocorticoids (usually dexamethasone or betamethasone) has been shown to reduce the incidence of respiratory distress syndrome and related complications in premature babies; the drugs are usually given as two doses 12–24 hours apart, with delivery 24 hours after the second dose if possible. The benefit is greatest at 30–32 weeks' gestation.

Problems/special considerations

Anaesthetic concerns are related to the underlying reason for steroid therapy, the presence of side effects of steroids and the requirement for supplementary steroids to cover the stress of delivery.

Reason for steroid therapy

This may be related to maternal disease or premature delivery, as described above.

Side effects

These are well known and no different in the pregnant state to those in the non-pregnant state, and they may be of relevance to the anaesthetist (e.g. electrolyte disturbance, osteoporosis). In general, hydrocortisone and prednisolone are about 90% metabolised by the placenta and therefore little reaches the fetus. However, maternal dosage above 10 mg prednisolone per day has been associated with neonatal adrenal suppression, and similar effects are theoretically possible in breastfed neonates, although reported measured concentrations of steroids in breast milk have been extremely low. There are unlikely to be adverse maternal effects of short-term administration of steroids given for premature delivery, although a raised white cell count is common and this may potentially cause confusion if infection is suspected. Transient reductions in fetal heart rate variability have been reported.

Steroid supplementation

Severe hypotension characterises the acute adrenocortical insufficiency of Addison's disease, and hypotension may also occur following surgery or trauma in chronic takers of steroids who do not receive supplementation, presumably as a result of suppression of the adrenals' ability to mount a stress response. This has led to the recommendation that all patients on steroid therapy should receive supplementation perioperatively; however the population at risk is uncertain, although most authorities would include all those with more than a week's steroid therapy within the last 3–6 months. If too much supplementary steroid is given, there is at least a theoretical risk of increased susceptibility to infection; in addition many patients dislike taking increased doses because depression and other mood changes may be apparent even after a short time, although other side effects typically take longer to occur. Finally, the amount of steroid reaching the neonate through breast milk should be kept to a minimum, even though small.

Management options

For general surgery, a more logical approach than the traditional '200 mg hydrocortisone 6-hourly' is to consider the normal endogenous response to surgery and to ensure that the equivalent amount of steroid is provided, e.g. 25–50 mg hydrocortisone for minor surgery, 75–100 mg for intermediate surgery and 100–150 mg for major surgery (N.B. 1 mg prednisolone is equivalent to 4 mg hydrocortisone). This daily amount is required for 1–3 days depending on the extent of surgery and should include any therapy the patient is already taking, e.g. maintenance dose.

The situation concerning labour and delivery is less clear; although caesarean section could be considered intermediate/major surgery, the stress of a prolonged and difficult labour is likely to be greater than that of a simple and rapid one. In general, the above plan may be adapted according to the particular circumstances of the case. If the patient is already taking adequate steroid to cover the daily requirement, no extra steroid should be required so long as the usual dose can be taken orally. If supplementation is necessary, it can be given as hydrocortisone intravenously divided into 2–4 doses per day or oral prednisolone, each tailing off after the required period.

Key points

- Steroids may be given for medical or obstetric purposes.
- Side effects may be important to the anaesthetist just as in the general population, although they are usually not a problem after administration for premature delivery.
- Steroid cover should be given according to the particular circumstances of the case but most patients require less than is traditionally given.

Further reading

Vidaeff AC, Ramin SM. Antenatal corticosteroids after preterm premature rupture of membranes. *Clin Obstet Gynecol* 2011; **54**: 337–43.

Trauma in pregnancy

Trauma during pregnancy may be coincidental or related to instability and difficulty moving, especially in the third trimester. It is a consistent cause of maternal death, usually associated with road traffic accidents but also including other forms such as violence, suicide and falls. Although the general principles are the same as in non-pregnant women, the physiological effects of pregnancy and the presence of the fetus impose particular conditions upon the presentation, assessment and management of injured mothers.

Problems/special considerations

- The increased metabolic demands of pregnancy make the mother less tolerant of hypotension, poor organ perfusion and hypoxaemia. Assessment of circulating volume status may be complicated by the increased cardiac output, pulse rate and blood volume of pregnancy and the potential for aortocaval compression. Injury to the abdomen and/or pelvis may result in fetal injury, maternal urinary tract injury or severe haemorrhage from the increased vascularity.
- Obstetric complications include premature rupture of membranes, premature labour and placental abruption, the last an especially common cause of fetal death. Fetomaternal haemorrhage may occur, with maternal sensitisation to fetal blood antigens if susceptible.
- The fetus is susceptible to the effects of drugs given to the mother.

Management options

General resuscitation is as for any injured patient, with the risk of aortocaval compression and regurgitation borne in mind. The choice of drugs administered to the mother will be influenced by the stage of the pregnancy. In the early stages of pregnancy, teratogenicity should be considered, and in the second and third trimesters the effect of the drugs on fetal growth and uterine function must be considered.

In the management of acute head injury, the normal blood gas values for pregnancy (arterial partial pressure of carbon dioxide approximately 4 kPa) must be remembered, especially if artificial ventilation is required. The risk of acid aspiration should be considered when airway reflexes are obtunded, and early intubation and ventilation may need to be considered.

Many of these women will require diagnostic radiological investigations, especially for head or spinal cord injury. Computerised tomography requires that the fetus is screened from the ionising radiation. Magnetic resonance imaging (MRI) requires an immobile patient, which may necessitate general anaesthesia with all its attendant risks. Aortocaval compression must be avoided at all times. Access to the MRI scanner may not be possible in an advanced state of pregnancy.

If indicated by the clinical condition, neurosurgical procedures can be performed in pregnancy.

The fetus should be monitored for at least several hours since abruption or fetomaternal haemorrhage may be delayed. In addition, the fetus may have suffered direct injury itself or be stressed by any concomitant hypotension, hypoxaemia or maternal therapeutic drugs or manoeuvres (e.g. inotropes, mannitol, furosemide, hyperventilation for control of intra-cranial pressure).

Caesarean delivery should be for obstetric reasons; epidural analgesia can be an integral part of the management of labour or operative delivery.

Key points

- General principles are as for non-pregnant patients.
- Pregnant women are more susceptible to the effects of hypotension and hypoxaemia.
- Aortocaval compression must be avoided at all times.
- Assessment may be complicated by the physiological changes of pregnancy.
- Placental abruption and fetomaternal haemorrhage are particular risks.

Further reading

Brown HL. Trauma in pregnancy. *Obstet Gynecol* 2009; **114**: 147–60.

Oxford C, Ludmir J. Trauma in pregnancy. *Clin Obstet Gynecol* 2009; **52**: 611–29.

Weinberg L, Steele RG, Pugh R, *et al.* The pregnant trauma patient. *Anaesth Intensive Care* 2005; **33**: 167–80.

Chapter

143

Malignant disease

There have been continuing improvements in the treatment of malignancies affecting children and young adults and in the management of reduced fertility that commonly follows such treatment. Thus, there are increasing numbers of women with treated (but not necessarily cured) malignant disease who become pregnant. In addition, malignant disease may occasionally present for the first time during pregnancy and may also be related to the pregnancy itself.

Problems/special considerations

General problems of malignancy

These may be local (compression effects, local invasion, scarring, etc.), metastatic (e.g. liver involvement, etc.) or general (malaise, anaemia, endocrine effects, weight loss and cachexia). There may also be problems relating to treatment, e.g. cytotoxic drugs, steroids, fibrotic effects of radiotherapy. There may be coagulation abnormalities or increased risk of deep-vein thrombosis necessitating anticoagulant therapy. Electrolyte disturbances may be a feature of the malignancy (e.g. hypercalcaemia) or its treatment.

Problems during pregnancy

Malignancies may be affected by the different hormonal profile of pregnancy and its effects on the tissues; this may make certain tumours more aggressive (e.g. breast cancer, melanoma). Some maternal malignancies may metastasise to the fetus or placenta (e.g. melanoma) although in general this is rare.

The patient's medication may need altering, especially in early pregnancy, since many cytotoxic drugs are harmful to the fetus. Similarly, there may be concerns about the use of radiotherapy or even surgery to treat malignancy during pregnancy, and the risks and benefits to both the mother and the fetus of administering or withholding treatment need careful consideration. In addition, the normal psychological stresses of pregnancy and delivery are especially intense if the mother has (or has had) cancer. The physiological demands of normal pregnancy may stress the more susceptible systems in the mother with malignant disease, e.g. anaemia may become more pronounced; mild cytotoxic-induced cardiomyopathy may become more severe. Finally, there may be direct effects of the malignancy or its treatment on the uterus and birth canal, e.g. cervical surgery and scarring, perineal scarring and abdominal adhesions.

A particular form of malignant disease affecting pregnancy is that arising from the placenta itself (gestational trophoblastic neoplasia), comprising hydatiform mole, invasive mole, choriocarcinoma and placental site trophopbastic tumour. It is more common at the extremes of reproductive age, in the Far East and Asia and if previous pregnancies have been affected. The pregnancy itself is non-viable and concerns about the fetus do not apply. These tumours generally respond well to chemotherapy, even if metastatic spread has occurred, with a mortality of $< 1\%$. Molar pregnancy may be associated with hyperemesis, hypertensive disease, anaemia, ovarian cysts and rarely hyperthyroidism. Surgical evacuation may be followed by pulmonary oedema or acute lung injury, possibly related to trophoblastic pulmonary embolism.

Management options

General care is directed towards the particular organs or systems affected by the malignancy itself and its treatment. Thus all mothers require careful antenatal assessment with particular attention to haematological, cardiac, renal and hepatic function, etc., with decisions concerning anaesthetic management made accordingly. Some mothers may knowingly have put their lives at risk in order to give the fetus the best chance of survival, and this must be respected when managing their analgesia and anaesthesia.

In trophoblastic neoplastic disease, uterine evacuation may be adequate surgical management but hysterectomy may be required in more invasive disease, especially in older women. Surgery may also be required for torsion of or haemorrhage into ovarian cysts. Chemotherapy may be required if human chorionic gonadotrophin levels remain elevated or in metastatic disease. In terms of anaesthetic management, the above considerations should be taken into account and appropriate measures taken regarding investigation (including liver and thyroid function blood tests and chest radiography), monitoring and management. General anaesthesia is usually recommended since uterine bleeding may be rapid and severe, and blood should be cross-matched and ready before surgery.

Key points

- Malignancies may be present before pregnancy, may develop or be diagnosed during pregnancy or may arise from the pregnancy itself.
- Problems may be related to general effects of malignancies or those related to the interaction between malignancy, its treatment and pregnancy.
- Gestational trophoblastic neoplasia represents a particular form of malignancy.

Further reading

Maxwell C, Barzilay B, Shah V, *et al.* Maternal and neonatal outcomes in pregnancies complicated by bone and soft-tissue tumors. *Obstet Gynecol* 2004; **104**: 344–8.

Morice P, Uzan C, Gouy S. Gynaecological cancers in pregnancy. *Lancet* 2012; **379**: 558–69.

Ward RM, Bristow RE. Cancer and pregnancy: recent developments. *Curr Opin Obstet Gynecol* 2002; **14**: 613–17.

Chapter

144

Transplantation

Advances in transplant surgery and in immunosuppressive drug treatment have led to increasing numbers of women with transplanted organs choosing to embark on pregnancy. Pregnancy following renal transplantation is now almost commonplace, and successful pregnancy following liver, heart and heart–lung transplantation has been reported. The major considerations for the medical staff caring for the pregnant transplant recipient are the effects of immunosuppressive therapy, the alteration in physiological function of the transplanted organ and the impact of the physiological changes of pregnancy.

Problems/special considerations

Immunosuppressive therapy

All transplant patients are at risk of organ rejection and therefore require long-term immunosuppressive therapy. There is no evidence that pregnancy itself increases the risk of rejection, which, in the case of renal transplants, is about 10% in the first year and up to 40% after 5 years.

Infections, both bacterial and viral, are more common because of the immunosuppressed state, with urinary tract infections (already more common during pregnancy) the most frequent infectious complication. The immunosuppressed patient is at risk of infection with uncommon pathogens, and it is therefore important to take appropriate cultures before beginning treatment.

Immunosuppressive drugs include cyclosporin, azathioprine and corticosteroids. Frequent monitoring of drug levels is required because of the changing blood volume during pregnancy, although in some cases the dose requirement may be reduced rather than increased.

Cyclosporin is associated with systemic hypertension (caused by activation of the sympathetic nervous system), and women with transplanted organs also have an increased risk of developing pre-eclampsia – an incidence of 30% has been reported. Pre-eclampsia may be difficult to diagnose because of the pre-existing hypertension and proteinuria. There have also been reports of thrombotic complications occurring in patients receiving cyclosporin, leading to recommendations that prophylactic heparin should be considered during pregnancy.

Azathioprine is associated with abnormal liver function tests and thrombocytopenia.

The problems associated with long-term corticosteroid therapy are well known; of specific concern during pregnancy are hypertension and glucose intolerance.

Immunosuppressive drugs are associated with a relatively low rate of fetal abnormality (cyclosporin is less teratogenic than azathioprine) but an increased rate of preterm delivery and intrauterine growth retardation.

Renal function

The background rate of deterioration in renal function following transplantation is about 10% per year, and this is not affected by pregnancy. It is important to monitor renal function closely throughout pregnancy; as with hypertension there may be difficulty with differential diagnosis if pre-eclampsia develops.

Heart and heart–lung transplant

The transplanted heart is denervated, and thus there are no vagal influences acting upon it. Adequate cardiac output is dependent on maintenance of adequate preload. Heart rate can increase in response to hypovolaemia or vasodilatation, but this response is delayed compared with that of the normal pregnant woman. There is considerable controversy regarding the response of the denervated heart to adrenergic agonists, with reports of both extreme hypersensitivity and blunted response. Likewise there have been reports of bradycardia and even sinus arrest following administration of neostigmine, despite theoretical grounds for believing that the drug should not alter the rate of the denervated heart.

Afferent denervation of the heart prevents the patient experiencing angina; the anaesthetist and obstetrician should be aware that the woman with a cardiac transplant is at increased risk of coronary artery disease (20% by one year post-transplant and up to 50% by 5 years), which can only be reliably detected by cardiac catheterisation.

Obstetric outcomes

Apart from the increased incidence of pre-eclampsia with cyclosporin, parturients who are recipients of transplanted organs have an increased risk of premature delivery, intrauterine growth retardation and the need for operative delivery. Surgery may be complicated by the previous transplant and the risk of postoperative infection is also increased. There is also a risk of transplant rejection during pregnancy, possibly related to the physiological changes in pregnancy and alterations in drug metabolism.

Management options

Most women are advised not to become pregnant for 18–24 months after transplantation, in order to allow organ function and immunosuppressive therapy to stabilise.

There are reports of successful vaginal delivery following renal, heart, heart–lung and hepatic transplants. As a general rule, caesarean section is only indicated for obstetric complications, although each case must be considered individually. The woman with a renal transplant can be treated as normal and may receive epidural analgesia and either regional or general anaesthesia. Particular attention should be paid to venous access, keeping cannulae as peripheral as possible and preserving any sites for shunts and fistulae.

Epidural analgesia has been used for heart transplant recipients in labour, and regional anaesthesia (both epidural and spinal) has been used successfully for operative delivery. It is important to avoid dehydration and to use adequate preloading, but the risks of catheter-related sepsis probably outweigh the benefits of central venous pressure monitoring in these patients. Ephedrine has been used in normal doses, but it is wise to use small increments because of the risk of exaggerated response to the drug.

Infectious complications remain one of the major risks for all transplant recipients, and scrupulous attention to aseptic technique is therefore vital.

Key points

- Immunosuppressive drugs are used by all transplant recipients.
- Cyclosporin is associated with systemic hypertension and proteinuria.
- Transplanted hearts are denervated and cardiac output is primarily dependent on preload.
- Successful vaginal delivery with epidural analgesia has been reported following organ transplantation.

Further reading

Armenti V, Constantinescu S, Moritz M, *et al*. Pregnancy after transplantation. *Transplantation Reviews* 2008; **22**: 223–4.

Cardonick E, Moritz M, Armenti V. Pregnancy in patients with organ transplantation: a review. *Obstet Gynecol Surv* 2004; **59**: 214–22.

Josephson MA, McKay DB. Pregnancy in the renal transplant recipient. *Obstet Gynecol Clin North Am* 2010; **37**: 211–22.

Kallen B, Westgren M, Aberg A, Olausson PO. Pregnancy outcome after maternal organ transplantation in Sweden. *BJOG* 2005; **112**: 904–9.

Critical care in pregnancy

Information about critical care in pregnancy is hampered by the lack of detail provided in published reports, differing admission criteria used by different units and the absence of systematic data collection schemes. The Confidential Enquiries into Maternal Deaths reports recognise the importance of adequate intensive care unit (ICU) provision and care, but since it focuses solely on deaths it does not give a complete picture of critical illness and pregnancy, although recent reports have included sections about ICU management. The need for adequate provision of ICU or high-dependency beds, especially in smaller delivery units, is repeatedly stressed. More recently, emphasis has been on providing 'intensive care' to the sick mother within the maternity unit – i.e. before she is actually admitted to the ICU.

Most series give an overall ICU admission rate of 0.2–9 per 1000 deliveries, although there is much variation between countries and even units as a result of differences in patient population and selection. The most common reasons for admission are haemorrhage and hypertensive disorders (including HELLP (haemolysis, elevated liver enzymes and low platelet count) syndrome). Other causes include respiratory failure and sepsis. Most patients stay in the ICU for less than 3–4 days. Mortality rates are difficult to estimate for the above reasons but are generally low overall (in the order of 3–4% in reported UK series) although they range from 0–20% in published series worldwide. Objective prediction of mortality is hampered by the relative inability of standard scoring systems (e.g. APACHE) to allow for the physiological changes of pregnancy or the particular spectrum of conditions seen in pregnancy (e.g. platelet count has greater importance in obstetric patients than in the non-pregnant population).

Problems/special considerations

A modification of the Department of Health's 2000 classification of critical care has been suggested for obstetrics:

- *Level 0:* Normal ward care of low-risk mother.
- *Level 1:* Additional monitoring or intervention, or step down from higher level of care (e.g. risk of haemorrhage, oxytocin infusion, mild pre-eclampsia, medical condition, e.g. congenital heart disease, diabetes).
- *Level 2:* Single organ support:
    - respiratory (e.g. requiring continuous oxygen, continuous positive airway pressure, bi-level positive airway pressure).
    - cardiovascular (e.g. pre-eclampsia requiring intravenous antihypertensives, arterial or central venous lines, cardiac output monitoring, intravenous antiarrythmic/ antihypertensive/vasoactive drugs).

- neurological (e.g. magnesium to control seizures, intracranial pressure monitoring).
- hepatic support (e.g. acute fulminant hepatic failure with consideration of transplantation).
- *Level 3:* Advanced respiratory support or two other organ systems support.

General ICU care is as for non-obstetric patients. Particular points to note are the risks to the fetus and the need for fetal monitoring (if antepartum); the requirements of the patient's partner and family; the midwifery care required in the puerperium (if postpartum); and the physiological changes of pregnancy. Of particular importance amongst the latter are the increased risk of aspiration; the increased oxygen demands and changes in respiratory function; the apparently increased propensity of critically ill obstetric patients to develop acute lung injury, susceptibility to aortocaval compression, increased cardiac output and other cardiovascular changes; and haematological changes including anaemia, increased risk of deep-vein thrombosis (DVT) and the readiness towards disseminated intravascular coagulation. These effects of pregnancy may be overlooked by staff unfamiliar with managing pregnant women. Finally, there may be psychological problems in the mother who is, or has been, critically ill, both before and after delivery. The fetus is likely to have been affected by her illness, increasing the stress upon her. The ICU environment is a far from ideal place to deliver or care for a baby.

Management options

Routine ICU support includes DVT and stress ulcer prophylaxis. Management of any associated organ failure is along standard lines. Premature labour is always a risk of severe maternal illness; however, the use of tocolytic drugs may be considered too risky for the mother. Aortocaval compression must be avoided at all times.

Caesarean section may be required in order to improve the mother's condition, e.g. in severe cardiac or respiratory disease or hypertensive disorders. Postpartum haemorrhage may be severe if a coagulopathy is present. Breast milk may be collected postpartum but may be unsuitable for use because of maternally administered drugs. If breast milk is not collected for neonatal feeding or to maintain lactation until the mother is well enough to nurse, lactation can be suppressed with bromocriptine although this is not recommended routinely (especially in pre-eclampsia) since hypertension, stroke and myocardial infarction have followed its use.

Good communication between all the involved clinicians (obstetricians, intensivists, etc.) and midwife/ICU nursing staff is vital to ensure that continuity of care is achieved with regards to treatment decisions and information given to relatives.

Key points

- About 0.2–9 per 1000 obstetric patients require intensive care.
- Hypertensive disorders and haemorrhage are the most common causes of admission.
- Basic principles apply but the special needs of the fetus/neonate, mother and family, and the physiological effects of pregnancy, must be remembered.
- Overall mortality of intensive care unit admission in UK series is 3–4%.

Further reading

Intensive Care National Audit and Research Centre. Female admissions (aged 16–50 years) to adult, general critical care units in England, Wales and Northern Ireland, reported as 'currently pregnant' or 'recently pregnant'. London: ICNARC 2009, http://www.oaa-anaes.ac.uk/assets/_managed/editor/File/Reports/ICNARC_obs_report_Oct2009.pdf.

Plaat F, Wray S. Role of the anaesthetist in obstetric critical care. *Best Pract Res Clin Obstet Gynaecol* 2008; **22**: 917–35.

Pollock W, Rose LN, Dennis CL. Pregnant and postpartum admissions to the intensive care unit: a systematic review. *Intensive Care Med* 2010; **36**: 1465–74.

Royal College of Anaesthetists/Royal College of Obstetricians and Gynaecologists. Providing equity of critical and maternity care for the critically ill pregnant or recently pregnant woman. London: RCoA 2011, http://www.rcog.org.uk/womens-health/clinical-guidance/providing-equity-critical-and-maternity-care-critically-ill-pregnant.

Chapter

146

Invasive monitoring

The increase in the number of pregnant women with significant co-existing medical disease has led to a need for high-dependency facilities during labour, delivery and the puerperium. In addition, women with complications of pregnancy such as pre-eclampsia may require high-dependency care. In these situations, an understanding of the pathophysiological changes that are taking place may be improved by the use of invasive monitoring.

Recent Reports on Confidential Enquiries into Maternal Deaths in the United Kingdom (CEMD) have recommended the more frequent and earlier use of invasive monitoring in the management of obstetric haemorrhage.

Problems/special considerations

Midwives are not intensive care nurses, and invasive monitoring may only aid management if the data obtained are reliable and correctly interpreted. All invasive cardiovascular monitoring has significant morbidity associated with its use, such as line sepsis, accidental arterial puncture, pneumothorax and even death. Insertion of pulmonary artery catheters is associated with a particularly high morbidity, and their use is rarely indicated nowadays.

The relative risks and benefits of invasive monitoring need to be assessed carefully – the difficulties of conducting labour and delivery on an intensive care unit may, in some circumstances, outweigh the potential benefits of such monitoring. The implications of the CEMD recommendations are that all obstetric units should be able to care for women with central venous pressure (CVP) monitoring, and that if not possible to do so, these women should be transferred to an intensive care unit.

Management options

It is now realised that cardiac output correlates better with uteroplacental perfusion than do heart rate and blood pressure. Thus non-invasive methods of cardiac output monitoring, such as transthoracic or transoesphageal echocardiography, suprasternal Doppler ultrasound and electrical bioimpedance, have been used in the obstetric setting. However, these techniques all have inter-observer variation and so are considered unsuitable for routine use, though they may be useful in specific cases (e.g. with severe cardiac disease) or as research tools.

Central venous pressure monitoring

Insertion of a central venous catheter to measure right atrial pressure may give valuable information in women with co-existing cardiac disease (see relevant chapters for further details). Most protocols for managing women with severe pre-eclampsia also suggest insertion of a CVP line to aid in fluid management, although it is important to realise that the information obtained (right atrial pressure) may not accurately reflect left atrial pressure.

The least invasive technique is recommended for women who are undelivered, i.e. use of a long line inserted from a peripheral vein (usually in the antecubital fossa). It may be technically difficult to cannulate the subclavian or internal jugular vein in the neck of a pregnant woman. She will be intolerant of the head-down position, and the need to adopt lateral tilt or the supine wedged position may distort the usual anatomical landmarks. The apprehension caused by attempting insertion of a neck line may provoke hypertension or arrhythmias caused by increased circulating catecholamines. In addition, the pre-eclamptic woman may have considerable soft tissue oedema of the face and neck and may also be thrombocytopenic.

A clear right atrial pressure waveform on a directly transduced trace may provide confirmation of correct placement of the line without the need for radiological confirmation, although the decision about whether to perform radiography should follow consideration of the relative risks and benefits. Chest radiography should be performed regardless of whether the woman is delivered if there is any anxiety about correct placement or complications of insertion.

Midwives should be able to look after women with CVP lines, and there should be continued education led by the anaesthetic team to ensure that new and existing staff are familiar with this aspect of care of high-risk patients.

Pulmonary artery catheterisation

Pulmonary artery catheterisation is becoming less common generally, since its use has been linked to increased mortality in some studies (although patient selection may be a confounding factor). In obstetrics, many authorities would reserve its use for extreme cases of impaired global cardiac function such as cardiomyopathy, or for severe pre-eclampsia with impaired left ventricular function. The risks are those of CVP monitoring plus the potential for pulmonary artery rupture and infarction, as well as technical problems such as knotting of the catheter.

Direct arterial pressure monitoring

Intra-arterial monitoring provides valuable information in conditions where even brief periods of hypotension may cause significant morbidity or mortality. Women with severe cardiac disease resulting in a fixed cardiac output require continuous blood pressure monitoring if epidural analgesia is used in labour, and before induction of either general or regional anaesthesia for operative delivery.

Direct arterial pressure monitoring is desirable in women with severe pre-eclampsia, or those receiving intravenous infusions of antihypertensive agents.

On rare occasions an intra-arterial cannula may be inserted to facilitate frequent arterial blood gas analysis in women with severe respiratory pathology.

Most midwives are not used to managing arterial lines, and it is therefore vital to ensure that the line is clearly labelled to minimise the risk of its being confused with an intravenous line. The insertion site must be readily accessible and kept visible at all times. It is sensible to explain the purpose of the line to the mother and to involve her in responsibility for its care.

New techniques

Arterial waveform analysis techniques have been suggested as alternatives in obstetric practice and include the LiDCO*plus* (LiDCO, Cambridge, United Kingdom) and PiCCO*plus* (Pulsion Medical Systems, Munich, Germany), and the uncalibrated Vigileo monitor (Edwards Lifesciences, Irvine, CA). These devices provide beat-to-beat data and are generally precise and reliable in terms of cardiac output measurement, and can thus monitor the patient's responsiveness to fluids and vasopressors. They are therefore thought to be more useful than the measurement of filling pressures.

Key points

- High-dependency care of women with co-existing medical disease or obstetric complications of pregnancy may require invasive monitoring.
- If appropriate monitoring cannot be provided in the maternity unit in which the woman is intending to deliver, arrangements should be made to transfer her care to another unit.

Further reading

Armstrong S, Fernando R, Columb M. Minimally- and non-invasive assessment of maternal cardiac output: go with the flow! *Int J Obstet Anesth* 2011; **20**: 330–40.

Fujitani S, Baldisseri MR. Hemodynamic assessment in a pregnant and peripartum patient. *Crit Care Med* 2005; **33** (10 Suppl): S354–61.

Morgan P, Al Subaie N, Rhodes A. Minimally invasive cardiac output monitoring. *Curr Opin Crit Care* 2008; **14**: 322–6.

Paech M, James M. Maternal hemodynamic monitoring in obstetric anesthesia. *Anesthesiology* 2008; **109**: 765–7.

147 Neonatal assessment

Formal assessment of the newborn baby is important: to allow documentation of the neonate's general state of wellbeing; as a prognostic exercise, to identify neonates at risk and focus medical attention on them; possibly as a means of following progress over time; and as a research tool for determining the effects of various interventions or conditions on neonatal outcome (e.g. drug therapy, anaesthetic techniques, epidemiological factors). Various methods have been described; as far as obstetric anaesthesia is concerned, the important ones are those that focus on the neonate's gross physiological status at or shortly after birth and those that assess its neurobehaviour.

Problems/special considerations

The easier the system for assessment (and therefore the more attractive it is to busy clinicians), the less its ability to discern subtle differences, and thus the less useful it is as a tool, especially when the effects being studied are likely to be small (e.g. a possible difference in effects of two similar drugs in labour). Conversely, tiny differences revealed by very sensitive measurements may be of uncertain significance clinically. In addition, factors that might ordinarily be prognostic may be susceptible to the actions of anaesthetic agents, e.g. ketamine may be associated with falsely high scores when using systems that rely heavily on muscle tone.

Methods of assessment
Measures of overall physiological status

- *Time to sustained respiration (TSR):* The time between delivery and sustained spontaneous ventilation is a very crude indicator of neonatal wellbeing, but does indicate babies that need special attention and attempts to quantify the degree of impairment. It does not distinguish between babies who are slow to breathe unsupported for different reasons (e.g. drugs, congenital defects) and is best suited to birth asphyxia. It is rarely performed routinely.
- *Apgar system:* Described by the American anaesthesiologist Virginia Apgar in 1953, the system comprises five variables, each scoring 0–2 (Table 147.1). The Apgar score is now a standard tool and is recorded routinely after virtually all deliveries. It is usually performed at 1 and 5 minutes after birth, although it may be repeated thereafter. A modified system, 'Apgar minus colour' (maximum of 8), has been suggested but is rarely used.

Table 147.1 Apgar scoring system

	0	1	2
Heart rate	Absent	<100	>100
Respiratory effort	Nil	Weak cry	Strong cry
Muscle tone	Limp	Poor tone	Good tone
Reflex irritability	Nil	Some movement	Strong withdrawal
Colour	Blue/pale	Pink body/blue extremities	Pink

Table 147.2 Effects of maternal anaesthetic and analgesic drugs on the neonate

Systemic drugs	Impairment is seen depending on the dosage and the test used: the more sensitive the assessment system, the greater the effect. Thus effects on alertness and responsiveness may be detected by using the NBAS and ENNS before respiratory depression is seen. Some effects of pethidine are apparent 24–48 hours postpartum, and subtle differences, e.g. in feeding, may persist for up to weeks
Regional anaesthesia	Lidocaine was suspected of impairing the ENNS in the 1970s (the 'alert but floppy baby') but this was not substantiated subsequently. There is no hard evidence of impairment after regional anaesthesia or analgesia for labour or caesarean section with various local anaesthetics or opioids. Although some studies have claimed to find differences, the difficulty of using adequate controls and conflicting results from other studies make these uncertain
	Hypotension lasting less than 2–3 minutes has not been associated with demonstrable effects, although Apgar score, acid–base profiles and crude neurobehavioural scores have been found to be affected if hypotension is prolonged
	The place of regional anaesthesia when the fetus is compromised is still debated by anaesthetists and others, most anaesthetists supporting its use
General anaesthesia	Its effects have been greater than those of regional anaesthetic techniques in most studies. Low concentrations of volatile agents are thought to have little effect

Tests of neurobehavioural status (sometimes referred to eponymously)

- *Neurobehavioural assessment score (NBAS):* Developed in 1973 by the British paediatrician Brazelton, the NBAS is the most commonly used of the detailed neurobehavioural assessment systems. It takes 45–60 minutes and requires trained staff to perform it.
- *Early neonatal neurobehavioural scale (ENNS):* Developed in 1974 by the American anaesthetist Scanlon, the ENNS is less complicated than the NBAS and therefore quicker to perform (about 5–10 minutes). It examines wakefulness, tone and the response to various stimuli, including the presence or absence of neonatal reflexes.

- *Neurological and adaptive capacity score (NACS):* Developed in 1982 by the paediatrician Amiel-Tison and anaesthetic colleagues in San Francisco, the NACS takes about 5 minutes to perform and is a relatively crude measure, mainly examining neonatal tone. It has been claimed that the NACS can distinguish between the effects of asphyxia and those of drugs, although this has been challenged. It is, however, widely used in obstetric anaesthetic studies because of its ease of use.

Effects of anaesthetic drugs

In general, the more gross an effect, the easier it is to show it; thus, for example, maternal pethidine can readily be demonstrated to suppress neonatal condition at birth and affect neurobehaviour and feeding for 1–2 days postpartum, by using relatively crude scoring systems. However, more subtle tools such as the NBAS are required to investigate smaller effects, and their significance may be disputed. Finally, the difficulty in conducting randomised studies, and the inadequate size of most studies that have looked at measures of neonatal assessment in depth, mean that no clear conclusions can be drawn in many cases. However, overall effects of anaesthetic and analgesic drugs are summarised in Table 147.2.

Key points

- The more complex the method used to assess the neonate's state, the more subtle the changes found.
- Anaesthetic and analgesic drugs have all been implicated in affecting neurobehaviour to some degree; this is generally agreed for systemic opioids and general anaesthesia but less certain for regional anaesthetic techniques, as long as hypotension is mild and limited.
- In terms of neonatal neurobehaviour, regional anaesthesia for delivery of the severely compromised fetus is thought by most anaesthetists to have advantages over general anaesthesia but this is still disputed.

Further reading

Littleford J. Effects on the fetus and newborn of maternal analgesia and anesthesia: a review. *Can J Anesth* 2004; **51**: 586–609.

Reynolds F. Labour analgesia and the baby: good news is no news. *Int J Obstet Anesth* 2011; **20**: 38–50.

Neonatal physiology and pharmacology

The physiology of the neonate is best considered in relation to the various body systems. Some of these are considered elsewhere in this book, but there follows a brief summary of the main points. Physiological factors that result in specific differences in drug handling by the neonate are also considered here. It should be remembered that functioning of the neonate's organ systems is closely related to the gestation at which it is born. Finally, factors that are important in the fetus may be equally important after birth; thus many of the following points refer to both the fetus and the neonate.

Circulatory system

In the fetus, oxygenated blood returning from the placenta is directed through the foramen ovale via the left atrium into the left ventricle, and thence preferentially to the brain. Deoxygenated blood from the brain passes via the right atrium and ventricle into the pulmonary artery; since the pulmonary vascular resistance is high, the blood passes through the ductus arteriosus into the aorta and thence via the two umbilical arteries (arising from the internal iliac arteries) to the placenta (Fig. 148.1). At birth, the systemic vascular resistance increases as the umbilical arteries close, whereas the pulmonary vascular resistance decreases as air is drawn into the lungs. Thus the circulation takes up the adult pattern, although the circulation remains transitional for about 2 weeks in term neonates, and fetal circulation may persist if pulmonary vascular resistance remains high (e.g. caused by hypoxaemia, acidosis, hypovolaemia and hypothermia). The neonate relies mainly on heart rate for maintenance of cardiac output, the stroke volume being relatively fixed.

Respiratory system

Two thirds of the pulmonary fluid is expelled from the chest by compression during delivery (reduced in caesarean section and if the neonate is small); remaining fluid is rapidly absorbed. Lung inflation is important to assist transition from the fetal to the adult circulation and to promote pulmonary surfactant production. Surfactant is required to enable alveolar expansion and is present in only small amounts up until about 34 weeks' gestation, although its production can be stimulated by maternal steroid therapy.

Fetal haemoglobin (containing α chains and γ chains) comprises about 80% of the circulating haemoglobin in the fetus. Its oxyhaemoglobin dissociation curve is shifted to the left compared with that of adult haemoglobin; thus transfer of oxygen from maternal to fetal blood is encouraged. Fetal haemoglobin normally persists for about 2–3 months after delivery, unless there is a haemoglobinopathy affecting adult haemoglobin.

The response of the neonate to hypoxia is discussed in Chapter 149, Neonatal resuscitation.

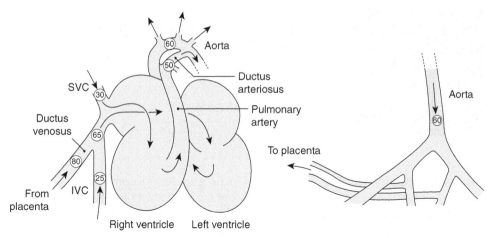

Fig. 148.1 Diagram of fetal circulation. IVC: inferior vena cava; SVC: superior vena cava. Arrows denote flow of blood. Figures refer to the approximate oxygen saturation.

Neurological system

The blood–brain barrier is generally accepted to be less complete in the neonate than in the adult, making the neonate more susceptible to depressant drugs, e.g. opioids. In premature babies, the fragile periventricular vessels are susceptible to fluctuations in arterial blood pressure and hypoxia, resulting in intraventricular haemorrhage.

Other systems

Heat production in the neonate is achieved by oxidation of brown fat, which results in increased oxygen requirements and may be inadequate if there has been growth retardation in utero. Thus, a warm environment for delivery is especially important.

Pharmacology

Uptake of drugs by the fetus is considered in Chapter 16, Placental transfer of drugs. The low plasma protein binding capacity of the fetus/neonate results in a greater amount of free drug in the plasma compared with that in the adult. Lipid-soluble drugs (e.g. anaesthetics) are extensively bound to fetal/neonatal tissues, offsetting this effect. Finally, fetal acidosis may result in the 'trapping' of drugs, which may persist postpartum if the neonate remains acidotic. The relative immaturity of both target organs (e.g. brain) and organs involved in metabolism (e.g. liver) make the neonate more susceptible to many drugs administered to the mother before delivery or directly to the neonate after delivery.

Key points

- Major circulatory and respiratory changes occur at birth.
- The neonate may exhibit the effects of intrapartum insults and remains susceptible to insults occurring postpartum.

Neonatal resuscitation

Published studies have reported some degree of resuscitation being required in up to 5–14% of neonates overall, although this may be higher in selected cases. Most neonates require assisted ventilation only. The need for resuscitation may often be predicted from the events and course of the pregnancy and labour (including the presence of meconium, the fetal heart rate and pH during labour and the mother's condition), although up to a third of cases occur after apparently normal labours. There has been a trend in recent years for paediatricians not to attend uncomplicated elective caesarean sections, since surveys have suggested the requirement for neonatal resuscitation is low in such cases, especially where the indication for caesarean section is previous operative delivery, and when regional anaesthesia is used. In such situations, anaesthetists should not take on the *responsibility* of resuscitating the neonate, since their primary responsibility is to care for the mother. However, all personnel in the delivery suite (including obstetric anaesthetists) should be competent at basic neonatal resuscitation.

Problems/special considerations
Cardiovascular
- The change from fetal to adult circulation normally accompanies delivery and the inspiration of air into the lungs. If there is poor lung inflation, high inflation pressures, hypercapnia, hypothermia or acidosis, the circulation (which remains transitional for about 2 weeks after birth in term neonates) may return to the fetal configuration.
- The neonate relies on a fast heart rate for cardiac output since stroke volume is relatively fixed. The neonatal heart responds to hypoxaemia with bradycardia, which in turn worsens oxygen delivery. The initial treatment is oxygenation.

Respiratory
- The squeezing of the chest during vaginal delivery helps to expel the fluid contained within the lungs in babies born this way. In babies born by caesarean section, this effect is absent and respiratory support is more likely to be required, especially superimposed on the underlying reason for emergency operative delivery. Uterine contractions themselves help to expel fluid, and even a short labour may be beneficial.
- The first breath needs to overcome the forces tending to keep the alveoli collapsed, and thus requires greater effort.
- If meconium is present, its dispersal throughout the lungs during resuscitation may result in the meconium aspiration syndrome.
- Hypoxaemia typically leads to vigorous respiratory efforts followed by a period of primary apnoea (accompanied by bradycardia), during which stimulation may provoke respiration.

After a few gasps a period of terminal apnoea ensues during which active resuscitation is required. It is possible for both stages to occur in utero if the fetus is hypoxic.

- Evidence of tissue damage (including brain tissue) caused by hyperoxia, especially after a period of asphyxia, has led to the avoidance of high concentrations of oxygen for neonatal resuscitation, with air being the gas recommended initially.

Management options

Appropriate equipment includes an oxygen source, funnel, bag and facepiece, suction, laryngoscopes, tracheal tubes (sizes 2.5–3.5 mm, non-shouldered) and a radiant heater. The laryngeal mask airway has been used for neonatal resuscitation and has been suggested as being faster, more reliable and thus safer than tracheal tubes, although its use is not yet widespread.

The latest Resuscitation Council (UK) algorithm is shown in Fig. 149.1.

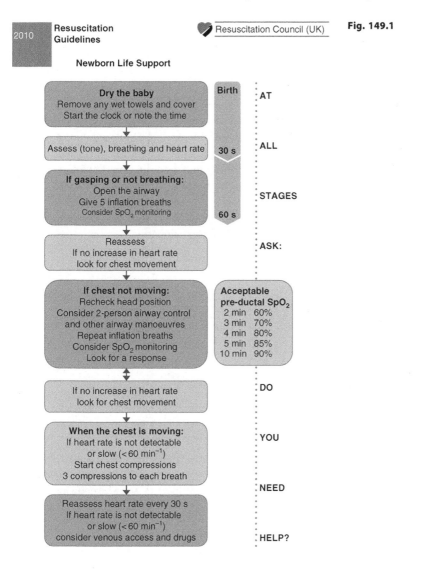

Fig. 149.1

Specific points:

- Basic principles of the 'ABC' of resuscitation apply.
- Vigorous oropharyngeal suction may cause apnoea. If meconium aspiration is suspected, direct laryngoscopy and pharyngeal/laryngeal suction under direct vision is preferred, with tracheal intubation if meconium is seen below the cords. Gentle suction and removal of meconium should take place before lung inflation unless the heart rate is under 60 beats/min.
- If controlled ventilation is required, the first breath should be held for 2–3 seconds to help expand the alveoli, with subsequent breaths lasting for 0.5–1.0 seconds. A maximum of 30–35 cmH$_2$O should be administered (20–25 cmH$_2$O if preterm). If heart rate does not increase or oxygenation (as indicated guided by oximetry) remains unacceptable despite effective ventilation, oxygen should be considered instead of air.
- Cardiac massage is performed either by encircling the baby's chest with the hands and compressing the sternum with the thumbs, or by using the index and ring fingers. The sternum should be depressed 1–2 cm. Compressions should occur at 120/minute, at a ratio of 3:1 with breaths.
- Intravenous access is usually obtained most easily with an umbilical venous catheter – the single umbilical vein is accompanied by two umbilical arteries, which aids its identification. Drugs are rarely required; doses are given in Table 149.1. The cannula should be flushed with saline after each drug is administered. The intraosseous route has also been used.
- The neonate should be kept warm and dry throughout resuscitation. Babies under 28 weeks' gestation should be wrapped up to the neck in plastic wrap or a bag.
- Therapeutic hypothermia should be considered for babies at term or near-term with evolving moderate or severe hypoxic–ischaemic encephalopathy.

Table 149.1 Drugs used in neonatal resuscitation

Drug	Dose	Notes
Naloxone	100 µg/kg i.m.	Should be considered if maternal opioids given
Adrenaline	10 µg/kg i.v. (0.1 ml/kg of a 1:10 000 solution) initially; 10–30 µg/kg i.v. if ineffective	If no significant cardiac output despite effective lung inflation and chest compression 50–100 µg/kg intratracheally is roughly equivalent to 10 µg/kg
Volume expansion	10–20 ml/kg	0.9% saline initially
Sodium bicarbonate 4.2%	1–2 mmol/kg i.v. (2–4 ml/kg)	High concentrations of bicarbonate have been associated with intraventricular haemorrhages

Key points

- Some degree of neonatal resuscitation is required in up to 5–14% of deliveries overall but the incidence is higher in selected cases.
- The anaesthetist's first duty is to the mother.
- It should be possible to predict two thirds of cases in which neonatal resuscitation is required before delivery.
- Basic principles are similar to those of adult resuscitation but with more emphasis on lung inflation and less on drugs.

Further reading

Guay J, Lachapelle J. No evidence for superiority of air or oxygen for neonatal resuscitation: a meta-analysis. *Can J Anesth* 2011; **58**: 1075–82.

Kattwinkel J, Perlman JM, Aziz K, *et al.* Neonatal resuscitation: 2010 American Heart Association Guidelines for Cardiopulmonary Resuscitation and Emergency Cardiovascular Care. *Pediatrics* 2010; **126**: e1400–13.

Resuscitation Council (UK). *Neonatal Life Support.* London: Resuscitation Council 2010, http://www.resus.org.uk/pages/nls.pdf.

Richmond S, Wyllie J. European Resuscitation Council Guidelines for Resuscitation 2010 Section 7. Resuscitation of babies at birth. *Resuscitation* 2010; **81**: 1389–99.

Chapter

150 Perinatal mortality

Perinatal mortality rate (PMR) is defined as the number of stillbirths plus the number of neonatal deaths within the first completed week of life, per 1000 total live births. It was proposed by the World Health Organization in 1975 as an international definition of late fetal and early neonatal loss and is a measure of antepartum care and wellbeing, care during delivery and immediate care postpartum. Perinatal mortality is thus generally accepted as a good indicator of general health and healthcare provision across different countries. In the developed countries it is about 6–12 per 1000 births, whereas in developing countries rates of up to 60 per 1000 births are reported, although many countries are unable to provide data. In England and Wales it has fallen from 32.8 per 1000 live births in 1961 to 7.8 per 1000 live births in 2009. In some countries, infant mortality rate (IMR; the number of deaths in the first completed year after delivery per 1000 total live births) is used as the

Table 150.1 Terms and definitions pertaining to perinatal mortality in England and Wales

Live birth	Expulsion from the mother after 24 weeks' gestation and the presence of breathing or any other sign of life, e.g. movement, heartbeat, etc.
Stillbirth	Expulsion from the mother after 24 weeks' gestation without breathing or any other sign of life
Early neonatal death	Death within the first 7 completed days after delivery
Late neonatal death	Death after the first 7 days, but before the first 28 completed days after delivery
Neonatal death	Early + late neonatal deaths
Perinatal mortality rate	Number of stillbirths plus number of early neonatal deaths per 1000 total live births
Infant mortality rate	Number of deaths in the first completed year after delivery per 1000 total live births

standard indicator; in the UK it was 4.6 in 2009 whereas in the developed countries generally it is about 3–8.

Problems/special considerations

Apart from difficulties collecting data, the figures are susceptible to variations in other definitions used; for example in the UK, an upward 'blip' in PMR was caused in 1991 when the definition of a live birth was changed from 28 weeks' to 24 weeks' gestation. Some of the definitions used are shown in Table 150.1.

Perinatal mortality has been found to increase with lower birthweight, lower gestational age, lower social class, age < 20 or > 40, parity < 1 or > 5, body mass index > 30 kg/m^2, presence of medical conditions, method of delivery, e.g. forceps and poor management of labour. It has been estimated that application of what is already known about good and poor practice would achieve a greater reduction in perinatal mortality than any other single measure.

For many years, the annual Confidential Enquiry into Stillbirths and Deaths in Infancy (CESDI) reported on causes of perinatal death and areas of suboptimal care, joining with the Confidential Enquiries into Maternal Deaths in 2003. CESDI's recommendations include establishing strategies and protocols for improving communication, training and peripartum clinical practice, appropriate involvement of senior medical staff and improvements in neonatal resuscitation. From 2012, the programme has been commissioned by the Healthcare Quality Improvement Partnership (HQIP).

Key points

- Perinatal mortality rate equals the number of stillbirths and neonatal deaths within the first completed week of life, per 1000 total live births.
- It represents the quality of provision of general healthcare for a particular country, as well as specific maternity and neonatal care.
- In the UK, perinatal mortality was 7.8 in 2009.

Further reading

Bell R, Parker L, MacPhail S, Wright C. Trends in the cause of late fetal death, 1982–2000. *BJOG* 2004; **111**: 1400–7.

Centre for Maternal and Child Enquiries (CMACE). *Perinatal Mortality 2009: United Kingdom.* London: CMACE 2011, http://www.hqip.org.uk/assets/NCAPOP-Library/CMACE-Reports/35.-March-2011-Perinatal-Mortality-2009.pdf.

Drife J. Can we reduce perinatal mortality in the UK? *Exp Rev Obstet Gynecol* 2008; **3**: 1–3.

Drugs and breastfeeding

Mothers often ask their anaesthetist for information about breastfeeding after anaesthetic and surgical interventions. The majority of drugs administered to the mother enter her breast milk but many are present in pharmacologically insignificant amounts and do not therefore pose a risk to the baby. The amount of drug that a breastfed baby receives is dependent on the concentration of drug in the milk and the volume of milk taken by the baby. In the first few days following delivery, the baby receives colostrum and then very small volumes of milk, so that any drug exposure is likely to be minimal. It is however common sense to administer drugs to the breastfeeding mother only if they are considered essential.

The *British National Formulary* (BNF) contains a comprehensive list of drugs that are known to be present in breast milk following maternal administration, but also points out that in many cases there are insufficient data to enable accurate information to be provided.

Breastfeeding and anaesthesia

Production of breast milk is dependent on adequate maternal hydration and regular stimulation (either by the baby feeding or by the mother expressing her milk). A mother scheduled for anaesthesia and surgery should be encouraged to feed her baby as near as possible to the planned time of surgery and also as soon as she feels able to postoperatively. In some cases it may be more appropriate for her to express milk in the early postoperative period.

There is some evidence to suggest that following a caesarean section under regional anaesthesia compared with general anaesthesia mothers are able to breastfeed more easily; this is intuitive but more research is required in this area. It has been proposed that babies born to mothers receiving epidural analgesia in labour are more likely to have delayed breastfeeding, but the evidence for this is extremely weak.

Intravenous agents

Both thiopental and propofol are found in breast milk in insignificant amounts following maternal administration. Levels of volatile agent excreted into breast milk are also negligible (most information relates to halothane, but extrapolation of data based on pharmacokinetic information suggests that isoflurane, sevoflurane and desflurane would be present in breast milk in even lower concentrations). Neuromuscular blocking agents are large, water-soluble, ionised quaternary ammonium compounds and therefore are not excreted into breast milk in any measurable quantity.

Analgesics

Transfer of non-steroidal anti-inflammatory drugs and opioids into breast milk has been extensively studied, and neither type of analgesic is present in clinically important quantities. Therapeutic doses of morphine and diamorphine given for postoperative analgesia (either following caesarean section or other surgical intervention) can be given to the mother as required. Maintenance on a methadone programme is not considered incompatible with breastfeeding, and there are no longer any restrictions on the maximum dose considered safe, although the lowest dose possible is generally recommended.

Antiemetics

All the commonly used antiemetics carry a manufacturers 'use with caution' or 'use only if essential' warning. Young women are at increased risk of oculogyric crisis with metoclopramide.

Benzodiazepines

Prolonged administration of benzodiazepines should be avoided. Diazepam is found in clinically significant quantities in breast milk and may cause hypotonia and impaired suckling in the baby. However, use of a single dose of temazepam or lorazepam as a premedicant drug is not contraindicated. Similarly, use of midazolam for intravenous sedation or during general anaesthesia is considered safe.

Other drugs

Anticoagulants

Warfarin and low molecular weight heparins are considered to be safe in breastfeeding mothers.

Antidepressants and anticonvulsants

The Report on Confidential Enquiries into Maternal Deaths has highlighted the risk of postnatal depression and its potential to lead to postnatal psychosis and suicide. There are numerous case reports offering conflicting advice about the use of psychotropic and anticonvulsant drugs in lactating women. Since the recommendations vary with each individual drug, specialist advice should be sought.

Antihypertensives

It is common for pre-eclamptic women to receive β-blocking drugs for several weeks following delivery. Atenolol is excreted in breast milk in measurable amounts, but there is no evidence that this is harmful to the infant.

Key points

- Most drugs are excreted into breast milk; information about the effect on the neonate is scarce.
- Commonly used anaesthetic and analgesic drugs can be safely used in breastfeeding mothers.

Follow-up

Follow-up of mothers after obstetric analgesia and anaesthesia is important for the individual anaesthetist, the hospital and obstetric anaesthesia as a whole. In an ideal world all anaesthetists would aim to follow up their own patients. This ideal is often not practical; therefore follow-up has to become part of the routine of an obstetric anaesthetic service. At national and international levels, data collection would enable anaesthetists to assess risk and monitor standards of care. At present there are very few data available at national or international level, and this is an area that comes more closely under the remit of audit.

Problems/special considerations

Follow-up of women who have had analgesia or anaesthesia administered by the anaesthetist should ideally be carried out within 24 hours. However, it may be difficult to see all women before they are discharged from hospital. This early discharge to the community means that anaesthetists must rely on midwifery, obstetric and general practitioner colleagues to refer back any problems. Areas that anaesthetists might wish to follow-up can be divided into:

- Anaesthetic interventions perceived to be uncomplicated
- Anaesthetic interventions where there was a problem.

Follow-up of the first group is important to ensure that women are satisfied with their treatment and, if not, why not. The follow-up interview gives the woman a chance to voice her opinion of the treatment she received. The anaesthetist should be responsive to criticisms of the service as a whole, since many women make their comments in order to help improve the service to others.

Suggested list of questions that may be asked at follow-up:

- *Relating to analgesia in labour:* Were you satisfied with the pain relief you received for the first and second stages of your labour? Were you able to mobilise during labour where appropriate? Has your sensation returned to normal? Have you a headache? Have you any comments about the care that you received?
- *Relating to regional anaesthesia:* Were you satisfied with the anaesthesia that you received? Did you feel any discomfort or pain at any time during the caesarean section? Have you had good postoperative pain relief? Are you mobile? Are you able to pass urine? Has your sensation returned to normal? Have you a headache? Have you any comments about the treatment that you received?
- *Relating to general anaesthesia:* Did you have a good sleep? Do you remember going to sleep? Do you remember waking up? Do you remember dreaming or waking up during

the operation? Do you have a sore throat, sore muscles or headache? Were you in pain when you woke up? Has the postoperative pain relief been adequate (at rest and on movement)? Have you had nausea or vomiting? Have you any comments about your treatment?

The most common problems associated with an anaesthetic intervention are:

- Difficulty in siting a regional analgesic
- Accidental dural puncture
- Paraesthesia during insertion of a spinal or epidural, and/or neurological symptoms afterwards
- Poor analgesia in labour (especially in the second stage if the epidural was inadequately topped up)
- Pain during caesarean section or operative delivery.

Patients with the above problems should always be followed up, ideally by a consultant obstetric anaesthetist. Continuity of care is important for these patients, and early involvement of other specialists, when appropriate, should occur at an early stage. For example, neurological consultation should be sought when there is any doubt as to the cause of a headache or neurological deficit. Early involvement of a clinical psychologist with a special interest in post-traumatic stress disorder following childbirth (if available) may be useful when there has been a painful experience during delivery.

Communication with the women, their partners and the midwifery and obstetric staff is essential to ensure that any problems, however small, are dealt with quickly and comprehensively. All women who have had a problem should have the opportunity to see the consultant obstetric anaesthetist after discharge from hospital. A follow-up visit at around 6–8 weeks post-delivery is useful for both the women and the obstetric anaesthetist. This consultation allows the lines of communication to remain open and offers the opportunity for a frank and open dialogue about any problems.

Key points

- Follow-up is important in both straightforward and complicated cases.
- Follow-up does not end when the woman leaves hospital.
- Consultant anaesthetic involvement is important.
- Communication is vital between all the professional groups involved.

Further reading

Cook TM, Counsell D, Wildsmith JAW, on behalf of the Royal College of Anaesthetists Third National Audit Project. Major complications of central neuraxial block: report on the 3rd National Audit Project of the Royal College of Anaesthetists. *Br J Anaesth* 2009; **102**: 179–90.

Jenkins JG. Some immediate serious complications of obstetric epidural analgesia and anaesthesia: a prospective study of 145,550 epidurals. *Int J Obstet Anesth* 2005; **14**: 37–42.

Nguyen T, Slater P, Cyna AM. Open vs specific questioning during anaesthetic follow-up after Caesarean section. *Anaesthesia* 2009; **64**: 156–60.

Maternal satisfaction

Maternal satisfaction has become a major outcome measure, mentioned in several import-ant documents and strategies concerned with childbirth. This means that providers of healthcare must pay attention to mothers' expression of satisfaction with their care during and after pregnancy. Anaesthetists have an important role to play in maternal satisfaction, since for many women aspects of their analgesia and anaesthesia can have an enormous effect on how they view their overall experience, in some cases irrespective of what happened in other areas of their care. Conversely, mothers' rating of their satisfaction with analgesia or anaesthesia in general, and different techniques in particular, may be affected by several factors unrelated to the anaesthetic itself. Despite this, studies comparing different techniques often quote measures of global satisfaction as evidence that one technique is superior to another. Similarly, obstetric anaesthetists are encouraged to assess and audit maternal satisfaction with the obstetric anaesthetic service as a marker of quality of performance, and patient feedback has been proposed as an important component in the process of consultants' revalidation.

Problems/special considerations

Apart from the confounding effects of various unrelated factors described above, another difficulty relates to the measuring tool used to assess satisfaction. Methods used have varied from simple 'satisfaction scales', e.g. visual analogue scale or verbal rating scale, to complex evaluations of different modalities that combine to produce a positive experience of childbirth such as fulfilment (e.g. happiness), lack of distress (e.g. pleasure) and physical wellbeing (e.g. lack of pain). The simpler systems will always be more attractive to busy clinicians such as anaesthetists than the more complex and time consuming ones, even though simple questions such as 'Are you satisfied?' or 'Rate your satisfaction on a scale of 1–10' are not very useful as objective outcome measures.

Studies suggest that factors associated with dissatisfaction include being excluded from one's care and decisions relating to it, poor communication and lack of information, bad outcome (although there may be strong satisfaction with the medical care if this is perceived to have been good) and being led to expect a particular event and then not experiencing it (e.g. receiving assurance that an epidural will be available but not receiving it because the anaesthetist is unavailable).

Despite initial assumptions that effective analgesia in labour automatically guarantees maternal satisfaction, this is not necessarily the case, and factors such as control and involvement in decision making may be more important. It is often suggested that satisfac-tion is increased when motor block is minimised by using low-dose epidural techniques or by the use of patient-controlled epidural analgesis (PCEA).

Management options

Until more work is done on the interplay between specific factors that contribute to maternal satisfaction, obstetric anaesthetists have to fall back on the use of vague and non-specific methods of assessing it. It is probably more important to assess dissatisfaction, which may indicate deficiencies in service, but any single measure of satisfaction is only as good as the methods used to obtain it. It is also important to ensure that if a mother has had a bad experience in childbirth but the anaesthetic care has been good and appropriate, her adverse opinion should not extend to include the anaesthetist. Sometimes attempts to prevent this are futile, especially when the opinions of other professionals on the labour ward towards anaesthetists are themselves adverse.

Attention meanwhile should be paid to those factors that have been shown to be important in promoting maternal satisfaction, such as involving the mother in decisions, keeping her informed, being prompt and courteous and other desirable general professional attitudes. Similarly, any expression of dissatisfaction should be taken seriously and an attempt made (and recorded in the notes) to discuss the particulars of the case, perhaps by offering an appointment at a later date. Medicolegal experience supports this approach as one of the most important factors in preventing subsequent legal action.

Key points

- Maternal satisfaction is an increasingly recognised but poorly defined measure of quality of care.
- Involving women in their care, good communication and honesty are important factors in increasing maternal satisfaction.
- Women expressing dissatisfaction should be identified and offered the opportunity to discuss their care further with a senior member of staff.

Further reading

Dickinson JE, Paech MJ, McDonald SJ, Evans SF. Maternal satisfaction with childbirth and intrapartum analgesia in nulliparous labour. *Aust N Z J Obstet Gynaecol* 2003; **43**: 463–8.

Hodnett ED. Pain and women's satisfaction with the experience of childbirth: a systematic review. *Am J Obstet Gynecol* 2002; **186**: S160–72.

Robinson PN, Salmon P, Yentis SM. Maternal satisfaction. *Int J Obstet Anesth* 1998; **7**: 32–7.

154

Antenatal education

Women preparing for childbirth make use of many sources of information. These will typically include discussion with other women, magazine articles, books and classes. Classes may be run by the GP practice or maternity unit, or by external bodies such as the National Childbirth Trust (NCT). Antenatal education is beneficial, since it has been shown that the well informed mother will cope better with labour, but it is important that the information received by the mother should be accurate, well balanced and relevant to local conditions (there is, after all, little point in discussing the virtues of epidural analgesia if no such service is available in the local hospital).

Much of the information given to mothers in the antenatal period is outside the control of the anaesthetist and may well be inaccurate or misleading; it is therefore particularly important for the anaesthetist to seek every opportunity to get his/her message across.

Problems/special considerations
Retention of information
The middle of a painful labour is the wrong time to attempt to provide quite complex information about regional analgesia. In addition to the pain itself and the inevitable tension, the mother may well be under the influence of powerful sedative/analgesic drugs. Theoretically, the antenatal period is the ideal time to educate mothers about pain relief and anaesthesia for caesarean section. Unfortunately, many studies have shown that the ability of patients to recall details of explanations is poor and that such information tends to be retained for the short term only. This problem is exacerbated by the fact that many primigravidae who have epidural analgesia in labour were not planning to use it; these women would be especially unlikely to recall information given in the antenatal period.

Written information
Poor recall of verbal explanations implies that antenatal classes should be supplemented with written information that mothers can take home and read at leisure; audiotapes and videos can also be very helpful. When preparing these sources, it is important to target them at a relatively low level of comprehension; it is all too easy to slip into medical jargon and unnecessarily complicated language. Studies have shown that written information for patients should be set at a reading age of about 12 years. The needs of mothers whose first language is not English should also be considered, and the Obstetric Anaesthetists' Association (OAA) has several translations of its information for mothers available on its website, including in smartphone/tablet format.

Content

Mothers need balanced information to enable them to make rational decisions; this is an essential element of the principle of consent. Talks, leaflets, videos, etc. need to present an unbiased view of the benefits and risks of the available alternatives and should be based on the best available evidence. Inevitably, material that is designed to inform a large number of women will be too complex for some and have insufficient detail for others; it is therefore essential that mothers should be able to discuss their concerns individually with an anaesthetist if necessary, and antenatal education should not be seen as a substitute for this facility.

Management options

Undertaking a regular antenatal class is a major (and almost certainly unpaid) commitment, often involving regular evening lectures. Equally, not every anaesthetist is suited to giving informal talks to large groups of mothers and fathers. In some circumstances, it is better to enlist the help of parentcraft teachers, who may be willing to put across the anaesthetist's message themselves. If this is to be done successfully, however, it is essential that the teachers fully understand and agree with the content and emphasis of the information. The anaesthetist should still attend the classes on a regular basis to ensure that the teacher is not going 'off-message', and must be available (not necessarily on the same day) to deal with any queries outside the teacher's experience. Audiovisual aids are useful, particularly as a prompt if the talk is delegated to someone else, but slides must be kept simple, jargon free and not gory.

The use of written/video material is worthwhile, but preparation to an acceptable standard is more difficult than might be imagined. Many hospitals have departments dedicated to provision of patient information, and their help should be sought at an early stage. Presentation in an attractive format is also important, and this will almost certainly require professional input. Production of high-quality leaflets is not cheap, and it is tempting to seek sponsorship from a company with a commercial interest in pregnancy or labour; however, many midwives are reluctant to distribute information that appears to endorse products, and their views should be sought before embarking on such a course. In general, the cooperation of midwifery staff is important in ensuring that the target audience is reached and they should therefore be involved at the preparation stage.

It is important to remember that antenatal education often misses the most socially deprived – and hence high-risk – mothers. The extent of this problem may be assessed by discussion with local community midwives, who may be willing to establish 'outreach' clinics for this vulnerable group.

Several national organisations have produced leaflets and videos about pain relief in labour, including the OAA. These provide an attractive way of informing mothers in the antenatal period, but care should be taken if using such material to ensure that the information given reflects local practice and experience.

Key points

- Antenatal education allows explanation of key facts in a low-stress environment.
- Retention of information given in the antenatal period is poor.
- Information should be accurate, locally relevant and carefully targeted.
- Leaflets/videos are useful supplements, but may be difficult to prepare.

Further reading

Bethune L, Harper N, Lucas DN, *et al*. Complications of obstetric regional analgesia – how much information is enough? *Int J Obstet Anesth* 2004; **13**: 30–4.

Broaddus BM, Chandrasekhar S. Informed consent in obstetric anesthesia. *Anesth Analg* 2011; **112**: 912–15.

Fortescue C, Wee MY, Malhotra S, Yentis SM, Holdcroft A. Is preparation for emergency obstetric anaesthesia adequate? A maternal questionnaire survey. *Int J Obstet Anesth* 2007; **16**: 336–40.

Obstetric Anaesthetists' Association. Information for mothers, http://www.oaaformothers.info/.

Chapter

155

Audit

Medical audit is a process by which certain aspects of practice are assessed and compared with predefined standards. If those standards are not met then the reasons for not meeting them are analysed and addressed; subsequent audits can be used to confirm that the situation has improved (thus completing the audit 'loop'). Audit should be distinguished from research, which seeks to determine what the standards should be; e.g. research might suggest that drug A is best for uterine relaxation in premature labour whereas audit determines whether drug A is in fact being used appropriately in a particular unit.

Audit is widely supported as a means of encouraging evidence-based medicine and improving standards of care.

Problems/special considerations

The best known and oldest obstetric audit is the Report on Confidential Enquiries into Maternal Deaths, in which obstetric deaths are analysed, their causes determined and management compared against 'best practice', and recommendations made about standards of care in maternity units. Anaesthetic aspects are considered by specific anaesthetic assessors. Other than this, there is no comprehensive national obstetric anaesthetic audit system, although most units have a system for collecting some measure of activity and outcomes. This causes problems with estimating true incidences of adverse outcomes, since the denominators are rarely known (e.g. the number of general anaesthetic caesarean sections in the UK), although there have been recent attempts by the Royal College of Obstetricians and Gynaecologists (and more recently, by anaesthetic organisations particularly the Obstetric Anaesthetists' Association) to collect these basic data. The third National Audit Project of the

Royal College of Anaesthetists provided national data on neuraxial analgesic/anaesthetic techniques relating to complications, and this included information from obstetric cases.

At unit level, rates of epidurals in labour, accidental dural punctures, anaesthesia for caesarean section and complications are commonly recorded. Whether this information is used for true audit as defined above is uncertain. In addition, definitions of these various terms may not be uniform amongst units (for example, should 'epidural rate' include spinals/ combined spinal–epidurals, and should the denominator be the number of women delivering, the number of women *in labour*, the number of *babies* delivered, etc?). Finally, the real impact of sometimes expensive audit on actual outcome of care has been repeatedly questioned.

It is important to perform audit with specific aims, rather than simply collect data for its own sake. Simple audit can easily be performed for particular aspects of care, e.g. to assess whether antacid prophylaxis is being given to all patients before elective caesarean section or to labouring mothers in high-risk groups, or whether appropriate investigations are being performed in pre-eclamptic patients before regional analgesia. Administrative aspects can also be audited, e.g. response times of anaesthetists on call or provision of adequate teaching on labour ward. The value of an audit is increased by concentrating on objective data, e.g. the measure of satisfaction is commonly done following obstetric anaesthesia, but data derived from vague satisfaction scales may be a poor reflection of quality of service.

Finally, if the data are unreliable the audit is worthless; thus each project should be planned carefully to ensure that high quality data are collected. During each cycle, the audit can itself be audited by sampling the data collected and checking it for accuracy and completeness.

Key points

- Audit comprises:

    1. Assessment of practice
    2. Comparison against 'best practice'
    3. Analysis of any shortcoming
    4. Correction of deficient practice
    5. Repeating the assessment.

Further reading

Cook TM, Counsell D, Wildsmith JAW, on behalf of the Royal College of Anaesthetists Third National Audit Project. Major complications of central neuraxial block: report on the 3rd National Audit Project of the Royal College of Anaesthetists. *Br J Anaesth* 2009; **102**: 179–90.

Holdcroft A, Verma R, Chapple J, *et al.* Towards effective obstetric anaesthetic audit in the UK. *Int J Obstet Anesth* 1999; **8**: 37–42.

Paech M, Sinha A. Obstetric audit and its implications for obstetric anaesthesia. *Best Pract Res Clin Obstet Gynaecol* 2010; **24**: 413–25.

Chapter

156

Labour ward organisation

Unplanned situations and emergencies inevitably arise in the best-managed obstetric units, but good organisation should be able to reduce these to a minimum. Anaesthetists are present in most labour wards for a majority of the working week, are involved in the care of the complex cases that test the organisational structure, and are accustomed to communicating with other medical and non-medical staff. They are therefore ideally suited to help in the planning of the various aspects of labour ward organisation.

Problems/special considerations

The labour ward is a potential hot-bed of organisational problems. Workload may vary suddenly and dramatically, and the urgent nature of many admissions makes forward planning very difficult. A variety of specialists are intimately involved with the care of the patients, and conflicts, although regrettable, are inevitable. Priorities are often difficult to establish, and prolonged periods of routine work may be suddenly interrupted by an extreme emergency. All of this makes careful organisation essential but very difficult.

Maternity care is by far the largest source of medicolegal litigation in Europe and the USA, and analysis of claims commonly implicates communication and other organisational factors – for example, failure to notify the anaesthetist of an impending caesarean section until the last minute, resulting in inappropriate anaesthetic decisions or excessive delay.

In many labour wards in the UK and elsewhere, midwives are taking an increasing role as lead clinicians, and so-called 'low-risk' mothers are frequently cared for solely by a midwife. This situation, although not hazardous in itself, calls for careful guidelines to ensure early communication of potential problems to relevant medical staff. The problem can be exacerbated if independent practitioners are allowed to admit their clients to labour ward.

Although the role of the anaesthetist is more widely appreciated by midwives and obstetricians than in the past, there is still a tendency in some units to regard him/her as an 'outsider', only to be summoned when required. This attitude fosters poor communication and should be discouraged.

Management options

There should be a consultant anaesthetist responsible for the provision of the obstetric anaesthetic service. A labour ward working party or equivalent, meeting on a regular basis, is an ideal forum in which to raise concerns and maintain communication, and there must be an anaesthetist on this body.

Guidelines and protocols should be drawn up to cover routine care, management of difficult cases, etc., and must be agreed by all parties involved. These guidelines should be updated frequently, be readily available on the labour ward and be distributed to all new staff, who should undergo a formal familiarisation programme before being allowed 'on-call'. Standards laid down in guidelines should be the subject of regular audit. Independent practitioners who require admitting rights must also agree to abide by the unit guidelines.

A formal scheme for reporting all critical incidents and 'near-misses' must be in place, and a blame-free culture established to encourage staff to utilise the system. Regular multidisciplinary morbidity meetings are useful to identify potential organisational problems. Information from these should pass to a risk management committee (also multidisciplinary), responsible for ensuring good practice and minimising risk to patients.

Good communication is the most important factor in a well-managed labour ward. A system should be in place to ensure that potentially difficult cases are referred to an anaesthetist early in the antenatal period, and that the anaesthetist is also notified when they are admitted. The anaesthetist should be familiar with all the patients on labour ward and this is best achieved by participating in joint ward rounds with the obstetricians and midwives. The duty anaesthetist must be rapidly contactable at all times; 'bleep' systems should not be relied upon as a sole means of contact. The names and methods of contacting consultant staff should be visible at the central desk. In general, anaesthetists should ensure that they are regarded as part of the 'team', rather than someone to be called when the situation is desperate.

Extreme emergencies such as cardiorespiratory arrest are very uncommon on the labour ward, but a successful outcome depends on a rapid, efficient response and this can be threatened by the very rarity of such events. The whereabouts of resuscitation equipment and drugs must, of course, be known to all staff, and regular 'drills' for emergencies such as maternal collapse and massive antepartum haemorrhage should be carried out to ensure that the system works smoothly.

Detailed guidelines covering the above points, and more, have been published by the Obstetric Anaesthetists' Association/Association of Anaesthetists of Great Britain and Ireland, and the Royal Colleges of Midwives and of Obstetricians and Gynaecologists. These documents serve as useful reminders of the various aspects of labour ward organisation that need attention, and also serve as tools for ongoing audit.

Key points

- Poor organisation results in unnecessarily hasty, and sometimes incorrect, decision making.
- Anaesthetists should be involved in labour ward management.
- Good, early communication will help prevent many disasters.

Further reading

Obstetric Anaesthetists' Association/Association of Anaesthetists of Great Britain & Ireland. *Guidelines for Obstetric Anaesthetic Services*, 2nd edn. London: AAGBI 2005, www.aagbi.org/sites/default/files/obstetric05.pdf.

Royal College of Anaesthetists, Royal College of Midwives, Royal College of Obstetricians and Gynaecologists, Royal College of Paediatrics and Child Health. *Safer Childbirth: Minimum Standards for the Organisation and Delivery of Care in Labour*. London: RCOG 2007, http://www.rcog.org.uk/files/rcog-corp/uploaded-files/WPRSaferChildbirthReport2007.pdf.

Midwifery training

Obstetric anaesthetists are part of the delivery suite team. This involves working closely with midwives who are often the lead professionals caring for the pregnant woman. It is therefore important to understand the training that midwives have received, and for senior anaesthetists to take responsibility for teaching obstetric analgesia and anaesthesia and the management of critically ill obstetric patients to midwives.

Training and regulation of midwives was formally established following passage of the Midwives Act in 1902, with the establishment of the Central Midwives Board (CMB). In 1983, the CMB was replaced by the United Kingdom Central Council for Nursing, Midwifery and Health Visiting (UKCC), whose functions were taken over by the Nursing and Midwifery Council (NMC) in 2002. The NMC register currently has ~629 000 nurses, ~28 000 midwives and ~12 000 dual-qualified nurse-midwives.

Problems/special considerations

Midwives working in the NHS have completed either a degree course in midwifery (usually three years) or a midwifery short programme (at least a year and a half) if they already have a nursing qualification.

Midwifery training usually requires the following topics to be covered:

- Biological sciences, applied sociology and psychology, and aspects of professional practice
- Pain in labour, the pain pathways involved, and pain relief (including both non-pharmacological and pharmacological methods)
- Anaesthesia; this includes both regional and general anaesthesia in pregnancy.

These modules do not have to be taught by obstetric anaesthetists, although in most training schools there is a good relationship between the midwifery tutors and obstetric anaesthetists, who may as a result be involved in many hours of teaching. This relationship has led to increasing awareness that anaesthetists are involved with the sick maternity patient and that they should be involved in teaching both high-dependency care and the recognition of clinical risk factors. Teaching of these skills is particularly important for the direct-entry midwives and has led to the following topics often being taught by obstetric anaesthetists:

- Postoperative and recovery skills
- Risk factors associated with women who have medical problems
- Care of the critically ill woman, e.g. high-dependency care for women who have pre-eclampsia or haemorrhage.

This extension of the teaching role of the obstetric anaesthetist may require around 18 hours of teaching to be given to each group of students. The students who have general nursing qualifications will require less time than the direct entry students.

Each training school has different courses that may culminate in a degree or diploma qualification. The length of training can vary between three and four years (shorter if the student is already qualified as a nurse), and the structure of the courses varies considerably, as does the obstetric anaesthetic involvement.

In order to practise, midwives must be registered with the NMC, which maintains a register. To remain registered they must maintain a professional portfolio as evidence of their keeping up to date, and notify the NMC annually of their intention to practise. Part of midwives' continuing professional development/training will include the practical management of epidural analgesia. The ability to administer epidural top-ups requires additional in-service teaching, which is usually done on the delivery suite. A certificate is issued to the midwife on completing the training satisfactorily. The exact requirements of the training differ depending on local practice and may require an update of resuscitation skills.

Anaesthetists are often involved in other areas of professional development, e.g. intravenous cannulation, resuscitation (adult and neonatal) and specific high-dependency training.

Key points

- It is important that obstetric anaesthetists are involved in midwifery training.
- Midwives require instruction during their midwifery training, as well as continuous education and maintenance of skills once qualified.

Chapter

Consent

158

Consent for treatment comprises a number of components:

- Provision of adequate information to, and its understanding by, the patient
- The ability of the individual to assimilate this information, weigh up the alternatives and consequences, and come to a decision (in ethical and legal parlance, 'capacity' and 'competence' respectively)
- Allowing adequate time for the process
- Voluntariness, i.e. no coercion by others.

Consent may be implied or expressed. Implied consent is usually assumed when a patient cooperates in allowing a minor procedure, such as venepuncture, to take place. The maintenance of a suitable posture; for example, epidural analgesia might be taken to imply consent to continue with the procedure, but it would be unwise to rely on this in the absence of a full discussion.

There is no legal difference between written and verbal consent. The only advantage of the former is that it provides concrete evidence that a discussion took place if a dispute arises.

Failure to obtain consent before performing a procedure could lead to an action against the anaesthetist for battery – the unlawful touching of another person. In practice, this is rarely, if ever, an issue in claims against doctors. Far more likely is the claim that a lack of informed consent resulted in a complication (if the patient had only been told of the risk, she would not have undergone the procedure) – i.e. a claim of negligence. (A 2005 House of Lords judgment means that a doctor may now be found negligent with respect to provision of adequate information to the patient even if this failure had no effect on the patient's decision to undergo treatment.)

The amount of information that a doctor must impart to a patient to aid her in making a decision has traditionally been based on the 'Bolam principle' from 1957; i.e. that an action – in this case the failure to mention a complication – is not negligent if it can be shown that the doctor has acted in accordance with a 'responsible body of medical persons skilled in that particular art'. However, this principle, which essentially allows the profession to set its own standards, has increasingly been challenged, probably most significantly by the 'Bolitho principle' from 1997, by which the views or practice of a body of medical opinion can only be considered as 'reasonable' or 'responsible' if it holds up against 'logical analysis'. Thus, for example, an anaesthetist who didn't explain the risk of nerve injury after an epidural might claim that many other anaesthetists would also not explain this (a defence based on Bolam) – but the Courts may decide that this is unacceptable practice nonetheless (Bolitho). Current guidance on informed consent is that each patient should be given the information that she herself would want, not what the treating doctor thinks she needs.

Problems/special considerations

The principles of consent to treatment in obstetric anaesthesia are essentially no different from those in any other field, the main distinction being that, in the often fraught circumstances that surround labour and delivery, they may be more difficult to apply:

- Prior information about epidural analgesia – e.g. in the antenatal clinic – is generally accepted as improving the consenting process, but it should be borne in mind that up to half of primigravidae who end up with an epidural were not intending to have one beforehand.

- Questions may arise over the issue of capacity when the mother is in the full throes of labour, especially when she is exhausted and/or has received powerful analgesic drugs. The practitioner treating the patient (in this case, the anaesthetist) is the person who must make the decision of whether or not the mother does have the capacity to understand what is being explained/proposed to her. If yes, then she is able to consent to (or refuse) treatment as in any other situation. If no, then the anaesthetist is obliged to treat her in her 'best interests' – which may not necessarily mean siting an epidural. A particular problem occurs when a woman has stated 'Under no circumstances am I to have an epidural, even if I scream for one during labour', or words to that effect, in her antenatal birth plan, and presents in labour screaming and begging for pain relief. In such a situation, the anaesthetist's first task is to establish whether she has capacity; if she does, then she is entitled to change her mind and so long as the anaesthetist is satisfied that the above components of consent are met, then it is appropriate to proceed with the epidural. On the other hand, if the anaesthetist assesses the woman as *not* having capacity, then the next decision is to determine what her best interests are. If, based on her birth plan and where possible, discussions with her partner and midwife about her prior views and strength of feeling, the anaesthetist has evidence to believe that she remains fundamentally opposed to epidural analgesia, then it would be incorrect to proceed with an epidural. If, however, such evidence suggests that she would be amenable to considering an epidural, given that the situation in labour is different to that when the birth plan was written, then it would be appropriate to proceed. Trainee anaesthetists would be well advised to consult with senior staff should such a situation occur. It is important in such circumstances to explain the difficulties of the situation to the woman's partner, to record the discussions in the patient's notes, and to visit her postpartum to explain events to her.

- Consent is ultimately a matter between the anaesthetist and the patient. However, the partner's views should not be dismissed summarily; he is an important participant in the birth process and should be encouraged to listen to the anaesthetist's explanation and accept the woman's decision. As outlined above, he also is a key provider of evidence as to what a woman's 'best interests' might be if she lacks capacity to give consent.
- The presence of the fetus does not interfere with the patient's right to make an autonomous decision about her own care, even if the decision taken will compromise the wellbeing of her unborn child. It is, of course, still very important that the risks and benefits to the fetus are also explained to the mother when seeking consent to a particular course of action.
- Patients whose first language is not English are as entitled as any others to an adequate explanation in their own language. The partner may act as translator in an emergency, but this is a very poor substitute for using an official interpreter. In hospitals where a substantial proportion of patients are from ethnic minorities, suitable interpreters should be made available at all times.

In difficult cases, it is wise to make sure that a witness (usually the midwife) is present, that all present agree on what has been said and decided, and that appropriate notes are made in the medical records, detailing the discussion and decision.

Management options

Good antenatal education about pain relief and anaesthesia, supported by booklets and/or videos, is an important part of the obstetric anaesthetist's job, and it is best not delegated to midwives unless the information that they disseminate is scrupulously checked.

Signed consent for epidural analgesia in labour is not currently considered necessary and in most units, verbal consent is taken only. What is important is to give an adequate explanation of the risks and benefits that are applicable to each particular woman making a decision in the prevailing circumstances. This will obviously vary according to the situation, but a note should always be made listing the matters discussed and identifying reasons why an explanation was brief or curtailed. If the procedure is difficult or prolonged, then verbal permission to continue must be sought at regular intervals.

For regional techniques, most obstetric anaesthetists would now consider, as a minimum, explanation of the risk of partial or complete failure of the technique, dural puncture and headache, motor block and neurological complications. An explanation of the risks of regional anaesthesia for caesarean section should always include the possibility of discomfort, pain and conversion to general anaesthesia. Failure to do this has resulted in many negligence suits against anaesthetists.

When offering anaesthetic options for elective caesarean section, it is perfectly reasonable to stress the maternal advantages of regional block, but there is no argument at present for insisting on this when there are no contraindications to general anaesthesia. A patient undergoing emergency caesarean section with a functioning epidural *in situ* is a different proposition entirely, and every effort should be made to encourage an epidural top-up, with refusal being carefully recorded in the notes.

Key points

- It is difficult to provide complex information to a woman in painful labour. Antenatal education makes this task much easier.
- Women with capacity are able to change their mind at any time; those without capacity should be treated in their 'best interests'.
- The risks and benefits discussed with the patient should always be recorded.
- A pregnant woman's autonomy is not affected by the fact that she is carrying a fetus.

Further reading

Association of Anaesthetists of Great Britain & Ireland. *Information and Consent for Anaesthesia.* London: AAGBI 2005.

Bethune L, Harper N, Lucas DN, *et al.* Complications of obstetric regional analgesia: how much information is enough? *Int J Obstet Anesth* 2004; **13**: 30–4.

Broaddus BM, Chandrasekhar S. Informed consent in obstetric anesthesia. *Anesth Analg* 2011; **112**: 912–15.

Kelly GD, Blunt C, Moore PAS, Lewis M. Consent for regional anaesthesia in the United Kingdom: what is material risk? *Int J Obstet Anesth* 2004; **13**: 71–4.

Middle JV, Wee MY. Informed consent for epidural analgesia in labour: a survey of UK practice. *Anaesthesia* 2009; **64**: 161–4.

Wheat K. Progress of the prudent patient: consent after Chester v Afshar. *Anaesthesia* 2005; **60**: 217–19.

White SM, Baldwin TJ. Consent for anaesthesia. *Anaesthesia* 2003; **58**: 760–74.

Medicolegal aspects

Obstetric anaesthetists may be involved in medicolegal issues in a number of different contexts, all of which have relevance or potential relevance to obstetric care, e.g. concerning consent and capacity (see Chapter 158, Consent); various statutes, e.g. the Mental Capacity Act, Mental Health Act, Data Protection Act, Human Tissue Act, Human Rights Act; involvement in coroners' courts; the risk of being accused of assault/battery; and claims of negligence. It is the last, however, that is by far the most likely reason for an obstetric anaesthetist to encounter the legal system.

Claims within the NHS are handled by the NHS Litigation Authority (NHSLA), although the named NHS body itself is the defendant, so that negligence claims are made against (and defended by) the trust and not the individual employees involved in the case. However, staff working outside the NHS may be personally named in negligence claims.

There is a general trend in the UK towards patients seeking redress in the courts when they think that they have been harmed as a result of a negligent act on the part of their medical attendants. In 2010–11, the NHSLA made payments in excess of £729 000 000 in respect of negligence claims, a 12% increase over the previous year (and a 90% increase since 2005–06). Since the Clinical Negligence Scheme for Trusts (CNST) started in 1995, surgery (41%) and obstetrics/gynaecology (21%) have been the most commonly involved specialties, with anaesthesia accounting for 2.4%. However, obstetrics/gynaecology accounts for almost half of the costs, and within anaesthetic claims, regional and obstetric anaesthesia accounts for ~40% of the costs of claims.

For a negligence claim to succeed, the patient has to demonstrate that the doctor had a duty of care towards her (normally not a matter for contention), that there was a failure of that duty of care (the standard applied here is that of the ordinary doctor professing skill in anaesthesia), and that she has suffered harm as a result. The test for causation is that were it not for the failure of care, the harm would not have occurred. However, a judgment in 2005 in the House of Lords relating to consent has established that, even were this not to apply, the doctor may still be found negligent.

Problems/special considerations

Consent

Consent is equally valid whether written or verbal, the only difference being that a record of the former is retained in the hospital notes as confirmation if a case comes to court after some years. Consent is only valid if it is informed, i.e. if the patient has been presented with enough information about the risks and benefits of the procedure to make a sensible choice. This can obviously be difficult in practice if a patient is in severe pain and under the influence of Entonox or opioids, as is often the case when epidural analgesia is needed in labour. It is generally agreed that provision of information in the antenatal period is best, although many women may not consider it applicable to them at this time. (See Chapter 158, Consent.)

Regional analgesia/anaesthesia

The extent of information required when seeking consent for regional analgesia/anaesthesia is controversial, although most surveys suggest that some women would wish to know most, if not all, complications. Most obstetric anaesthetists would now consider as a minimum, explanation of the risk of partial or complete failure of the technique, dural puncture and headache, motor block and neurological complications. Signed, written consent is not considered necessary currently although a list of the pertinent aspects of the discussion should be recorded, and a note made if the patient's condition does not allow for a full explanation. Antenatal access to an anaesthetist should be available for women who have particular concerns.

Pain during caesarean section

Pain felt during caesarean delivery under spinal or epidural anaesthesia is the most common source of successful litigation against UK obstetric anaesthetists. In practice, a pain-free procedure cannot be guaranteed, and the anaesthetist must mention this possibility when obtaining consent. The level of block must be carefully checked before starting the operation, and recorded, along with the sensory modality used. Any complaint of pain should be taken seriously, documented and treated.

Headache

Headache following accidental dural puncture is a common source of complaint. Dural tap is not, in itself, enough to demonstrate negligence, as long as it is correctly managed. This means that good analgesia should be established for labour and the patient followed up daily while in hospital. Any complaint of headache, neck pain or visual disturbances should be documented and definitive treatment, in the form of epidural blood patch, offered early. Any mother who has suffered a dural tap or postdural puncture headache should be encouraged to contact the hospital if there is a recurrence/worsening of symptoms. These patients should be routinely followed up at 6–10 weeks postpartum.

Backache

Claims are often made for backache after epidural analgesia, but few, if any, succeed. Prospective studies have shown that new, long-term backache is common following childbirth but is not related to whether or not regional analgesia has been used.

Management options

It is far easier to minimise the risk of litigation than to deal with it once it arises. Sensible guidelines for management of common obstetric anaesthetic situations are essential. Good communication with patients and relatives, and keeping them informed, will ensure them of one's good intentions – very few patients institute proceedings against doctors who have communicated well. Most hospitals now have an efficient risk-management procedure with a rapid response to complaints and so patients, most of whom only want an explanation of what went wrong and an apology, will often be content without needing to take more formal action. Complaints from mothers or their partners, however informal, must be handled at a senior level.

If, despite these precautions, legal action ensues, then good record keeping will help the anaesthetist to recall what happened long after the case has faded from memory. Even if it was always an individual anaesthetist's routine practice to give a test dose after performing an epidural, for example, it will be difficult to convince a judge of this fact without documentary evidence. The same applies to the explanations given when obtaining consent for a procedure. A case of negligence will often come down to the anaesthetist's recollection versus that of the patient – needless to say, she will remember the whole incident perfectly, while the anaesthetist may have performed many similar procedures since. The need for accurate records is particularly important when the complaint is of a subjective nature, such as pain or awareness during caesarean section. (See Chapter 160, Record keeping.)

An accusation of negligence is a very painful and traumatic experience for a doctor, and it is important to seek support from peers and seniors, especially those who have experience of medicolegal practice.

Key points

- Negligence claims against obstetric anaesthetists are increasing.
- Good relations should be maintained with patients and their relatives.
- Any complaint should be dealt with promptly.
- Full records are the best defence and should include details of explanations before consent.

Further reading

Cook TM, Bland L, Mihai R, Scott S. Litigation related to anaesthesia: an analysis of claims against the NHS in England 1995–2007. *Anaesthesia* 2009; **64**: 706–18.

NHS Litigation Authority. Claims (including factsheets), http://www.nhsla.com/Claims/.

Szypula K, Ashpole KJ, Bogod D, *et al*. Litigation related to regional anaesthesia: an analysis of claims against the NHS in England 1995–2007. *Anaesthesia* 2010; **65**: 443–52.

Wheat K. Progress of the prudent patient: consent after Chester v Afshar. *Anaesthesia* 2005; **60**: 217–19.

Record keeping

The increase in negligence litigation against doctors in general, and obstetric anaesthetists in particular, has led to increased concerns about the standard of record keeping in hospitals. Many hospitals now have clinical risk managers, and one of the main tasks of these individuals is to ensure that records are clear, complete and retrievable. Many practitioners criticise the current medicolegal climate as leading to the practice of 'defensive medicine', but in the area of record keeping at least, the benefits for practitioner and patient alike are clear – there is no doubt that record-keeping has often been poor in the past and that this has led to delays, unnecessary repetition of investigations and breakdowns in communication.

Increasingly, certain aspects of medical record keeping are being done electronically (e.g. prescribing, recording of intraoperative observation) but the particular features of obstetric analgesia and anaesthesia make such systems difficult to design and implement in the maternity setting.

Problems/special considerations

Legibility

Although it is not always easy to maintain good legibility in the emergency situation, every effort should be made to ensure that entries in the notes, and particularly signatures, can be read. While most doctors can read their own handwriting, this is not always true 20 years later, and it should be borne in mind that the interpretation will often be made by someone other than the writer. Each signature in the notes should be followed by the author's name in capital letters.

Hospitals rarely release original notes, and solicitors usually receive a photocopied bundle of records, often prepared in haste by the most junior office assistant. Therefore, black ink (it photocopies better) should be used, and notes should not be written in the extremes of the margin (often missed in the photocopying process).

Contemporaneity

The courts appreciate that it is often impossible to deal with a crisis and keep good, contemporaneous records. It is perfectly in order, for example, to copy a series of blood pressure results from the monitor 'trends' screen into the record after an operation. Similarly, it is quite reasonable to sit down after a dangerous situation has been stabilised and make a retrospective record of what happened – in this instance, however, the time at which the record was written should be included in the entry. It is even acceptable to go back and alter or add notes some time after the event – as long as the alterations are honest – but it must be made very clear in the notes that these are later additions. In general, complex notes should be made as soon as possible after the event, while the memory is fresh.

Completeness

While it may be one's standard practice to warn of the risk of headache before siting an epidural or to assess the level of block after instituting spinal anaesthesia for caesarean section, it is prudent to note that this has been done in each individual case – and ideally, this record should include the incidence quoted. An anaesthetist's actions may be queried many years after the event, by which time he/she will have no recollection of the individual case; the patient, on the contrary, will remember it as if it were yesterday. In this situation, the defence that something must have been done, because it was one's routine practice always to do so, does not carry much weight if there is no mention of it in the notes. Reasons for making clinical decisions – such as withholding a blood patch for a postdural puncture headache because it seems to be improving – should always be carefully noted, especially when the decision deviates from standard guidelines. Finally, all entries should be dated, timed and signed legibly.

The maintenance of complete records can be encouraged by developing forms with prompts for commonly omitted data, such as level of block and mode of testing after regional anaesthesia. Good record keeping can also be encouraged by stressing its value in departmental guidelines. One of the most effective methods for ensuring standards is to incorporate a review of clinical records into the audit programme.

Retrievability

The best records in the world will be of no help if they cannot be found. Anaesthetic notes, especially epidural forms, are often made on sheets that do not form part of the main record. There must be a system in place for incorporating these into the bound folder, preferably not by just inserting them into a pocket in the back.

Obstetric litigation may arise up to 21 years after the birth of the child. Maternity records must be kept for at least this long, and this often causes considerable logistic problems, as does the difficulty in tracing the practitioners involved after such a long period.

Key points
- Notes should be written clearly and legibly in black ink.
- The date, time and the author's name should be included.
- Even if a practice is routine, details should be noted.

Minimum standards, guidelines and protocols

Recent years have seen a proliferation of documents aimed at standardising and improving medical care. These are variously known as standards, guidelines and protocols and are developed at local, national and even international level. There are no firm, accepted definitions of these terms, and in practice, they are often used interchangeably. However, the term 'minimum standards' tends to be used for establishing general standards of services/care to which practitioners/units should aspire, while 'protocols' tends to refer to specific management of a particular condition or group of condition. 'Guidelines' is commonly used in both contexts.

Such documents are increasingly used throughout medicine since they are seen as an efficient way of maintaining good practice although they may have some disadvantages (Table 161.1). They are generally seen as an important part of risk management.

Current national standards and guidelines

In the UK, the Association of Anaesthetists of Great Britain and Ireland has promulgated a series of standards and guidelines over the past 15–20 years. In the field of obstetric anaesthesia, the Obstetric Anaesthetists' Association (OAA) produced its *Recommended Minimum Standards for Obstetric Anaesthesia Services* in 1994. In 1998, both organisations jointly produced *Guidelines for Obstetric Anaesthesia Services*, which was updated in 2005, and which is again being currently updated. This important document specifies recommendations for: staffing levels; acceptable response times; monitoring during regional analgesia and caesarean section; theatre, recovery, high-dependency and intensive care unit facilities; availability of blood; consent; support services; assistance and departmental guidelines. In addition, it has a section on professional relationships with midwives and obstetricians.

In 1999, the Royal Colleges of Midwives and Obstetricians and Gynaecologists published *Towards Safer Childbirth – Minimum Standards for the Organisation of Labour Wards*, setting out recommendations for organisational aspects of maternity services and risk management, which has also been updated in 2007.

In the USA, the American Society of Anesthesiologists produced its *Guidelines for Regional Anesthesia in Obstetrics* in 1988 and amended them in 1991. *Practice Guidelines for Obstetrical Anesthesia*, the report by the ASA's Task Force on Obstetrical Anesthesia, was produced in 1999 and updated in 2005; it aims to be evidence based, covering most aspects of obstetric anaesthetic practice. The ASA's *Guidelines for Regional Anesthesia in Obstetrics* and *Optimal Goals for Anesthesia Care in Obstetrics* (the latter produced jointly with the American College of Obstetricians and Gynecologists) were published in 2000, and have been subsequently replaced by a new document published in 2009 by the ACOG and the ASA entitled *Optimal Goals for Anesthesia Care in Obstetrics*.

Table 161.1 Advantages and disadvantages of minimum standards, guidelines and protocols

Advantages	Can support local departments/units in their argument for adequate resources/facilities
	Encourage practitioners/units to examine their own practice and establish good risk management procedures
	Represent an overview from established authorities
	Increase uniformity of practice, especially where there is a large turnover of staff
	Allow better adherence to evidence-based medicine
	Improve management of rare but serious conditions, e.g. anaphylaxis, major haemorrhage
	Can be used for teaching and training of staff
	May reduce the risk of medicolegal claims
	Required by most accreditation/assessment authorities as an indicator of good risk management
Disadvantages	Require continuous updating and removal when obsolete
	Lay the organisation or individuals open to potential criticism if not adhered to or if badly written
	May be ignored if the targets set are seen as unduly unrealistic
	May restrict clinical freedom
	May result in blind adherence to a set management path, even though it may be inappropriate in certain circumstances
	May remove the incentive to 'think for oneself'
	Require continuous updating and removal when obsolete
	Lay the organisation or individuals open to potential criticism if not adhered to or if badly written
	Rely on consensus; if opinions vary widely the resultant protocol may be too loose to be useful

Local protocols and guidelines

It is important that these are written clearly and unambiguously. Once a protocol has been written, it becomes an important legal document (e.g. in future claims that negligence occurred) even if it has not yet been formally introduced, since merely by existing it demonstrates that any other management is suboptimal. This potential exposure to criticism and possibly legal action has deterred some clinicians from utilising protocols more widely.

Each version of a protocol should be dated and previous ones removed in order to maintain consistency throughout the unit. Obsolete ones should be stored since subsequent legal actions may refer to guidelines that were in force at the time of the supposed mismanagement.

Although there have been calls for national protocols that can be used by all units, most prefer to alter basic schemes to suit the local circumstances.

Writing a protocol requires the clinical problem or procedure to be carefully defined at the start. It is important that protocols are written by multidisciplinary groups and that all individuals involved are consulted before their introduction, since the protocols must be willingly followed by all clinicians unless specific exclusion criteria are met. Management of cases meeting exclusion criteria should also be covered. It is equally important that adherence to the protocol is audited to ensure consistency of management.

Medicolegal considerations

As a method of protecting the practitioner from legal actions for negligence, documents of this type are obviously a double-edged sword, since they could be a useful weapon for lawyers when the stated standards have not been achieved.

In practice, however, standards and guidelines have not been afforded a great deal of weight in courts of law in the UK or USA. This is partly because, although they may reflect the views of a group of senior and respected practitioners, they are rarely firmly based on good scientific evidence, and there is often an equally respectable opinion that would support a different course of action or standard of care. Furthermore, since such documents and their authors cannot be cross-examined in court, greater weight is often attached to the evidence given directly by expert witnesses.

Key points

- Minimum standard documents provide a useful reference when developing local protocols and are an impetus to improving and maintaining the quality of medical care.
- Local protocols and guidelines can improve clinical management and form an important part of risk management.
- Many potential problems can be avoided by careful writing and achieving consensus.
- Each copy should be dated, and obsolete versions removed from all clinical sites and kept for future reference.

Further reading

ACOG Committee on Obstetric Practice. ACOG committee opinion No. 433: optimal goals for anesthesia care in obstetrics. *Obstet Gynecol* 2009; **113**: 1197–9.

American Society of Anesthesiologists Task Force on Obstetric Anesthesia. Practice guidelines for obstetric anesthesia: an updated report by the American Society of Anesthesiologists Task Force on Obstetric Anesthesia. *Anesthesiology* 2007; **106**: 843–63.

McGarrity L, O'Connor R, Young S. A national survey of obstetric anaesthesia guidelines in the UK. *Int J Obstet Anesth* 2008; **17**: 322–8.

Obstetric Anaesthetists' Association/Association of Anaesthetists of Great Britain & Ireland. *Guidelines for Obstetric Anaesthetic Services*, 2nd edn. London: AAGBI 2005, http://www.aagbi.org/sites/default/files/obstetric05.pdf.

Royal College of Anaesthetists, Royal College of Midwives, Royal College of Obstetricians and Gynaecologists, Royal College of Paediatrics and Child Health. *Safer Childbirth: Minimum Standards for the Organisation and Delivery of Care in Labour*. London: RCOG Press 2007, http://www.rcog.org.uk/files/rcog-corp/uploaded-files/WPRSaferChildbirthReport2007.pdf.

Risk management

Risk management is a process by which adverse outcomes are minimised by analysing their causes and instituting preventative steps, thus reducing both the chance of an adverse event occurring and its cost (both clinical and financial), should it occur. Although it may involve audit, the emphasis is based more on the analysis of individual real or potential adverse events rather than assessment of standards of practice generally. This approach is widely used throughout (and outside) healthcare to reduce risk and also liability.

Problems/special considerations

- Traditionally, anaesthetic risk has been seen as individual-based (e.g. arising from human error), but recent emphasis has focused on risk being operating room based (arising from the interaction between anaesthetists and their working environment, in this case labour ward) and most recently system based (human actions superimposed on inherent flaws in a system or process). Examples of system-based errors might include the patient with pre-eclampsia who presents unbooked late in pregnancy, requires emergency caesarean section but is not given antacid prophylaxis because her drug chart is missing; she is anaesthetised by a junior trainee, aspirates on induction and is transferred to another hospital because of a shortage of intensive care beds.
- Important steps in the development of a risk management programme include:
  - Analysis of risks (e.g. morbidity and mortality meetings, critical incident reporting schemes).
  - Prevention of risks associated with routine activities (e.g. proper training and supervision, provision of trained anaesthetic assistants).
  - Avoidance of particularly high-risk practices (e.g. general anaesthesia for caesarean section).
  - Minimising the severity of adverse events should they occur (e.g. having an antacid prophylaxis protocol in place).
  - Risk financing (e.g. indemnity).
  - Having a system in place for dealing with disasters and complaints: this may reduce both psychological sequelae and legal proceedings.
  Such a programme has implications for training, purchase and upkeep of equipment and other potentially costly processes but should ultimately reduce costs related to legal actions.
- Relatively simple measures can be taken to reduce the risks attached to specific activities, such as analysing a single procedure (e.g. caesarean section) at all its stages or focusing on a specific complication (e.g. dural tap) and working back. A climate in which

mistakes and critical incidents can be openly discussed without fear of retribution is important. More formal analytical techniques (e.g. root cause analysis) can be used to reveal underlying weaknesses in systems; such methods may have a role in helping to predict incidents but are usually employed to analyse incidents once they happen.

- Once a risk management programme is instituted, specific audits can then be performed to highlight areas where inadequacies still exist. Protocols are generally seen as a way of reducing risk if they are widely circulated and followed (itself a worthy subject of audit). Wider use of critical incident reporting schemes has been suggested as a more effective means of improving service than traditional reliance on outcome studies (e.g. looking at mortality), firstly because serious adverse outcomes are rare, and secondly because a proactive approach is inherently more attractive than a reactive one.

Within the NHS, the NHS Litigation Authority (NHSLA) handles claims against NHS bodies. Through its Clinical Negligence Scheme for Trusts (CNST), NHS bodies are encouraged to improve their structure and processes through financial incentives; the costs of the scheme are met by the bodies themselves according to whether they meet required CNST standards of organisational structure, routine and high-risk clinical care, and communication. Trusts may meet none (level 0), some (levels 1 or 2) or all (level 3) standards, and their contributions are adjusted accordingly.

Key points

- Risk may involve human actions and/or an underlying flawed system.
- Management includes:
  - Analysis
  - Reduction of risk attached to routine activities
  - Avoidance of high-risk activities
  - Damage limitation
  - Risk financing.

Further reading

Boothman RC, Blackwell AC. Integrating risk management activities into a patient safety program. *Clin Obstet Gynecol* 2010; **53**: 576–85.

Mann S, Pratt SD. Team approach to care in labor and delivery. *Clin Obstet Gynecol* 2008; **51**: 666–79.

NHS Litigation Authority. Risk management, http://www.nhsla.com/RiskManagement/.

Pettker CM, Thung SF, Norwitz ER, *et al.* Impact of a comprehensive patient safety strategy on obstetric adverse events. *Am J Obstet Gynecol* 2009; **200**: 492.e1–8.

Post-crisis management

Obstetric anaesthesia is a particularly stressful subspecialty of anaesthesia. It is important that all staff are aware that there are times when colleagues may need someone to talk to and they may need support in communicating with the patient and other colleagues. It is also clear that proper debriefing after catastrophes is an important part of risk management.

A crisis may be precipitated by a variety of factors, some obvious and others less obvious (Table 163.1).

Problems/special considerations

The reasons for the stress are many:

- The anaesthetist is looking after two people – the mother and the baby – during an important life event. There is therefore much at stake should things go wrong.
- Both mother and fetus are physiologically stressed and thus have less reserve than healthy patients. When adverse events occur, they often do so rapidly and without

Table 163.1 Causes of major stress when support and counselling of colleagues may be required

Serious adverse outcome	Maternal death or severe impairment Fetal death or severe impairment
Unexpected crisis	Anaphylaxis Failed or difficult tracheal intubation Shoulder dystocia Sudden severe maternal haemorrhage Maternal cardiac arrest
Complication of technique	Accidental dural puncture Neurological deficit following regional analgesia and anaesthesia
Failure of technique	Awareness during general anaesthesia for caesarean section Pain during regional anaesthesia for caesarean section Failed regional analgesia for labour
Human error	Giving the wrong drug or blood Not checking a blood result
Other	Letter of complaint from patient or solicitor Formal complaint from other hospital staff Violence from patient or relative/partner Coincidental professional or personal crisis

warning, with little time to treat them before irreparable damage occurs. Obstetrics thus represents a truly 'high-risk' area of medical practice.

- Pregnancy is perceived as a normal physiological function in which the outcome should be safe and happy. The public expectations are very high and it is inevitable that these high expectations may sometimes not be met.
- It is obvious that a maternal death will be a very traumatic event, but less obvious that a junior anaesthetist will be very upset by causing an accidental dural puncture. As maternity units are often very busy places and turnover of staff is high, there may not be a suitable opportunity to discuss potential problems with colleagues.
- Maternity units are areas where different professional groups (anaesthetists, obstetricians and midwives) work closely together, with sometimes different priorities. Therefore, it is important to ensure good communication within this multidisciplinary group.

Management options

Failure of communication is one of the main reasons for complaint, and it is important that the anaesthetist continually informs the patient and her relatives when there are problems.

Communication between staff is also crucial. Trainees must always feel able to discuss a problem with their senior colleagues, without embarrassment, and must feel that they, as a trainee, are part of the team whose aim is a high standard of care to all the women. Recent emphasis on teamworking (e.g. the World Health Organization's surgical safety checklist) has highlighted the need for proper communication between team members.

It is important that there is regular multidisciplinary discussion and that staff do not automatically blame each other when outcomes are bad. Senior staff of all disciplines should ensure that each major catastrophe is fully discussed in an open fashion, and that all staff involved with the case have a chance to discuss it. Counselling should be made available if required by any staff.

When any member of staff is worried that there has been a problem, it is often helpful to seek advice from their medical protection organisation. It is also useful to go back to the medical record and, where appropriate, expand the account of the events and keep a full copy for personal use.

Post-crisis management also includes identification of any legal and/or financial threats to the hospital and taking steps to avoid or reduce them.

Key points

- All staff are vulnerable to experiencing a catastrophe in the maternity unit.
- Communication with all levels of staff and a non-judgmental approach are essential.
- All members of staff involved in a catastrophe should be offered support and, if necessary, counselling.

Further reading

Association of Anaesthetists of Great Britain & Ireland. *Catastrophes in Anaesthetic Practice*. London: AAGBI 2005, http://www.aagbi.org/sites/default/files/catastrophes05.pdf.

McCready S, Russell R. A national survey of support and counselling after maternal death. *Anaesthesia* 2009; **64**: 1211–17.

Research on labour ward

Research involving pregnant women has particular ethical and practical issues. Perhaps partly because of this, much of obstetric and anaesthetic practice on labour ward was traditionally based on little available evidence or else little attention was paid to what evidence there was. Fortunately, there has been increasing reliance on published studies in guiding management, although in the quest for 'evidence-based' decisions, it is often forgotten that the best evidence there is may be far from perfect, i.e. the ideal randomised controlled trial (RCT) has not been done. For example, the question of whether loss of resistance to air is indeed associated with a greater incidence of accidental dural tap than loss of resistance to saline would require a huge study, which would involve more centres and take more time than is practicable. In this situation one is left with methodologically weak studies (e.g. retrospective reviews), which may suggest a causal link but no more.

In the generally quoted hierarchy of evidence, the best of all is the systematic review, in which all known RCTs are screened for correct methodology and the results pooled to increase power. Next, prospective RCTs themselves are still considered the gold standard for comparing different treatments or courses of management (particularly relevant to obstetric anaesthetic practice) if of adequate size; in descending order come non-randomised, single group, cohort or case-control studies; non-experimental studies; and finally case reports and 'expert' opinions.

Problems/special considerations

- Ethical issues are related to: the special vulnerability of pregnant women who are going through an intensely emotional time; the increasing involvement of mothers in decisions affecting their pregnancy and thus exposure of them to many potentially difficult choices already; the fact that many drugs in current obstetric anaesthetic practice are not licensed for use in pregnancy (largely related to the cost to manufacturers of separate trials in this group); and to the often uncertain effects of experimental drugs and procedures on the pregnancy, labour or fetus.
- The care of pregnant women has traditionally been something of a battleground between various medical and non-medical staff, and the risk that a well intentioned study may be viewed as an intrusion into a normal process should not be taken lightly. Courtesy dictates that the obstetrician, under whose care potential subjects are, should be informed of the study protocol. The situation of independent midwives caring for women with epidurals, without the input of an obstetrician, is already a controversial one, and there may potentially be conflict if such mothers are approached for enrolment into an anaesthetic study.

- The issue of consent may be cause for discussion. It has been argued that a woman in labour is unable to give truly informed consent for inclusion in a study (or even for a procedure such as an epidural) because of the pain and distress she may be suffering, especially if drugs such as pethidine have been given. This makes studies of epidural techniques especially difficult, since it may not be possible to identify in advance women who might go on to request epidural analgesia. An especially controversial area concerns the calls for randomised studies of epidural versus non-epidural analgesia, in order to assess side effects in particular; some would consider it unethical to withhold the only really effective form of analgesia from mothers, whereas others claim it is unethical not to do so if it is the only way of properly evaluating the effects of epidurals.

- Practical difficulties of conducting obstetric anaesthetic studies relate to: the obtaining of consent, discussed above; the defining of a homogenous group of subjects (the 'standard primip' was suggested by Crawford over 25 years ago as suitable for the majority of studies; women in this category are aged 25, healthy, with a full-term normal singleton pregnancy and no malposition or malpresentation); the fact that labouring women in particular are demanding in terms of requesting information and determining their own management; and the largely unpredictable nature of the workload. In addition, since all subjects must have the right to withdraw from any study at any time without penalty, randomised studies may suffer from considerable drop-out rates (e.g. those studies of epidural versus non-epidural analgesia). Since a mother's situation may change suddenly during labour, this may further increase the drop-out rate. Finally, the records relating to the research may easily become lost amongst the voluminous paperwork that passes through labour ward.

Management options

Apart from the considerations mentioned above, research methods are as for any other clinical situation. The practicalities of labour ward research preclude many topics from being suitable for study, even though they may be of interest and clinical value. Many potential or actual studies suffer from either too few subjects or too rare an outcome, or both; thus, for example, many complications that are relatively uncommon can only be meaningfully studied in multicentre trials (e.g. dural taps, neurological complications). Studies comparing different regional anaesthetic techniques are relatively easy to conduct in a single unit, since so many anaesthetic interventions involve regional techniques.

As for any project, an obstetric anaesthetic RCT requires appropriate consideration of: the primary hypothesis (what question is the study asking – and is it worth asking?); the subjects to be studied (inclusion and exclusion criteria); the type of data collected (what is being measured and how); the methods of analysis (which statistical tests to use); and the overall power of the study (related to the number of subjects per group, the size of the difference between the groups and the statistical test used).

Finally, it should be remembered that a statistically significant result may not be *clinically* significant (e.g. a 30-second difference in onset of epidural block), and also that a statistically significant result found in a single study may still be a chance finding (albeit with a likelihood of less than 5% if a probability of 0.05 was taken to denote 'statistical significance'). Conversely, just because the evidence supporting a particular course of action or management may be overwhelming, it does not necessarily follow that clinicians will adhere to it.

Key points

- For research on labour ward, basic ethical considerations apply.
- Subjects are especially vulnerable but may be especially demanding.
- Practical difficulties include obtaining consent and the unpredictability of labour.

Further reading

American College of Obstetricians & Gynecologists. Ethical considerations in research involving women. *Obstet Gynecol* 2003; **102**: 1107–13.

Lupton MGF, Williams DJ. The ethics of research on pregnant women – maternal consent sufficient? *BJOG* 2004; **111**: 1307–12.

Yentis SM. Ethical guidance for research in obstetric anaesthesia. *Int J Obstet Anesth* 2001; **10**: 289–91.

Chapter

165 Obstetric anaesthetic organisations

Several organisations and societies relevant to obstetric analgesia and anaesthesia exist. In the UK, there are many regional societies and groups, some involving non-anaesthetists as well as anaesthetists. National organisations exist in many countries but not all. There are no separate international organisations (the European Society of Obstetric Anesthesia (ESOA) was active for a few years in the late 1990s but is now inactive), although the European Society of Anaesthesiologists (ESA) has an Obstetric Committee and the Obstetric Anaesthetists' Association (OAA), which represents obstetric analgesia and anaesthesia in the UK, has many members from overseas.

Obstetric Anaesthetists' Association

The OAA was formed in 1969 to promote the highest standards of anaesthetic practice in the care of the mother and baby, and has an international membership in the order of 2000. It provides a focus for all anaesthetists who want to improve the care and safety of women in childbirth. The OAA has charitable status, supports a research fellowship and offers annual research grants and bursaries. It also offers prizes for trainees for research presented at the annual scientific meeting.

The OAA holds three main meetings a year: in March, a one-day meeting in London on cases and controversies in obstetric anaesthesia; in the spring, a two-day meeting at different venues in the UK on current research and practice; and in late autumn, a three-day course in London presenting the latest academic and clinical views on modern obstetric anaesthesia and analgesia. Further smaller refresher courses and meetings on various topics are also held.

The *International Journal of Obstetric Anesthesia* (*IJOA*) is the official Journal of the OAA, carries OAA notices, and is included in the annual subscription. The OAA also supplies educational videos and publications; details are available from:

Obstetric Anaesthetists' Association, 21 Portland Place, London, W1B 1PY, UK.

Website: www.oaa-anaes.ac.uk.

Society for Obstetric Anesthesia and Perinatology (SOAP)

Outside Britain, SOAP is the biggest and most active group for obstetric anaesthetists. It was founded in the USA in 1968 to provide a forum for discussion of problems unique to the peripartum period. SOAP comprises anaesthetists, obstetricians, paediatricians and basic scientists who share an interest in the care of the pregnant patient and the neonate; membership currently numbers approximately 1000.

The mission of the society is to promote excellence in research and practice of obstetric anaesthesia and perinatology. Through its newsletter, internet site and annual meetings, SOAP allows practitioners of several specialties to meet and discuss clinical practice, basic and clinical research and practical professional concerns. SOAP has a travelling scholarship programme, allowing overseas anaesthetists from developing countries to travel to the annual meeting and to spend one week at a centre of excellence in the USA. The society awards an annual research fellowship and a smaller research starter grant is also offered. The address of SOAP is:

Society for Obstetric Anesthesia and Perinatology, 520 N. Northwest Highway, Park Ridge, IL 60068-2573, USA.

Website: www.soap.org.

Chapter 166

Vital statistics

In the UK, figures are collected by three main mechanisms:

- Statutory reporting schemes (e.g. registration of births to the Office of National Statistics (ONS) by the parents; birth notification to the Director of Public Health by midwives or medical staff; reporting of congenital abnormalities to ONS).
- Non-statutory but obligatory schemes (e.g. those organised for accreditation and training by the Royal Colleges; the Confidential Enquiries into Maternal Deaths).
- Specific projects, which may or may not be supported by national or professional bodies (e.g. surveys carried out by the Audit Commission or National Birthday Trust; hospital- or department-based projects; Obstetric Anaesthetists' Association (OAA) or Association of Anaesthetists projects).

Anaesthetists may be involved in some of the above schemes and the information gained may be of interest to obstetric anaesthetists in particular. There may be considerable overlap between the information gained for public health or political purposes and that gained for research or audit purposes; there may also be conflicting interests of the bodies supporting them. Specific schemes related to obstetric anaesthesia are few and far between.

Some of the national figures from recent years are provided in Table 166.1.

Problems/special considerations

As with all large information-gathering schemes, there may be inaccuracies in the figures collected, which in turn can be interpreted in different ways. It is also generally easier to collect information about outcome events than about denominators, e.g. the total number of births is known but the total number of pregnancies is not (it is estimated from the number of births, the number of ectopic pregnancies and the number of legal and spontaneous abortions from hospital data systems and morbidity reports). There may also be discrepancies between data collected for the UK and its composite parts. There are also considerable differences between the ability to collect information, and thus contribute to the various reporting schemes, of the approximately 320 National Health Service and independent units in the UK in which babies are born. Finally, centrally collected and administered schemes invariably report several years after the period of interest.

Table 166.1 UK maternity statistics (per year). Figures are from Confidential Enquiries into Maternal and Child Health and/or Department of Health/OAA statistics

Total no. live and stillbirths	~723 000 in 2010 (680 000–790 000 over past 20 years)
General fertility rate	~55–60 live births per 1000 woman aged 15–44 over the past 20 years (was ~90 in the late 1950s–early 1960s)
Total no. pregnancies (estimated)	900 000–1 000 000
Legal abortions	~189 000
Mothers < 20 years old (2008–2010)	7–9%
Mothers > 35 years old (2008–2010)	22–30%
Gestation < 37 weeks or > 41 weeks	5–7% each
Caesarean section rate (England)	24–25% since 2006 (emergency rate 14–15% and elective rate 9–10%) (see Chapter 31, Caesarean section)
General anaesthesia for caesarean section	9–12% in 2007–08 (> 50% in 1989–90)
Forceps or ventouse delivery (England)	12%
Induction rates (England)	17–20%
Epidural rate in labour	22–47%

Key points

- Collection of maternity and related data may be a statutory requirement, an obligatory professional requirement or a non-obligatory but desirable practice.
- A number of national data collection schemes produce reports of interest to anaesthetists.
- Intervention rates are increasing steadily.

Further reading

Hospital Episode Statistics. http://www.hesonline.nhs.uk/Ease/servlet/ContentServer?siteID=1937&categoryID=1475.

Chapter 167

Historical aspects of obstetric analgesia and anaesthesia

Knowledge of the major developments in obstetric anaesthesia and analgesia helps to put modern obstetric practice into context. The following brief summary outlines some of these developments and also those in general anaesthetic practice who have had profound effects on the subspecialty.

General

- Ancient methods of pain relief included various plant-derived sedatives, acupuncture and physical methods such as binding.
- 1881: Matrons' Aid Society founded (becoming the Midwives' Institute and later College of Midwives).
- 1929: British College of Obstetricians and Gynaecologists founded (granted a Royal Charter in 1947).
- 1932: Association of Anaesthetists of Great Britain and Ireland founded.
- 1933: Grantly Dick-Read, English obstetrician, published his book *Natural Childbirth*, followed in 1944 by *Childbirth Without Fear*. He proposed a link between fear, tension and pain, suggesting that the cycle could be broken by abolishing fear.
- 1941: College of Midwives founded (granted a Royal Charter in 1947).
- 1948: Faculty of Anaesthetists of the Royal College of Surgeons of England founded.
- 1952–54: the period covered by the first Report on Confidential Enquiries into Maternal Deaths, published by the Department of Health.
- 1953: Virginia Apgar, anaesthesiologist at Columbia University, described her scoring system for assessing neonates.
- 1958: Ferdinand Lamaze, French obstetrician, published his book *Painless Childbirth*, in which he suggested that pain was a conditioned reflex triggered by uterine contractions, and that a period of unconditioning followed by reconditioning (psychoprophylaxis) could reduce pain.
- 1969: Obstetric Anaesthetists' Association founded.
- 1975: Frederick Leboyer, French obstetrician, published *Birth Without Violence*, in which he advocated delivery in a quiet, darkened room, with minimal stimulation.
- 1988: College of Anaesthetists founded (granted a Royal Charter in 1992).
- 1993: the Department of Health's Expert Maternity Group published its report *Changing Childbirth* (the Cumberledge Report), which placed the expectant mother at the centre of care, emphasising her right to choose and signalling a formal move away from the traditional paternalistic 'medical' approach.

Systemic analgesia

- 1902: morphine and hyoscine first used in labour.
- 1940: pethidine first used in labour.
- 1950: pethidine approved by the Central Midwives Board.
- 1970: pethidine patient-controlled analgesia (PCA) described.
- 1999: remifentanil PCA described.

Inhalational analgesia

- 1847: James Young Simpson, Professor of Midwifery at Edinburgh University, administered the first obstetric general anaesthetic using ether. Considerable opposition came from religious leaders for going against the Bible and from medical authorities for compromising safety. Simpson went on to advocate chloroform in preference to ether, having used it the same year. He was a major influence in British obstetrics and also designed obstetric forceps, which bear his name.
- 1853: John Snow, London physician, generally considered the father of British anaesthesia, delivered Queen Victoria's eighth child (Prince Leopold) under chloroform, putting an end to the above objections. Snow is also famous for his part in ending the London cholera epidemic of 1854.
- 1881: Stanislav Klikovitch, Russian physician working in St Petersburg, described the use of nitrous oxide (80% with 20% oxygen) for labour, noting its lack of effect on the uterus and the requirement for inhalation before each contraction started.
- 1936: Minnitt's nitrous oxide/air apparatus approved by the Central Midwives Board.
- 1961: Michael Tunstall, Aberdeen anaesthetist, described the use of premixed nitrous oxide and oxygen in labour. The mixture was marketed 2 years later in the UK as Entonox. Tunstall also described the isolated forearm technique for detecting awareness, developed the Entonox demand valve (from diving equipment) and advocated the 'failed intubation drill' in obstetrics.

Regional analgesia

- 1884: Carl Koller, German ophthalmologist, used cocaine for eye surgery.
- 1885: James Leonard Corning, New York neurologist, produced spinal and epidural blockade in dogs.
- 1899: August Bier, German surgeon, used spinal anaesthesia for surgery. Bier described postdural puncture headache for the first time.
- 1901: Jean-Athanase Sicard and Fernand Cathelin, French neurologist and urologist respectively, introduced caudal analgesia.
- 1921: Fidel Pages, Spanish surgeon, used lumbar epidural blockade for surgery.
- 1931: Eugen Bogdan Aburel, Romanian obstetrician, described continuous caudal plus lumboaortic plexus blocks in labour.
- 1933: John Cleland, American obstetrician, described paravertebral block in labour.
- 1942: Robert Hingson, American obstetrician, described continuous caudals in labour.
- 1949: Cleland described continuous lumbar epidural block in labour.

- British pioneers: Andrew Doughty (Kingston; 1960s–1970s); J. Selwyn Crawford (Birmingham; 1960s–1980s); Donald Moir (Glasgow; 1960s–1980s); Barbara Morgan (Queen Charlotte's, London; 1980s–1990s).
- More recent developments:
  (i) Pencil-point spinal needles first described in 1920s but advances in their manufacture resulted in their wide availability in the late 1980s/early 1990s.
  (ii) Combined spinal–epidural technique first described in the UK in 1981–82; popularised in obstetrics in the 1990s; 'mobile epidural' combined spinal–epidural technique popularised at Queen Charlotte's Hospital by Barbara Morgan.
  (iii) Microfine spinal catheters used in the late 1980s/early 1990s; withdrawn in the USA by the Food and Drug Administration in 1992.
  (iv) Patient-controlled epidural analgesia (PCEA) used in the 1990s.
  (v) More sophisticated methods of epidural analgesia (e.g. programmed intermittent bolus, computer-integrated PCEA) described in the mid–late 2000s.

General anaesthesia for caesarean section

- 1945: Curtis Mendelson, American obstetrician, described the syndrome of acid aspiration both clinically and experimentally, distinguishing it from upper airway obstruction caused by inhalation of large pieces of food.
- 1961: Brian Sellick, London anaesthetist, described cricoid pressure as a means of preventing aspiration of gastric contents.
- 1960s: the problem of intraoperative awareness became topical, with up to 9% of mothers who received thiopental, nitrous oxide and neuromuscular blockade, remembering intraoperative events. Donald Moir, Glasgow anaesthetist, described a technique of halothane 0.5% with 50:50 nitrous oxide:oxygen in 1970, with no recall. Tunstall described the isolated forearm technique as a means of monitoring consciousness during general anaesthesia, in 1979.

Index

Page numbers in *italics* refer to information in figures or tables.